Off-the-Shelf Natural Health

Off-the-Shelf
Natural Health

How to Use Herbs and Nutrients to Stay Well

From Energy Boosters to Smart Drugs to Longevity Aids:
The Handbook of Natural Substances for Everyday Benefits

Mark Mayell

BANTAM BOOKS

NEW YORK · TORONTO · LONDON · SYDNEY · AUCKLAND

OFF-THE-SHELF NATURAL HEALTH

A Bantam Book / October 1995

Library of Congress Cataloging-in-Publication Data

Mayell, Mark.
Off-the-shelf natural health : how to use herbs and nutrients to stay well : from energy boosters to smart drugs to longevity aids : the handbook of natural substances for everyday benefits / by Mark Mayell.
p.   cm.
Includes index.
1. Self-care, Health.   2. Herbs—Therapeutic use.   3. Dietary supplements.
4. Homeopathy.   I. Title.
RA776.95.M28   1995
613—dc20   95-14937
CIP

ISBN 0-553-37457-5

Published simultaneously in the United States and Canada

Bantam Books are published by Bantam Books, a division of Bantam Doubleday Dell Publishing Group, Inc. Its trademark, consisting of the words "Bantam Books" and the portrayal of a rooster, is Registered in U.S. Patent and Trademark Office and in other countries. Marca Registrada. Bantam Books, 1540 Broadway, New York, New York 10036.

PRINTED IN THE UNITED STATES OF AMERICA

FFG   10 9 8 7 6 5 4 3 2 1

Contents

Contents

ONE

Introduction
to Natural Health

1

Natural Health
and Natural Medicines

The current crisis in American health care seems to pose an unsolvable riddle. Given the fact that Americans face some of the highest medical costs in the world, causing us to spend more of our hard-earned dollars on health than virtually any other society, why do we not live as long and as healthfully as the citizens of most other industrialized countries, many of whom have per capita health-care costs considerably lower than ours? Much of the debate about this important public issue focuses on ways to trim, add on to, or streamline the current medical system. How can we offer more procedures for more people, or fewer procedures for more people, or pay less for the same procedures?

Yet it is possible that the riddle can be solved merely by questioning the unspoken premise at its very heart. Simply put, the premise is that curing disease is the essence of health. As evidence accumulates that modern medicine is not as good at curing today's killer diseases as society is at creating them, more and more people are calling for a restructuring of our health-care system to reflect a more useful approach to health and wellness, one that emphasizes prevention as much as treatment.

Unfortunately, many of the practitioners of modern medicine are not particularly inclined to consider radically new approaches. To some extent, they are prisoners, as many people are, of their background, training, and information sources. In the United States, disease prevention gets little attention in medical-school curricula. Therapeutic nutrition remains an elective in almost all major medical schools. Some studies indicate that medical doctors are more strongly influenced by drug companies than by professional societies, scientific journals, or even their medical-school education.

Thus it should come as no surprise that the majority of doctors continue to wield the hammers of conventional medicine—drugs and surgery—against the health-care crisis. They believe that if we can just slug away at cancer or AIDS or diabetes, eventually we'll find easy, reliable (though probably expensive) cures, and be on the way to ensuring longer, healthier lives for all.

Americans for the most part accept this approach, gobbling down an average of 25 million pills per hour, including more than 50 million aspirin tablets and 30 million sleeping pills per day. Adverse drug effects now rank among the top ten causes of hospitalization and account for as many as 50 million hospital patient days a year. Twenty percent of all Americans are destined to have surgery of some kind this year. Some medical authorities admit that one in five of these operations may be unnecessary, including half of the cesarean sections (which now account for 23 percent of births in the United States); one quarter of the 650,000 hysterectomies; one third of the 400,000 coronary bypasses; and, medically speaking, virtually all of the 1.5 million circumcisions. One estimate is that the total number of avoidable deaths in the United States each year from dangerous and unnecessary surgery is between 50,000 and 100,000.

Figures such as these suggest the reason why doctors' strikes such as those in Israel in 1973 and Los Angeles in 1976, in which doctors stopped doing elective surgery, led not to the predicted health-care crisis but to actual drops in the local death rate. They also suggest why the number of operations performed in a given locale has been proven to be a function not of the health of the population but of the number of surgeons in practice. Even preventive medicine, which until recently focused on individual diet and lifestyle changes, is increasingly becoming an area where doctors intervene with invasive and often dangerous drugs and surgery. Double mastectomies to prevent breast cancer are the most dramatic examples of this trend, although more widespread is the prescription of cholesterol-lowering drugs of questionable overall effectiveness.

While drugs and surgery remain the medical standard, an increasing number of Americans are choosing to opt out of this system. A noted study published in 1993 in the *New England Journal of Medicine* found that many of today's health consumers are as likely to see an acupuncturist, chiropractor, herbalist, or other practitioner of natural medicine for relief from common ailments as they are to turn to an internist or other M.D. The researchers found that in 1990 Americans made an estimated 425 million visits to practitioners of natural medicine, almost 40 million more visits than they made to all types of conventional primary-care doctors.

Many people are also accepting more responsibility for their own health and paying more attention to diet, exercise, and emotions. They are slowly but surely making the switch to a new set of medicinal substances—herbs and nutrients that work with the body to keep it well. While many of these natural substances are useful for *treating* conditions, often this is not their sole appeal. Unlike some conventional drugs, which may relieve certain symptoms but otherwise leave you feeling drugged and confused, the natural substances presented here are qualitatively different. Especially when used to help prevent disease or to aid in relaxation, digestion, or other bodily processes, herbs, vitamins, and nutritional supplements are safer and cause fewer side effects. They're likely to make you feel better, more alive, more alert, maybe even smarter. They're an important part, though admittedly not the whole, of the *active prevention* approach to staying well, an approach that may well be the answer not only to our nation's health-care crisis but to your very personal health-care needs.

The Healing Herbs

Herbs are natural remedies derived from whole plants as well as plant roots, leaves, seeds, stems, and other parts. Herbs were probably humanity's first medicines; the traditional therapeutic use of herbs in China, India, and Greece dates back millennia. Many of the early herbalists used plants—aloe for wound healing, ginger for digestive upset—for the same purposes we use them for today. Frequently, though not uniformly, scientific research has validated the wisdom of ancient herbalists.

Consider the example of ephedra. Use of this stimulating herb dates back as far as five thousand years ago, when Chinese herbalists began to prescribe one of its species, ma huang (*Ephedra sinica*), for relief of congested breathing passages. Chemical analysis has shown that the stems and branches of ma huang contain compounds, particularly the alkaloids (nitrogen-containing substances) ephedrine and pseudo-ephedrine, with proven pharmacological effects. Millions of Americans still use pseudoephedrine (though now mostly synthetically derived) for some of the same conditions that prompted the ancient Chinese herbalists to recommend ma huang. Anyone who has taken

Sudafed or one of the many similar over-the-counter (OTC) decongestants has in effect experienced this herb's power to dilate bronchial tubes and free breathing.

Some of the other notable plants that have yielded healing compounds widely used in conventional modern medicine include:

White willow and meadowsweet. The bark of the former (*Salix alba*) and the leaves and flowers of the latter (*Filipendula ulmaria*) contain salicin, a compound originally used (circa 1850) in the synthesis of that well-known painkiller acetylsalicylic acid—aspirin.

Purple foxglove. The leaves of this toxic plant (*Digitalis purpurea*) contain glycoside components now widely prescribed, as the drug digitalis, for certain serious heart conditions. Foxglove's use as a heart remedy goes back to at least the late eighteenth century.

Cinchona. The bark of this South American "fever tree" (*Cinchona succirubra*) is the original source of the alkaloid quinine, which was used for over three hundred years to both prevent and treat malaria. (Quinine has now been mostly replaced for this purpose by synthetic drugs.)

Indian snakeroot. This is a popular plant (*Rauwolfia serpentina*) used in Ayurveda, the traditional medicine of India. The compound reserpine, isolated from its root, is used as a drug to treat hypertension.

Opium poppy. A whole class of potent (and addictive) pain-killing, sleep-inducing drugs, the opiates (codeine, morphine), are derived from alkaloids of this plant (*Papaver somniferum*).

Jimson weed. This is a highly toxic plant (*Datura stramonium*) that nevertheless has yielded medicinally potent alkaloids, including atropine and scopolamine, useful in the treatment of eye diseases, motion sickness, and other conditions.

Research into plant-derived compounds regularly turns up exciting new possibilities for therapeutic uses. Just recently extracts from the roots and flowers of kudzu (*Pueraria lobata*), the fast-growing vine imported from Asia that has plagued the South in recent years, were found to offer tremendous potential in the treatment of alcoholism. Kudzu has long been used for this purpose (and others) by practitioners of traditional Chinese medicine. An animal study confirmed that kudzu could quickly and dramatically reduce the appetite for alcohol, according to a report in the *Proceedings of the National Academy of Sciences*. The early indications are that kudzu extracts work better at curbing alcohol consumption than Antabuse or any of the other conventional pharmaceuticals currently used for that purpose.

Herbalists can identify at least 120 commercially sold drugs, accounting for about one in every four prescriptions issued every year in North America, whose origins can be traced to plants and herbs. Three fifths of these drugs were made possible because of the way traditional herbalists and other natural healers were using the plants. In recent years, the efforts to discover plant molecules with therapeutic applications have spread to all corners of the globe, as medical researchers have realized that deforestation and other factors threaten to remove permanently many plant species from the list of potential medicines. "Species are disappearing and taking with them valuable genetic and chemical information before we even know what we're losing," says Thomas Eisner, a biologist at Cornell University.

Less than one half of 1 percent of the 265,000 flowering species from around the world have been studied for their chemical composition and medicinal value, according to a recent report by ethnobotanists Paul Alan Cox of Brigham Young University and Michael J. Balick of the New York Botanical Garden. They estimate that today a hundred or so projects are under way hunting for new drugs from the rain forests. The biological basis for all this interest, they contend, probably has to do with plants' adaptability. "Plants have been a rich source of medicine because they produce a host of bioactive molecules, most of which probably evolved as chemical defenses against predation or infection," they note. Studies suggest that these same defensive actions can be used by humans to help ward off our disease-causing enemies, from microorganisms to harmful free radicals.

"Mother Nature is the supreme chemist, and I say this with great respect for chemists at the bench," says Gordon Cragg, in charge of the National Cancer Institute's natural-products branch. "It's very difficult to dream up these fantastic molecules." Let's hope we don't have to. It would be ironic if some of these plant species, after surviving hundreds of thousands or even millions of years by developing compounds that also happen to be of tremendous potential benefit to humans, were to be wiped out by humans before these compounds could be identified and put to use.

The Essential Nutritional Substances

Ancient peoples were also aware of the web of connections among individual foods, diet, and personal health. Egyptian healers, Greeks such as Hippocrates, and practitioners of traditional Chinese medicine believed food to be the root of much disease as well as humanity's best medicine. Writers such as Luigi Cornaro, author of a mid-sixteenth-century book on diet and longevity, also remarked upon how everyday foods influenced health. (Cornaro apparently practiced what he preached, for he lived to the then—and now—incredible age of 99.) By the late eighteenth century, scientific pioneers such as the French chemist Antoine-Laurent Lavoisier (also called the father of modern nutrition) had begun to explain important dietary and nutritional concepts such as respiration, metabolism, and digestion, and the differences between carbohydrates, fats, and proteins.

Lacking scientific methods for analyzing foods, the actual compounds within foods essential to health remained a mystery. Scientists of the eighteenth and nineteenth centuries thought at first that the essential components of foods were merely the carbohydrates, fats, and proteins. Various scientists tried experiments in which they fed animals synthetic milk or other artificial mixtures of these macronutrients. For the most part they succeeded only in killing off test subjects with alarming frequency. Clearly, some food elements not yet identified were crucial to overall health.

Clues had already begun to accumulate, for those who could notice. Since 1700 or so, some sailors had suspected that eating limes and other citrus fruits could prevent scurvy, a common seagoing-related condition characterized by bleeding gums, loose teeth, and swollen joints. Scurvy was a serious medical problem not only for sailors but also for soldiers and, until the twentieth century, large segments of any society suffering from disasters that interrupted the supply of fresh fruits and vegetables (scurvy has even been detected in the skeletal remains of prehistoric humans). The Scottish naval surgeon James Lind confirmed during a long cruise in 1746 the power of lemon juice to prevent scurvy, and published his findings in 1753. Researchers in the early 1800s also discovered that iodized salt could help prevent goiter.

These vital elements in foods did not begin to be isolated and identified, however, until the end of the nineteenth century. In 1882 a Japanese naval doctor found that he could prevent beriberi by adding vegetables and milk to peasants' normal diet, which consisted mostly of polished rice. Five years later researchers determined that they could cause beriberi in chickens by restricting their diet to polished rice. Extracts of rice polishings, capable of curing the deficiency, were the source of the first identified vitamin, thiamine (B_1). A flurry of similar animal experiments at the beginning of the twentieth century identified a string of nutrients, named "vitamines" in 1912, capable of preventing specific diseases, from vitamin D for rickets to vitamin B_{12} (finally isolated in the late

1940s) for pernicious anemia. The Hungarian-born American biochemist Albert Szent-Györgyi synthesized the first vitamin (C, the antiscurvy agent) in 1932. Over the next two decades scientists synthesized other vitamins, thus making possible the food-industry practice of adding vitamins to foods as well as the pharmaceutical practice of formulating vitamins into supplements.

Scientists now realize that vitamins are compounds needed by the body in small amounts for normal growth, development, and functioning. In the body, vitamins work with enzymes and other bodily compounds to help produce energy, build tissues, and remove waste products. In recent years research has focused on the role that vitamins, minerals, and other nutritional substances play in maintaining health, not only preventing obvious deficiency diseases but acting to ensure optimal functioning of all bodily organs and systems. Studies have shown that nutritional substances can lower the risk of major diseases such as heart disease and cancer. They can also boost immunity, stimulate learning and memory, enhance sexual performance, and affect a host of other actions that we'll look at in more detail in subsequent chapters.

Minerals are metals and other inorganic compounds. They function much as vitamins do, promoting and regulating various bodily processes. Minerals also provide much of the structure for teeth and bones. Minerals include the major minerals (needed in quantities of over 100 mg per day: calcium, phosphorus, potassium, sodium, chloride, magnesium, and sulfur) and the minor minerals, or trace elements (needed in quantities of less than 100 mg per day: chromium, zinc, selenium, silicon, and a half-dozen others).

In 1941 the Food and Nutrition Board of the National Research Council established the first set of Recommended Dietary Allowances (RDAs) for vitamins and minerals. These are nutrient levels that are estimated to be adequate for almost all healthy people. With periodic revisions, the RDAs have gained widespread acceptance as benchmarks for nutritional health, though their purpose has always been more to prevent overt nutritional disease than to maximize health. The Food and Drug Administration (FDA) develops its own related set of recommended nutrients and intake levels for use on food labels. Its U.S. Recommended Daily Allowances (U.S. RDAs) differ only slightly from the RDAs set by the NRC, chiefly in providing a single suggested nutrient level rather than a range based on the person's age and sex. Altogether, these federal agencies have determined recommended dietary allowances for some twenty nutrients, including the vitamins

A, D, E, K, B_1, B_2, B_3, B_6, B_{12}, folic acid, biotin, pantothenic acid, and C, and the minerals calcium, phosphorus, magnesium, zinc, iron, iodine, copper, and selenium.

With a few exceptions, essential nutrients are not manufactured in the body and must be obtained from foods or supplements. Many nutritionists and dietary counselors contend that most Americans routinely do not obtain sufficient nutrients from diet alone and would benefit greatly from supplementation. Studies confirm that fewer than one in ten Americans consumes the five to ten servings of fruits and vegetables per day recommended by health authorities. In addition, studies have shown that illness, strenuous exercise, high stress levels, injury, drug use, and various other factors can substantially increase the body's need for certain nutrients.

So-called natural vitamins and supplements have some minor but noteworthy differences from conventional brands. The natural form of a few vitamins, notably vitamin E, differs slightly from their synthetic form. The research is not complete, but there is some indication that the natural form may present advantages in terms of factors such as bioavailability, the rate at which the nutrient enters the bloodstream and is circulated to specific organs. In most cases, however, supplement producers use the same synthetically derived compounds for the principal ingredient of natural and conventional tablets. Supplements may differ significantly, however, in the other ingredients that make up a vitamin or mineral tablet, such as the binding and preserving agents. Natural supplements in general have no artificial colors, flavors, or sweeteners, and no synthetic binders or preservatives. In some cases natural supplements are strictly vegetarian, avoiding the animal-based gelatin used to make capsules, for instance.

With minor exceptions (particularly potassium tablets containing more than 99 mg), vitamins, minerals, and other micronutrients do not require a doctor's prescription. They are widely available over the counter in drugstores and health- and natural-food stores, and by mail order.

Today, nutritional supplements constitute a $4-billion-per-year industry. Approximately half of all Americans now take vitamins, minerals, and other dietary supplements to boost their overall health. The industry has expanded in recent years to include not only vitamins and minerals but important vitaminlike substances such as coenzyme Q10, the essential fatty acids, amino acids, and even medicinal mushrooms (though these could also be considered as belonging to the herb category).

The Potent Essential Oils

Essential oils are a growing category of natural medicines, attracting increased attention for their ability to affect both the mind (especially when dispersed in the air and inhaled) and the body (particularly when diluted and applied topically). Until a few years ago they were sold only as single-source, concentrated liquids. Today essential-oil producers are making a wide variety of essential-oil-based health-care and body-care products, from skin-care lotions to fragrance-emitting candles. Innovative producers have also begun to market combination remedies with names, such as Tranquility and Euphoria, that suggest their potential uses.

Essential oils are concentrated liquids derived from the leaves, bark, roots, flowers, resin, or seeds of some seven hundred plants. Essential oils may be thin or thick, clear or colored. Unlike greasy and fatty vegetable oils, essential oils are volatile, quickly evaporating from the skin. They are usually derived from steam distillation of plant parts, though some are cold-pressed, as are vegetable oils. Pure essential oils are typically sold in quantities of an ounce or less. Because essential oils are so potent, only a few drops at a time are used to produce the desired effects.

Aromatic plants, gums, and oils were used for culinary, cosmetic, and spiritual purposes by various ancient civilizations, including the Chinese, Egyptians, Greeks, and Romans. There is also some evidence for early medical applications of essential oils, including their use on battlefields to heal wounds. Over the past thousand years essential oils' popularity has risen and fallen depending upon factors that include technology, trade, and the philosophy of medicine. The great Arab physician Avicenna (980–1037) refined the distillation process and produced essential oils of high purity. The use of these oils in Europe increased after the Crusades. Along with herbs, essential oils were an integral part of Western medicine until the development of synthetic drugs in the nineteenth and twentieth centuries. Though the medicinal use of essential oils declined, they continued to be used in cooking and cosmetics.

Despite the long history of essential oils, the word *aromatherapy* is relatively new, having been coined by the French cosmetic chemist Dr. René-Maurice Gattefossé in the late 1920s. He began to investigate the healing effects of essential oils after he burned his hand and on an impulse plunged it into a container of Lavender oil. He subsequently experienced an accelerated, complete healing.

Aromatherapy aptly suggests the intimate connection between the sense of smell and healing functions, but it should not be taken to imply that the *only* effect that essential oils have on the body comes through their being inhaled through the nose. In minute amounts, taken orally or diluted and applied to the skin, they affect the body in the same ways as do conventional drugs, herbs, and nutritional supplements. Herbalists and aromatherapists often recommend applying essential oils topically (by massage, compresses, and baths, for example) for everything from skin conditions to aching muscles to headaches. It is crucial to work with a knowledgeable practitioner if you want to take essential oils orally, since many can be toxic even in small doses.

The body's sense of smell has been shown to have close connections to mood, emotions, and even sexual desire. These connections have long been recognized and exploited by the perfume industry, a major producer and buyer of essential oils until the advent of synthetic fragrances around 1930. Essential oils are also inhaled to address respiratory ailments and nervous problems. Common methods include putting a few drops of essential oil on a cotton cloth and then holding the cloth up to the nose to smell, and dispersing the oil throughout a room by means of vaporization.

Some aromatherapists prefer to explain how essential oils work by referring to the "vital energy" of the whole plant. Aromatherapists and scientists with a more analytic and reductionistic approach focus on essential oils' chemical constituents and how they affect the body. These chemical constituents can be extremely numerous and complex. Scientists have isolated some 160 components of the essential oil of Lavender, and they do not think they have found them all. Certainly at this point the components of essential oils and the mechanisms by which they act on the body are only partially understood.

Homeopathic Remedies

The German physician Samuel Hahnemann (1755–1843) is credited with being the founder of homeopathy. Even Hahnemann admitted, however, that he borrowed elements of the new medicine from the ancient Greeks and others, particularly the central idea of working with nature's healing powers rather than against them.

The word Hahnemann devised to describe the practice, *homeopathy,* reflects how it works. Homeopathy joins the Greek words *homoios,* meaning "like, similar," and *pathos,* meaning "suffering." This distinguishes the theory and practice of homeopathy from *allopathy,* whose

Greek root, *allos,* means "other." Hahnemann claimed that an illness can be cured by giving patients minute doses of drugs (derived from plants, animal products such as bee venom, and minerals) that in a healthy person would produce symptoms like those of the particular illness. He called this idea, that like cures like, the "law of similars." It is fundamentally opposed to the theory and practice of allopathy, which provides the philosophical foundation for conventional medicine. Allopathy posits that the best treatment of disease is by using drugs that produce effects opposite to (other than) those produced by the disease.

Hahnemann's ideas quickly gained adherents in the nineteenth century, when conventional "heroic" medicine was often characterized by the use of extremely toxic drugs and procedures (bloodletting, for example) now recognized as dangerous and ineffective. Homeopathic medical schools were founded in the United States, and the practice flourished. By the early twentieth century, an estimated one in seven medical doctors were homeopathic physicians, and homeopathic remedies were available at over a thousand homeopathic pharmacies.

Various factors led to homeopathy's decline, starting in the late nineteenth century. The advances made in scientific medicine and the development of the bacterial theory of disease were important, though unfair competitive practices by the practitioners of conventional medicine also played a part. In some ways allopaths learned from homeopaths. Homeopaths paid close attention to the individual and his or her unique symptoms. Homeopaths' thorough case studies, matching of conditions and treatments, and emphasis on testing drugs on healthy patients to discover the drugs' effects were picked up by allopaths. Allopaths also began to recognize the wisdom of using less-toxic drugs, though they never accepted the homeopathic practice of using extremely small dosages.

Within the past two decades homeopathy's fortunes have reversed in the United States, and its popularity has begun to increase. Still, medical doctors who practice homeopathy, in whole or in part, remain a tiny percentage of all M.D.'s in the United States. Homeopathy in Europe maintained a much stronger position throughout the early twentieth century, and remains a popular medical practice there. Britain's royal family, for example, uses homeopathic medicine.

The FDA takes the position that homeopathic remedies are safe and nontoxic, though the agency avoids entering the debate about whether the remedies are effective. The FDA has recognized and regulated homeopathic remedies since 1938, when it declared that they were to be treated as prescription drugs. It put virtually no effort, however, into enforcing a prescription-only policy until the mid-1980s. That was when the agency became concerned about some homeopathic remedies being marketed for serious illnesses such as cancer and heart disease. So in 1988 the FDA issued new labeling and packaging guidelines that said, in effect, that those homeopathic remedies marketed for self-limiting conditions (those that normally go away without treatment), such as colds and headaches, can be sold as OTC medicines, available without a prescription.

A homeopath typically conducts an extensive interview with and examination of a patient to try to find the one remedy that most closely matches all of the person's physical, mental, and emotional symptoms, signs, and characteristics. Thus, two people who seem to have the same illness may be prescribed different remedies, depending on whether the individual feels better in the morning or evening, is experiencing throbbing or burning pain, is thirsty for cold or hot drinks, and so forth.

Such "classical" homeopathic practice is part art and part science. It is time-consuming and requires much study to perform correctly. Though a few dozen individual remedies are common ones, used repeatedly, there are more than a thousand remedies to choose from, each slightly different in appropriateness for any individual's condition. The best classical homeopaths have studied for years to learn how to match single remedies to people's illnesses.

The painstaking practice of classical homeopathy has its limits, though. Often a professional homeopath is not in the area, or a condition is not serious enough to warrant an office visit. In such cases combination remedies are a convenient and dependable alternative to single remedies.

Homeopathic manufacturers formulate combination remedies by trying to include the various single remedies that are most often used for any particular symptom, thus increasing the likelihood that you'll get exactly the right remedy that you need. For some symptoms, almost all of the combination remedies contain two or three of the same ingredients. (A good example is combination remedies for teething, most of which contain *Chamomilla, Belladonna,* and/or *Calcarea phos.*) In other categories of combination remedies, the ingredients used by producers are much more diverse. (For example, one cold remedy may have ten ingredients, another four, with none of the fourteen ingredients being the same.) Thus, if a combination cold and flu remedy doesn't help your cold, you can try another and it may have the effect you need.

Most homeopathic manufacturers make both types of remedies. Single and combination remedies look the same, coming in small tablets or pellets. Remedies are also combined to make ointments, lotions, and tinctures for external application.

How Safe Are Natural Substances?

The relative safety of herbs, vitamins, minerals, amino acids, and other nutritional supplements has been the subject of an acrimonious debate in recent years, involving consumers and public-interest groups, the FDA and other federal regulatory agencies, supplement-industry trade groups, and practitioners of both conventional and natural medicine. With the passage of the Dietary Supplement Health and Education Act of 1994, the federal government has begun to set official safety standards for dietary supplements. Currently, natural substances can be sold as OTC remedies if they do not pose a "significant or unreasonable risk" of injury if used as directed. Moreover, the makers of new products have to show the FDA proof that the products are safe 75 days before they go on the market, giving the FDA an opportunity to regulate any supplements it identifies as posing a health hazard.

Is all this concern about safety much ado about nothing? Yes and no. In general, natural substances are much safer than prescription drugs and at least as safe as over-the-counter drugs. (One report prepared from data collected by the American Association of Poison Control Centers compared fatalities over the seven-year period between 1983 and 1990 that were caused by prescription and over-the-counter drugs to fatalities over the same period from vitamins. The result: over 2,500 deaths from conventional pain-killers, sedatives, antidepressants, and so forth, compared to one death from vitamins.) On the other hand, adverse reactions are possible, and natural substances should not be used indiscriminately.

Herbs. Plants are hardly safe just because they are natural—some of the most toxic substances known to humanity are compounds from plants, including some herbs and mushrooms. Herbal medicine is, however, thousands of years old, and responsible herbal practice makes use of plants with established safety records. Though herbal products sold in natural-food stores are essentially safe and nontoxic, herbs should be used with knowledge and caution.

According to fourth-generation herbalist Christopher Hobbs, "Although the charge is often made that herbalists say that all herbs are safe, no responsible herbalist would ever make such a claim. Herbs are often very safe, usually much safer than synthetic drugs, both for the person taking them and on our environment and energy resources. But herbs are complex mixtures of chemical compounds that can heal, change different body processes, and sometimes cause side effects, especially when overused or used without proper knowledge and awareness of an herb's total impact on health."

Herbal authority Mark Blumenthal notes that the American Association of Poison Control Centers gathers so few reports of adverse reactions to herbs that they have no category in their computer database for herb-related incidents. Plant-related poisonings that do get reported to them are almost always cases of children eating the leaves of poisonous houseplants, such as dieffenbachia and poinsettia. "As with most things in life," Blumenthal says, "moderation and the proper information are critical. . . . Most herbs found in the marketplace are in fact quite safe; they have withstood the test of hundreds of years of usage, many as food products. It is this long history of use combined with current scientific validation that has spurred the increase in popularity of herbs."

Paul Bergner, a widely published herbal writer and the editor of *Medical Herbalism,* adds that "many herbs that are safe for regular use may pose risks during pregnancy." Check with an herbalist or knowledgeable practitioner of natural medicine if you are pregnant and unsure of an herb's safety.

Nutritional substances. Taking large doses of some vitamins (particularly the fat-soluble ones, vitamins A, D, E, and K) over extended periods of time can cause adverse health effects. Even the water-soluble vitamins, such as B and C, can on occasion cause adverse reactions. Taking high levels of one B vitamin, for example, can cause an imbalance in other B vitamins. And taking high doses of C for an extended period of time and then abruptly stopping all C supplementation may cause a type of rebound deficiency. Large doses of some supplements should also be avoided by pregnant and lactating women, infants, and people with certain illnesses. In general, vitamins, minerals, and nutritional substances such as coenzyme Q10 and essential fatty acids are completely safe and nontoxic at levels many times those suggested in this book.

Too much protein, in the form of mixtures of amino acid supplements, may be toxic over the long term to the liver and kidneys.

Taking single amino acid supplements for an extended period of time may cause an imbalance in other amino acids or affect their function. It should also be noted that even the safety of regular doses of single amino acids has been brought into question by the more than three dozen deaths caused by tryptophan in the late 1980s. There is, however, good reason to believe that the danger of occasional use of single amino acids (and tryptophan in particular) has been overstated (see the discussion of tryptophan in Chapter 12).

Essential oils. Properly used, essential oils have few side effects. As a rule, however, essential oils are extremely potent, more so than most of the other natural remedies discussed in this book, and must be kept out of the reach of children. Essential oils are used in minute amounts for healing purposes. Measurement is by the drop, and most essential oils should be diluted before being applied to the body or taken internally. Topically, some can cause allergic reactions and photosensitivity, so it is a good idea to do a patch test on the skin before applying any oil to large areas of the body. Certain oils should be avoided if you're pregnant, have a seizure disorder, or have high blood pressure.

Homeopathic remedies. Because they are so dilute, homeopathic remedies are among the safest medical substances on record. Indeed, some homeopathic remedies are so dilute they probably contain no molecules of the original plant, animal, or mineral substance. From the homeopathic point of view, it must be noted, these extremely dilute remedies are actually the most potent ones, since they've gone through the greatest number of succussions (the process of diluting and shaking the mother tincture that is said to "energize" or "potentize" the remedy). From either the biochemical viewpoint or the homeopathic one, the remedies that are commonly sold in natural-food stores are safe and nontoxic.

Using Natural Substances Responsibly

The two most basic guidelines for safely using natural substances are based on common sense.

• Pay attention to potency, dosage level, frequency of use, and body size. The higher the potency and the dosage level, the more likely it is that an herb or nutritional substance can have druglike effects.

• It is best always to check with a knowledgeable practitioner if you have a special health condition, are pregnant or breast-feeding, or are unsure about the safety of a supplement program.

The supplement levels suggested throughout this book are safe and nontoxic for the vast majority of adults. If you suspect an herb or nutritional substance is causing an adverse reaction, stop using it and try something else that is better suited to your body and its needs.

How to Use This Book

Though it contains some valuable therapeutic information, this book is not a guide to healing medical problems with natural substances. If you want to know how to treat your asthma or lower a fever or heal a burn using herbs or nutrients, a number of excellent texts can guide you. (See Chapter 19, "Resources," for the names of a few of the more comprehensive books in this category.) This book is not focused on or organized around medical conditions in part because there already exist so many worthwhile books on natural health that are oriented toward curing disease. Treatment is undoubtedly a worthwhile focus, and it is one for which natural remedies offer many advantages.

This book, however, takes a different approach. This chapter and the next make up Part I, which introduces the most popular types of natural substances. It also provides background on the twenty most popular herbs, vitamins and minerals, nutritional substances, amino acids, and medicinal mushrooms that have disease-preventive, health-promoting, or psychoactive properties.

The fifteen chapters of Part II make up the bulk of the book. These chapters are organized by the actions or purposes associated with natural substances—boosting your immunity, increasing your energy levels, elevating your mood, stimulating your sexuality, lowering your risk of cancer, and so forth. Each chapter discusses how specific natural substances can benefit almost anyone on an everyday basis, whether you are ill or healthy, young or old, male or female, active or sedentary.

Part III emphasizes the need to use supplements in a way that complements rather than substitutes for a healthful lifestyle. It also offers a wide range of resources for finding further information on natural substances and for obtaining them.

Here are some general guidelines for getting the most out of the information presented here:

• Because the most versatile herbs and nutrients have numerous benefits, a number of these popular natural substances appear in three or more chapters. The earliest mention will contain the most detailed background information on the product's history, derivation, traditional use, cautions, and so forth. While the background information on these substances is not repeated each time they are mentioned, every effort has been made to make certain that the safety cautions are.

• Suggested dosages are provided each time a substance is discussed in connection with a particular use. For some natural substances, dosages are identical for various purposes. For others, such as the amino acids, dosages frequently differ somewhat depending upon the purpose.

• As a general rule, the most popular, effective, and scientifically validated remedies are given their own subhead and listed first in the discussions of each category of remedy. Thus, for example, valerian comes first in the discussion in Chapter 12 of the calming herbs. It is the most widely recognized and thoroughly studied of the sedative herbs, and it is the one herb that is almost always included in combination products for relaxation or insomnia.

• In a few cases a common use of a natural substance has been discussed but suggested dosages have been intentionally omitted. This may be due to unresolved safety concerns, or because the substance should be taken as part of a therapeutic program devised and supervised by a knowledgeable practitioner.

• Every effort has been made to cite scientific studies when they have confirmed—or disputed—a substance's effects. A lack of scientific proof, however, has not automatically disqualified a substance from inclusion herein. When a substance's purported action is validated primarily by traditional use or anecdotal evidence, it is so mentioned.

• Most of the chapters offer up to two dozen or so natural substances from which to choose. Obviously, you wouldn't need or want to take all of these. See the short sections on "How to Choose" and "Where to Start" for help in identifying the best substances for you.

• Combining substances—this herb with that vitamin, an amino acid with a homeopathic remedy—is part art and part science. Unfortunately, the scientific investigation of natural medicine is still in its infancy. Many individual herbs and nutrients have been researched for their effects on the body, but combinations in general have not been. Thus, for example, individual studies on vitamin C, on zinc, and on the herb echinacea have suggested that timely ingestion of these nutrients may help to prevent or shorten the duration of colds. Yet to date no studies have looked at what, if anything, might happen if you took optimal levels of all three of these substances at the first sign of a cold. Even lacking specific studies, many practitioners of natural medicine feel that it is a reasonable assumption that such a combination may work as well as, or even better than, any single substance, with similar levels of safety.

• Experiment with single substances before you do begin to combine them. Taking a specific herb or nutrient for a week or so allows you to identify any effects it may have on you physically, mentally, and emotionally. It also allows you to determine whether you are allergic to it or have some other adverse reaction.

• Look to the natural-products industry for help with combinations. Your local natural-food store carries a diverse supply of combination remedies for stimulation, relaxation, longevity, and so forth. In every chapter, I mention the brand names of typical products. These are representative rather than exhaustive lists. Also, do not interpret these lists as endorsements of specific products—you need to make an independent evaluation as best you can. Nevertheless, many people find that buying natural combination products is much easier than formulating one's own remedies. If you do choose to formulate your own remedies, commercial natural products can serve as valuable models for ingredients and dosage.

• First and foremost, do no harm. This age-old advice underlies all of the suggestions in this book. As with any reference guide, every contingency cannot be covered nor can an individual's own circumstances be considered. If you have a concern about the safety of any substance, check with your doctor or health practitioner. Of course, you should regularly consult your personal physician or primary care practitioner in matters relating to your own health, particularly with respect to any symptoms which may require diagnosis or medical attention. Furthermore, if you're on a prescription drug, you must not stop taking it without first consulting with your doctor.

The Top Twenty Natural Substances

Setting up your natural stay-well remedy chest is an important first step toward optimal health. Just as the well-stocked medicine chest contains pain relievers, anti-inflammatories, decongestants, and wound healers, your stay-well remedy chest should contain substances to boost immunity, prevent heart disease and cancer, promote relaxation, and keep all your body's systems functioning well. Following is a list of the top twenty most commonly used natural substances mentioned throughout the book for these purposes.

Herbs

Garlic
Ginkgo
Ginseng
Siberian ginseng

Vitamins and Minerals

Vitamin A/beta carotene
Vitamin C
Vitamin E
Calcium and magnesium
Chromium
Zinc

Nutritional Substances

Choline
Coenzyme Q10
Essential fatty acids
Polyphenols and flavonoids
Beneficial live bacteria
Melatonin

Amino Acids

Phenylalanine
Tyrosine

Medicinal Mushrooms

Reishi
Shiitake

Though they are not used as frequently for stay-well purposes as the above natural substances, two other categories of medicinal agents—essential oils and homeopathic remedies—are represented in forthcoming chapters and are worth mentioning here.

A Note on Plant Names

Because some plants play an important role in different branches of natural medicine, it is important to distinguish how the plant has been prepared for its use as a remedy. For instance, both herbalists and homeopaths use chamomile to make tablets, tinctures, lotions, and other types of preparations. There is also an essential oil of Chamomile, used by herbalists and aromatherapists. The level of active chemical constituents and the potency of these preparations vary dramatically. The essential oil is the most concentrated form in terms of chemical constituents, and in general essential oils are not taken orally and need to be diluted before they can safely be applied to the skin. Some homeopathic preparations, on the other hand, may not have even a single molecule of chamomile. Thus, the recommendation "use chamomile for insomnia" is unclear, since it doesn't specify the type of preparation. The convention we'll follow will be to:

- Refer to herbal remedies using lowercase letters in a roman typeface: chamomile tablets, chamomile tincture
- Refer to homeopathic remedies using an initial capital and italics: *Chamomilla* ointment

• Refer to the medicines in the form of essential oils using an initial cap and roman typeface: Chamomile

The first time a plant is mentioned, the most widely accepted scientific classification for the genus and species will be provided, to avoid the confusion that sometimes arises from the multitude of common names. For instance, comfrey (*Symphytum officinale*) is sometimes called boneset, a name shared by a different plant (*Eupatorium perfoliatum*). Consumers should be aware of this potential for misidentification of plants when they purchase remedies at natural-food stores or Oriental pharmacies.

Also note that unless stated otherwise, the dosage suggestions for herbs and supplements in this book are for average-sized adults. Children's dosages are usually one half of the adult dosage (for 10- to 14-year-olds), one third of the adult dosage for 6- to 10-year-olds, or even less, depending on the child's size. Check with a knowledgeable practitioner if you have any doubts about the safety of an herb for your child.

The Herbs of Health

Some herbs are as easy to use as aspirin: open the jar and pop a pill. In many cases, though, a somewhat different form will help speed the herb's healing ingredients to where they're most needed. Here's a rundown of the most common ways herbs are prepared and used.

Fresh or dried plant. This is the herb in its most natural, unprocessed forms. The fresh herb is the recently picked leaves, stems, flowers, roots, or bark of a plant. These begin to dry immediately upon being picked, so most fresh herbs are obtained from growing your own or wildcrafting it (picking it in the wild), rather than purchasing it at the natural-food stores. Herbal manufacturers pick the fresh herb and dry it. They then lightly pulverize it and package it in bottles or plastic bags. Herbs lose potency over time. Look for a fresh smell and taste, and natural-looking colors that are not washed out.

Tea. Start with about ¹/₂ to 1 ounce, or 1 teaspoon, of dried herb, or 3 teaspoons of fresh herb per cup of water. Pour boiling water over the herb and steep for 5 minutes or so before straining. Only the herb's water-soluble elements will be present.

Infusion. Prepare a tea but steep it longer, for 10 to 20 minutes, so it becomes considerably darker and more potent. Like a tea, it may be bitter and need to be sweetened before drinking. An infusion has a limited shelf life in the refrigerator, so most people make only as much as they need at the moment. Teas and infusions are appropriate for herbs in which the upper parts of the plant, the flowers and leaves, contain the active ingredients.

Decoction. This is essentially an infusion that is boiled instead of steeped. A decoction is used for hard, woody herbs in which the roots and bark harbor the main healing chemicals. Prepare as you would an infusion, cutting the herb into small pieces or grinding it into a powder, and adding it to boiling water. But instead of turning off the heat and steeping the herb, cover the pot and keep the water boiling at a simmer for 10 to 20 minutes. Strain while still hot. Making a decoction helps to break down the tougher cell walls of bark and roots, allowing the transfer of the active chemicals. Unfortunately, the high heat does tend to destroy some of the herb's volatile oils.

Tinctures, concentrated drops, and liquid herbal extracts. These are generally made by adding the whole or powdered herb to an alcohol-water mixture and letting it sit for days or weeks, or using special extraction machines. The process extracts and concentrates various plant constituents. This is a more involved task, and most people prefer to buy ready-made liquid concentrates at the natural-food store. The use of alcohol allows you to extract more of the plant's active ingredients, and preserves the solution so that it has a longer shelf life. Absorption into the bloodstream is quicker than with tablets and capsules. Because some people want to avoid even the small amounts of alcohol found in tincture products, in recent years many herbal companies have begun to offer alcohol-free liquid extracts or herbal glycerites.

Dosages of liquid concentrates are usually given in drops (for example, 30 to 60 drops), dropperfuls, or teaspoons (it takes approximately 3 dropperfuls to equal a teaspoon). You can swallow the liquid directly, though with many herbs the taste may be unpleasant. Most people prefer to dilute liquid concentrates in a few ounces of water, herbal tea, or juice.

Solid and standardized extracts. Solid extracts are often made by evaporating the tincture to obtain a gummy residue, which is dried and then used to make tablets or capsules. Solid extracts may be identified by a ratio such as 5:1, referring to the number of parts of herb used for every part of solvent. Standardized liquid extracts contain certain (though not all) of the active ingredients of the whole plant in specified concentrations.

Tablets, capsules, and lozenges. These are the familiar pill forms, which may contain anything from the dried herb to a standardized extract. A tablet is simply an herb powder and a base compressed into a small ball or other shape, sometimes with added binders and stabilizers. A capsule is a container (usually gelatin) filled with the herb in the form of a powder, juice, or oil. And a lozenge is the powdered herb or oil combined with sugar and mucilage or gum into pills that are meant to be sucked.

Essential oils. Some plants can be processed to yield pure essential oils, aromatic liquid concentrates of most of the important chemical constituents. (See Chapter 1 and the discussion below for more information on essential oils.)

The Herbal Favorites

The following four herbs are among the most valuable, versatile, and historically rich plant remedies known to humanity.

Garlic

Garlic is a widely venerated food and medicinal herb. It is not a root but a bulb (comprising a number of cloves) that forms on the stem of the plant. Along with some 450 other species, including onions, leeks, shallots, and chives, garlic (*Allium sativum*) is a member of the lily family. As a food, it is a rich source of protein, vitamins A, B complex, and C, and various trace minerals. Garlic figures in a seemingly endless array of folk remedies for everything from insect bites to fever as well as a lengthening list of scientifically validated treatments for conditions including heart disease and intestinal ailments.

Garlic has a history of medicinal use that goes back at least five thousand years. Garlic's medicinal value was known by the ancient Egyptians, as evidenced by carvings of garlic found in pharaohs' tombs as well as a medical papyrus (circa 1500 B.C.E.) that recommends using garlic to relieve headaches and other ailments. Phoenician and Viking sailors took garlic along on voyages to treat ailments. Greek athletes took garlic in the earliest Olympics to improve their performance. Garlic was also well known to practitioners of the traditional medicines of China and India. More recently the Russian army used garlic at the front lines during the two world wars to dress wounds (until it was supplanted by penicillin), and Albert Schweitzer used garlic to treat amebic dysentery and cholera in Africa.

Garlic is among the oldest cultivated plants in existence. The alliums are thought to have originated in Central Asia sometime prior to the advent of written history. They can survive in a variety of climates, and today are grown throughout the world, with China and Spain leading producers. The Japanese are one of the few cultures that avoid garlic, in contrast to the Koreans, who love it.

Garlic research has become a minor industry in the past two decades, with more than seven hundred scientific studies completed. The evidence indicates that garlic is one of the best natural products for the prevention and treatment of a variety of conditions. Garlic is a reliable agent for inhibiting the growth of microorganisms such as bacteria and viruses. Its antibacterial properties were clinically observed as long ago as 1858, in a study done by Louis Pasteur. Its antifungal activity has prompted people to use it to combat skin infections such as athlete's foot and ringworm. It can also kill intestinal parasites and worms.

Garlic's popularity in Mediterranean countries that have relatively low rates of heart disease has led researchers to explore its effects on the circulatory system. There is growing evidence that it can prevent heart attacks by lowering the levels of blood fats, including triglycerides and cholesterol (see Chapter 8). Numerous studies indicate that garlic can also help to prevent cancer; a recent Chinese study suggests it may reduce the risk of stomach cancer (see Chapter 9). Studies also indicate that garlic can boost immunity, balance blood sugar levels (see Chapter 13), and help prevent digestive ailments (see Chapter 16). Japanese researchers have found that garlic can trap toxic lead and mercury in the body and remove them, possibly by helping the liver to neutralize them and other poisons and chemical pollutants.

Garlic is also an effective antioxidant (see Chapter 10), capable of protecting the body against the effects of free radicals—unstable, reactive atoms or molecules (from chemicals, smoke, fatty foods, and other sources) that are damaging to living cells. Antioxidant nutrients such as vitamins A, C, and E can combine with and neutralize free radicals without themselves becoming unstable, thus defending the body against harmful effects that may range from cancer to aging.

The herb is a reliable source of amino acids, certain plant compounds known as flavonoids, and various vitamins and minerals. Scientists have discovered more than two hundred additional compounds in garlic, including about three dozen sulfur compounds rarely found in most other plants. Many garlic researchers believe that the principal medicinal ingredients are the same sulfur compounds as those responsible for garlic's characteristic smell. When garlic is crushed or chopped, chemical constituents such as alliin start to convert into allicin, an unstable substance that in turn breaks down into diallyl disulfides and other organic sulfur compounds, which account for the pungent smell. This may be a protective mechanism for the plant, discouraging bacteria and pests from preying on it. This same protective action may be the source for much of the alliums' medicinal properties.

Garlic is widely used in cooking, though heat inactivates its enzymes and significantly reduces its medicinal effects. Garlic supplements are now a major industry in the United States, where garlic is available fresh or juiced as well as in powders, tablets, capsules, concentrated drops, tinctures, and extracts. Leading brands of garlic supplements include Garlicin, Kwai, Pure-Gar (Quintessence), and Kyolic. Mushrooming consumer interest and new formulations in which garlic is combined with ginkgo, echinacea, or a wide variety of other herbs, as well as various nutrients, have made garlic one of the fastest-growing product lines in the supplement industry. Garlic supplements are now even available in chewable forms for children.

According to herbal authority Varro E. Tyler, Ph.D., Sc.D., author of *Herbs of Choice,* "Most authorities now agree that the best measure of the total activity of garlic is its ability to produce allicin, which, in turn, results in the formation of other active principles. This ability is referred to as the allicin yield of the garlic preparation." Unfortunately, commercial garlic products vary considerably in their levels of sulfur compounds, depending upon growing techniques, mode of preparation, and other factors. A recent study, for example, found that the allicin content in some commercial garlic preparations was six times that found in others. Garlic supplement producers are increasingly standardizing their products for desirable garlic compounds, principally allicin but also alliin, diallyl disulfides, total sulfur, and other components such as s-allyl cysteine.

Most scientists believe that as allicin decays over time it loses its medicinal values. Though some also believe that if there is no smell, there is no therapeutic value, there is solid evidence that "odor-free" and "odor-controlled" garlic products release allicin during digestion and do have significant health effects.

The strength of garlic products is often described in terms of mg of pure or concentrated garlic, mg of "fresh garlic equivalent," or micrograms (mcg) of allicin. Commonly suggested daily dosages are 600 to 1,000 mg of garlic extract or concentrate, or 1,800 to 3,000 mg of fresh garlic equivalent. These doses are approximately equal to eating one clove of fresh garlic. An average recommended daily dose for allicin is 1,800 to 3,600 mcg.

Ginkgo

Ginkgo preparations are derived from the fan-shaped leaves of one of world's most ancient tree species (*Ginkgo biloba*), often termed a living fossil. Christopher Hobbs, herbalist and founder of the Institute for Natural Products Research in Capitola, California, also calls ginkgo "a biological supertree." He notes that as a species, ginkgo has survived almost unchanged for more than 150 million years and that individual trees have lived for more than a thousand years. Ginkgo trees were widespread until the last ice age, when they were wiped out everywhere except in parts of Asia. They have been grown in North America and elsewhere as ornamentals for more than two hundred years.

The Chinese have used both the small, pungent-smelling fruits and the leaves for thousands of years to treat various conditions, including asthma, allergies, and coughs. In the West, ginkgo-leaf preparations are gaining popularity for their reputed ability to improve brain function and boost memory (see Chapter 11) and stimulate alertness (see Chapter 5). Researchers say that ginkgo stimulates circulation in the brain and ears and thus may help prevent dizziness, hearing loss (see Chapter 14), tinnitus, stroke, and depression (see Chapter 6). Ginkgo acts as an antioxidant (see Chapter 10). Studies indicate it has potential use in the treatment of impotence (see Chapter 7), varicose veins and other circulatory conditions (see Chapter 8), and Alzheimer's disease. It is now among the most widely recommended herbal medicines in Europe.

Ginkgo is rich in flavonoids, including quercetin, and in unusual compounds, such as the ginkgolides, apparently unique to the vegetable kingdom. According to herbalist Steven Foster, "As far as we can ascertain, virtually all of the nearly 250 pharmacological and clinical studies published in the last 15 years have involved a specific standardized extract developed and researched in Germany. It is subject to a complex extraction process and standardized to 24 percent flavone glycosides, as well as possibly being further calibrated for, among other constituents, ginkgolides and bilobalide." This 24-percent-flavoglycoside standardized extract is the form of ginkgo commonly found for sale in North American natural-food stores. The usual dosage recommendation is 40 mg three times daily.

Ginseng

Ginseng is an elusive, human-shaped root that is one of the most popular healing herbs in the East and in the West. It includes species from Asia (*Panax ginseng,* usually called Chinese or Korean ginseng) and North America (*Panax quinquefolius,* called American ginseng). Siberian ginseng is not in the *Panax* genus, though it is in the same plant family (Araliaceae) as the ginsengs and has effects and uses somewhat similar to theirs.

The names *panax* and *ginseng* point to this herb's revered status in the East: *panax* combines the same Greek derivatives (*pan-* for "all" and *akos* for "remedy") found in the English word *panacea,* "cure-all." In China, where they have been using ginseng for more than three thousand years, *ginseng* means basically the essence (*seng*) of man (*gin*). "The ancient Chinese believed that the root of the ginseng plant was the crystallization of the essence of the earth in the shape of a man and that ginseng had rejuvenating, recuperative, revitalizing, and curative actions," note T. B. Ng and H. W. Yeung, the authors of the monograph "Scientific Basis of the Therapeutic Effects of Ginseng."

Along with garlic, ginseng is among the most widely studied herbs. Scientists worldwide have written an estimated three hundred original scientific papers on (primarily Asian) ginseng over the past ten years; some three thousand scientific studies have focused on ginseng within the past 50 years. Researchers have determined that some of the active elements in ginseng have a chemical structure that resembles the structure of certain steroids and hormones. It is also a source of vitamins, amino acids, and trace elements, including germanium.

Ginseng has been shown to act on both the cardiovascular and central nervous systems. It helps to regulate blood pressure, maintain blood-glucose levels (a traditional use is in the control of diabetes), and support the thymus and spleen (thus boosting immunity). Ginseng constituents such as the ginsenosides may affect the nervous system, blood flow to the brain, and certain brain neurotransmitters.

People from all walks of life are now using ginseng for a variety of functions, including to

- Improve athletic performance and endurance (see Chapter 4)
- Stimulate the nervous system and boost energy levels and alertness (see Chapter 5)
- Strengthen the sexual system (see Chapter 7)
- Lower blood-cholesterol levels and possibly other factors that can reduce the risk of heart disease (see Chapter 8)

- Protect cells from damage due to radiation and exposure to toxic substances, thus encouraging longevity (see Chapter 10)
- Enhance memory, concentration, and learning (see Chapter 11)
- Normalize physical functioning and help lessen the effects of stress (see Chapter 13)

"Countless studies have proven that ginseng, when used properly, is completely safe and nontoxic," says Mark Blumenthal, executive director of the American Botanical Council in Austin, Texas. He says that reports of "ginseng abuse syndrome," characterized by irritability, nervousness, insomnia, and other adverse effects, are essentially mythical, a "common misconception that continually gets regurgitated into both the lay and scientific press . . . [It is] more aptly termed the 'press abuse syndrome.' "

Ginseng comes in a wide variety of forms, from the whole root to standardized extracts. Potency varies considerably, depending on the type, how it was cultivated, its place of origin, storage factors, and preparation. A recent analysis of 50 commercial ginseng products published in the British medical journal *The Lancet* found tremendous variations in ginsenoside content, from 0 percent (in six of the samples) to 9 percent. Steven Foster and Yue Chongxi, authors of *Herbal Emissaries: Bringing Chinese Herbs to the West,* recommend that for the most predictable results consumers purchase the whole roots or potent standardized products, such as those standardized to 7 percent ginsenosides. Look for brands of standardized extracts such as Ginsana and Ginsun.

Dosages depend upon the purpose for which it is being taken; see specific chapters for recommendations. In general, higher dosages are used when use is occasional (such as to stimulate energy or sexuality) rather than ongoing (such as to extend longevity).

Siberian Ginseng

Also referred to as eleuthero, Siberian ginseng is a popular herb derived from the roots or leaves of a northern shrub (*Eleutherococcus senticosus;* Chinese scientists prefer another name: *Acanthopanax senticosus*) from the Far East. It was a lesser-known strengthening or "tonic" herb of Russian and Chinese folk tradition until Russian scientists of the 1940s and 1950s focused on it as a more widely available (and considerably cheaper) substitute for *Panax ginseng*. Studies on Siberian ginseng by Russian scientists and others have shown that it has considerable promise as an agent to increase longevity and improve overall health. Like other ginsengs, it is an adaptogen, a substance that strengthens, normalizes, and regulates all of the body's systems (see Chapter 13). It supports the workings of the adrenal glands and prevents the worst effects of nervous tension. It tends to increase energy, extend endurance, and fight off fatigue. Siberian ginseng boosts overall immune function (see Chapter 3) and may play a role in the treatment of hypertension, blood-sugar irregularities, and depressed mood and other psychological ailments (see Chapter 6). Studies indicate that Siberian ginseng stimulates circulation, dilates blood vessels, protects cells from free radicals, and boosts cellular oxygen use.

Chemical analysis has isolated various compounds in Siberian ginseng that may affect the body, including the eleutherosides. These differ from the ginsenosides isolated from the *Panax* ginsengs. I. I. Brekhman, one of the Russian scientists who pioneered research into Siberian ginseng, says that the pure, isolated eleutherosides do not have the same strengthening and balancing effects on the body as the whole plant.

Adverse side effects from using Siberian ginseng are very rare. It is considered to be safe for daily consumption even in relatively large doses. Herbal producers often combine it with other adaptogenic herbs such as ginseng and schisandra. Siberian ginseng is usually less expensive than other ginsengs. Adulterated and/or mislabeled products have been identified in recent years; purchase from reputable, quality producers. An average dose is 250 to 500 mg once or twice daily, or 1 to 2 dropperfuls of the concentrated drops or tincture two to three times daily.

Vitamins and Minerals

All of the following vitamins and minerals are readily available both singly and in combination products. Multinutrient tablets, capsules, powders, and liquids offer the advantage of being easy to use. The supplement producers have selected the nutrients for you and combined them in a balanced formulation. Many people prefer taking a "one-a-day" to taking a variety of individual tablets or capsules.

The drawback to the one-a-day approach is that such supplements can offer only a limited amount of certain minerals, such as calcium and magnesium, that have large molecular structures. A true one-a-day supplement can offer 100 percent or higher of the RDA for many but not all nutrients before it just becomes too large to swallow.

Furthermore, more and more progressive nutritionists and natural practitioners are recognizing the inadequacy of RDAs. RDAs are "the nutritional equivalent of the minimum wage," says nutritional researcher Alexander Schauss, Ph.D. Along with a growing number of others, such as the late Nobel Prize–winning scientist and vitamin C proponent Linus Pauling, and clinical nutritionist Shari Lieberman, R.D., coauthor of *The Real Vitamin & Mineral Book,* Schauss says that the "outmoded RDAs" should be scrapped in favor of an entirely new scale for nutrient levels. These "optimal nutrient levels" reflect nutrient intakes that not only prevent obvious deficiency conditions, but actively promote increased health and longevity. Schauss notes that the optimal-nutrient approach is supported by a 15-year study of 13,500 American men and women, led by Drs. Emanuel Cheraskin and W. M. Ringsdorf, Jr., of the University of Alabama School of Medicine. Their study compared nutrient consumption with subjects' health and found that those people with the highest nutrient intakes from diet and supplements were the healthiest individuals.

Admittedly, research on optimal nutrient levels is in its infancy. No universal level exists such that scientists can say, for instance, everybody should take 500 mg of vitamin C daily. Some people require higher or lower nutrient levels than others. Those who generally need higher than average nutrient levels include people who:

- Drink alcohol to excess or smoke
- Live in polluted areas or in areas where food is grown in nutrient-depleted soil
- Are ill, inactive, or have a small appetite
- Are overweight or trying to lose weight (one study of 11 weight-loss diets found that they all fell short of at least one RDA)
- Are pregnant or breast-feeding
- Are elderly
- Have poor intestinal absorption

Those who may need lower-than-average supplemental nutrient levels include individuals who for most of their lives eat diverse and healthful diets with, for example, numerous servings per day of dark-green leafy vegetables and other nutrient-dense foods, don't drink alcohol to excess or smoke cigarettes, experience low levels of mental stress, are not overweight, and get regular exercise or are physically active. If you're not among this select group (and just the first criterion narrows the field considerably: fewer than one in ten Americans is thought to eat the recommended minimum of five servings of vegetables and fruits per day), consuming optimal nutrient levels will probably boost your health.

The optimal nutrient levels suggested for the following vitamins and minerals are well below any known toxicity levels. Optimal levels are generally a number of times higher than either RDAs or U.S. RDAs, though for some nutrients (zinc and calcium, for instance) they're quite close.

To obtain optimal intake levels, you'll need to take either individual vitamin and mineral supplements or any of the many supplements that offer optimal vitamin and mineral levels by means of a dosage that requires taking two or more capsules per day. Formulas requiring four to six tablets or capsules per day are common.

Vitamins and minerals are widely available not only in natural-food stores but in pharmacies, supermarkets, and drugstores. Prices vary considerably, but you can take even a wide variety of high-quality supplements at a cost of only a few dollars per day. You can safely and effectively take the following optimal levels of nutrients for short periods or indefinitely.

Vitamin A/Beta Carotene

Vitamin A, or retinol, is a fat-soluble micronutrient essential for healthy vision, cell reproduction, wound healing, and other crucial bodily functions. In its preformed state it is derived from animal sources; beta carotene is a plant-derived vitamin A precursor. In addition to its role as a vitamin A precursor, however, beta carotene and other related carotenoids are increasingly being recognized as having further important health-related roles in the body.

Vitamin A's ability to boost the immune system (see Chapter 3) has been well established by scientific studies. Vitamin A improves resistance to infection and may play a role in the prevention or treatment of respiratory infections, diarrhea, and measles. Some researchers say vitamin A and vitamin A derivatives may also help prevent or treat cancer (see Chapter 9). Vitamin A supports the functioning of the eyes and ears (see Chapter 14). Dermatologists use vitamin A derivatives to renew aged skin and treat acne (see Chapter 15).

Beta carotene is the most well known of the almost six hundred carotenoid pigments that have been identified in plants. Carotenoids give cantaloupes, carrots, sweet potatoes, and other fruits and vegetables their yellow-orange color. Various carotenoids in addition to beta carotene also occur naturally in dark-green leafy vegetables and other foods rich in chlorophyll.

Your liver and intestines convert beta carotene to vitamin A with a high degree of efficiency. Beta carotene is apparently the most bioavailable of the sixty or so carotenoids that act as precursors to vitamin A. Beta carotene is also the carotenoid found in the highest amounts in the foods we eat. Recent studies have found, however, that other carotenoids may have preventive and therapeutic effects that equal or surpass beta carotene's. Many carotenoids that are not vitamin A precursors are powerful antioxidants (see Chapter 10). Carotenoids such as lycopene may help to prevent cancer; the carotenoid lutein may protect against cataracts. Alpha carotene, after beta the most common carotene, is less potent than beta as a vitamin A precursor but, like beta, may be a powerful cancer controller. Many nutritional researchers expect that future studies will identify other carotenes that are similarly important for promoting bodily health.

It is likely that carotenoids act much more effectively together than individually. Currently, most supplements contain only beta carotene, though some manufacturers are beginning to include alpha carotene. Supplements rich in a number of the other carotenoids as well are principally the concentrated green foods, such as spirulina and blue-green algae, and the dried juice of young shoots of cereal plants such as barley and wheat grass. As whole-food concentrates, these offer relatively low levels per dose of any one carotenoid. Eating a diverse, carotenoid-rich diet supplies an estimated 5 to 10 mg of beta carotene daily; average adult consumption of beta carotene on the standard American diet is much lower, at 1 to 2 mg daily.

Most nutritionists consider beta carotene to be as effective as preformed, meat-based vitamin A yet much less toxic. Taking high doses of preformed vitamin A, such as 100,000 International Units (a measure of provitamin A activity) daily for months, or 500,000 to 1,000,000 IU daily for two to three weeks, can allow it to accumulate in the body and cause potentially serious adverse health effects. On the other hand, the body converts to vitamin A only as much beta carotene as it needs. Extra beta carotene is stored, but the only apparent adverse effect of such storage is a slight orange tinge to the skin. Thus, many people prefer to take vitamin A supplements in the form of beta carotene.

It is also possible, however, that preformed vitamin A combines with beta carotene and other carotenoids to produce synergistic effects. Most supplement manufacturers offer mixed vitamin A–beta carotene supplements. A single supplement may provide, for example, 5,000 IU of vitamin A (usually derived from cold-water fish liver oil) and 15,000 IU vitamin A activity from beta carotene (derived either synthetically or from carrots or algae). Pure beta carotene supplements are usually in the form of tablets or capsules (either dry or oil-filled). Potency typically ranges from 10,000 to 50,000 IU, though products such as Mega Carotene Caps provide as much as 83,000 IU per capsule.

Because of the recent studies identifying positive health benefits from carotenoids other than beta carotene, and the fact that one study found that consuming high levels of pure beta carotene can depress blood levels of other carotenoids, a consensus is building that taking mixed carotenoid supplements is probably even safer and more effective than relying on pure beta carotene. Within the past year or so a number of producers have started to offer mixed carotenoid supplements, with and without beta carotene. These supplements often include alpha and gamma carotene and such carotenoids as lycopene, lutein, and cryptoxanthin. Look for supplements such as Extension Carotenoids and CAROTeam.

The U.S. RDA for vitamin A is 5,000 IU. An optimal daily dose for adults is 5,000 to 10,000 IU of preformed vitamin A plus 25,000 to 50,000 IU of beta carotene or, preferably, beta carotene plus mixed carotenoids. (Beta carotene is sometimes measured in milligrams rather than International Units. Since 1 mg approximately equals 1,667 IU, 25,000 to 50,000 IU is equivalent to 15 to 30 mg.)

Vitamin C

Vitamin C was involved in one of the earliest scientific inquiries into the role of nutrients. In 1746 the Scottish physician James Lind demonstrated that lemon juice could prevent scurvy, though the active ingredient (ascorbic or "antiscurvy" acid, also known as vitamin C) was not isolated until 1932. Studies have since shown that vitamin C strengthens the walls of blood vessels, helps the body resist infection, and protects other vitamins from oxidation. Vitamin C is crucial to optimal immune-system function (see Chapter 3) and has been shown to reduce the symptoms of colds, asthma, and allergies. Vitamin C also plays a central role in the healing of wounds and broken bones and in recovery from surgery, in part because it is vital to the formation of collagen, a fibrous tissue found throughout the body. Adequate vitamin C intake will contribute to healthy collagen formation in the skin, thus protecting blood vessels from the effects of trauma and bruising (see Chapter 15). High blood levels of vitamin C have been tied to improved athletic performance (see Chapter 4), mood (see Chapter 6), cardiovascular health (see Chapter 8), cancer prevention (see Chapter

9), longevity (see Chapter 10), brain function (see Chapter 11), and sense functioning (see Chapter 14).

Vitamin C is concentrated in certain fruits and vegetables, with the highest levels in dark-green leafy vegetables, broccoli, Brussels sprouts, cauliflower, potatoes, strawberries, and grapefruit. It is the most widely taken vitamin in supplement form. The adult RDA is 60 to 95 mg, though this is a fraction of what many people take to optimize their overall health.

Supplement manufacturers offer vitamin C in tablet and capsule sizes ranging all the way from 250 mg to 1,500 mg. You can also find vitamin C in a wide variety of chewable or time-release tablets, buffered capsules (with added calcium, for example, to reduce C's natural acidity), powders, liquids, and even chewing gums.

Vitamin C is nontoxic at levels far in excess of the RDA. If you take approximately 2 to 5 g or more per day, you may develop diarrhea or loose stools. Many alternative practitioners of natural medicine call this a person's "bowel tolerance" and recommend that vitamin C be taken at dosages lower than those that cause overt symptoms. You can determine your bowel tolerance by taking 1 g daily of vitamin C, in divided doses, for three to four days, noting the condition of your stools, and then increasing your daily dose to 2 g, again for three to four days, and so on, up to 5 g, if the stools stay normal. Megadoses beyond 2 to 3 g may increase the risk of kidney stones in some people and the risk of miscarriage in pregnant women.

An optimal dose of vitamin C is 250 to 500 mg two to three times daily.

Vitamin E

First isolated in 1936, vitamin E is a powerful antioxidant that plays a crucial role in promoting overall health. By protecting the body against the harmful effects of free radicals, vitamin E reduces the risk of health problems ranging from cancer (see Chapter 9) to the effects of aging (see Chapter 10). Vitamin E is used by most of the tissues of the body. It protects vitamins A and C from destruction and aids in the formation of red blood cells, muscles, and other tissues. Studies suggest that oral doses of vitamin E can help eliminate exercise cramps and nighttime leg cramps. Vitamin E may also boost immunity (see Chapter 3), enhance athletic performance (see Chapter 4), promote virility (see Chapter 7), protect against heart disease (see Chapter 8), and aid the senses (see Chapter 14).

Vitamin E oil applied to the skin (just break open the oil-filled capsules) seems to accelerate the healing of burns. It nourishes the skin (see Chapter 15) and benefits a range of skin conditions, such as canker sores, nipples that are sore and cracked from breast-feeding, and diaper rash. Vitamin E applied to a closed wound helps prevent a scar from forming.

The highest levels of vitamin E are found in vegetable oils, including safflower, wheat germ, and corn. The best food sources are dark-green leafy vegetables, whole grains, vegetable oils, wheat germ, nuts, seeds, and legumes. Meat and dairy products usually have low amounts. Vitamin E supplements most commonly are oil-filled capsules. The naturally occurring forms of vitamin E, designated by the prefix D- (as in D-alpha tocopherol), are somewhat more absorbable than the synthetic DL- forms (DL-alpha tocopherol) of the vitamin.

The U.S. RDA for vitamin E is 30 IU. Some people may experience dizziness, elevated blood pressure, decreased blood coagulation, or other side effects at daily dosages of 1,200 to 1,600 IU. An optimal supplement level is 400 to 600 IU daily, a safe and nontoxic dosage for long-term consumption.

Calcium and Magnesium

Calcium is a well-known mineral that plays an important role in a variety of essential bodily functions, including building of bones and teeth, transmitting nerve messages, regulating heartbeat, and coagulating blood. It is recommended in the treatment or prevention of osteoporosis, heart disease, problems of menopause, and certain cancers. Taken before bed, calcium and magnesium may have a slight sedating effect (see Chapter 12). Calcium supplements are derived from a variety of sources, including dolomite, oyster shells, and bone meal. It is also produced in different chemical forms, with calcium citrate and calcium carbonate noted for being highly absorbable.

Magnesium is an essential major mineral found primarily in dark-green leafy vegetables, soybeans, and nuts and seeds. Magnesium is required for strong, healthy bones, and is concentrated in the body in the bones and teeth. It is important to a variety of other bodily processes: It helps keep cells electrically stable and, with calcium, regulates the body's energy levels and maintains normal heart function (see Chapter 8) and neurotransmission. A magnesium deficiency can cause muscle tremors, convulsions, and possibly psychiatric problems. Supplements are used to treat premenstrual syndrome (PMS), high blood pressure, anxiety (see Chapter 6), osteoporosis, fatigue (see Chapter 5), and diabetes. Calcium and magnesium may enhance athletic performance (see Chapter 4), lower cancer risk (see Chapter 9), boost brain power (see Chapter 11), and protect the skin (see Chapter 15). Some therapists use magnesium supplements to treat convulsions in pregnant women. Magnesium is probably the safest mineral, with no record of toxicity from supplements.

These two minerals work closely with each other in the body and are sometimes combined in supplements. Many nutritionists suggest taking these supplements in a ratio that approximates 2:1, as in 750 mg calcium and 375 mg magnesium.

The adult RDA for calcium is 800 to 1,200 mg; for magnesium, 280 to 400 mg. An optimal daily intake is 800 to 1,500 mg of calcium and 450 to 650 mg of magnesium.

Chromium

In the 1950s chromium was wildly popular among auto makers as the source for the shiny alloy chrome, but it was considered toxic by nutritionists. Today auto makers shun it, but fans of nutritional supplements have made it a hot item in natural-food stores. The whims of Detroit are mysterious, but there are good reasons why nutritionists now consider chromium an essential mineral. In the late 1950s Dr. Walter Mertz discovered that chromium was needed for insulin to maintain its effectiveness. Because insulin is crucial for regulating the metabolism of proteins, carbohydrates, and fats, when the body is given insufficient chromium all sorts of health problems often follow, from blood-sugar imbalances to obesity and diabetes. In recent years more and more people are taking chromium to reduce the risk of heart disease (see Chapter 8), help control blood-sugar levels (see Chapter 13), and reduce the risk of vision problems (see Chapter 14). Athletes and others have also been turning to chromium for help in lowering body-fat levels and encouraging muscle development (see Chapter 4) and controlling hunger and weight (see Chapter 17).

There is no established RDA for chromium. The National Academy of Sciences considers 50 to 200 mcg safe and adequate. Dietary surveys done by the U.S. Department of Agriculture and others indicate that 90 percent of Americans get insufficient chromium from their diet. The USDA estimates that Americans consume an average of only 25 to 33 mcg of chromium daily. (Similar deficiencies have also been identified in England and Finland.) Most foods are low in chromium; the best food sources are brewer's yeast and organ meats, while shellfish, whole grains, potatoes, and wheat germ may also provide reliable amounts. Foods that have been processed usually lack chromium. Strenuous physical activity increases an individual's requirement for chromium; mental stress and eating large amounts of sugary foods depletes your body's chromium stores.

Chromium is one of the safest nutritional supplements known. It does not cause side effects at levels up to 100 times greater than the average adult dose, and can be taken on a daily basis indefinitely. Diabetics taking insulin, however, should consult with a physician before taking chromium supplements.

Chromium is sold in a number of forms and under a variety of brand names. Because elemental chromium, like the chrome used on car bumpers, cannot be absorbed by the body, supplement manufacturers use biologically active trivalent chromium. The form of chromium that researchers have determined has the most effect on insulin function, and which is found naturally in brewer's yeast, is called glucose tolerance factor (GTF), an organic chromium complex that contains niacin as well as cysteine and other nutrients. Chromium polynicotinate is also a niacin-bound form of chromium. Another well-absorbed form of chromium is chromium picolinate, a patented synthetic compound sold under various brand names.

Some chromium supplements combine GTF chromium, chromium picolinate, and other nutrients. Chromium supplements available in stores include Chromoplex, Chromium Complex, and Performance Picolinate. They are widely available in tablets and capsules (usually 100 to 200 mcg), and liquids. An optimal daily dose for adults is 200 to 400 mcg.

Zinc

Zinc is a trace mineral essential for proper wound healing, immunity (see Chapter 3), male sexual potency (see Chapter 7), liver detoxification, and numerous other bodily functions. Zinc is necessary for the sense organs that provide proper vision, hearing, taste, and smell (see Chapter 14). Its potential therapeutic uses include treatment of acne and other skin diseases and injuries (see Chapter 15), colds, infertility, eye disorders, ulcers, and alcoholism. It is often taken before and after surgical operations to speed recovery. In the body it is found in the greatest concentrations in semen, the eyes, the heart, and the brain. Zinc supplements may help to lower cancer risk (see Chapter 9), boost brain power (see Chapter 11), balance blood sugar (see Chapter 13), and assist in weight loss (see Chapter 17).

Zinc is found naturally in animal foods, oysters, whole grains, and some seeds and nuts. Increased food processing and declining soil levels of zinc have made marginal deficiencies of the mineral more prevalent. Zinc supplements come in tablets, capsules, and lozenges. It is frequently combined with other minerals and vitamins—taking high levels of only zinc can lead to copper, selenium, or iron deficiency. Most people experience no adverse effects from taking up to about 150 mg per day (six to nine times the optimal dose) of zinc; a few people experience side effects such as gastrointestinal irritation. Dosages on the order of 2,000 mg are toxic enough to cause vomiting.

The adult RDA is 12 to 19 mg; an optimal dose for most adults is 17 to 25 mg daily.

Nutritional Substances

Some nutritional substances have nutrientlike effects that rival those of the vitamins and minerals. Whether substances such as choline, coenzyme Q10, essential fatty acids, and flavonoids actually should be considered vitamins is the subject of some debate in the nutritional field. Two other natural substances, the beneficial live bacteria and the hormone melatonin, are not essential micronutrients, yet when they are lacking or out of balance, overall health can be undermined.

Choline/Phosphatidylcholine/Lecithin

Choline is a nutrient that some nutritionists now consider to be a B-complex vitamin. Though no RDA has been established, recent research indicates that choline, in conjunction with nutrients including other B vitamins and vitamin C, plays an important role in the metabolism of fats (see Chapter 17), proper liver function, and the workings of the nervous system. Choline is necessary for the healthy functioning of cell membranes, nerves, and the brain. Deficiencies have been linked to certain neurological disorders, such as Parkinson's disease and tardive dyskinesia, that are characterized by convulsive muscular movements. Research is underway that may establish choline's protective effect against heart disease and some forms of liver disease.

Choline is intimately involved in the synthesis or release of certain neurotransmitters, particularly acetylcholine, that affect mood (see

Chapter 6), sexuality (see Chapter 7), and memory and learning (see Chapter 11). When some types of neurons are deprived of adequate acetylcholine, the result may be memory loss or even the development of conditions such as Alzheimer's disease that are usually associated with aging. A number of studies have indicated a potential role for choline supplements in the prevention or treatment of Alzheimer's.

Some choline is synthesized in the body; breast milk is a rich source. Choline is also a component of lecithin, a fatty acid found in a variety of foods. Particularly rich sources of lecithin include egg yolks, soybeans, oatmeal, seed oils, peanuts and other legumes, seafood, and certain vegetables such as cabbage and cauliflower. Marginal choline deficiencies may be increasing, according to some nutritionists, as people cut back on lecithin-rich foods such as eggs, peanuts, and oils because of their high cholesterol or fat content. (Prolonged exercise can also reduce blood levels of choline.) The food industry adds lecithin to products such as mayonnaise to act as an emulsifier, thickener, or stabilizer, though not in levels that are dietarily significant. Many people take lecithin in liquids, granules, and capsules for the choline content.

The word *lecithin* really has two meanings. To scientists, it is a technical term referring to phosphatidylcholine, a natural choline-containing compound. Nutritional-product manufacturers and the general public, however, use the term to refer to supplements that contain pure phosphatidylcholine as well as other substances such as the amino acid serine.

The many names and forms of this nutrient are a source of confusion when determining dosage. To make matters worse, the level of pure choline in a lecithin or phosphatidylcholine supplement may not be readily evident from the product label. For many lecithin supplements, a rule of thumb is that the lecithin/phosphatidylcholine/choline ratio is approximately 50:10:1. Thus, for example, 1,200 mg of lecithin yields 240 mg of phosphatidylcholine yields 24 mg of choline. Some lecithin products offer higher percentages of phosphatidylcholine and thus choline. Phosphatidylcholine supplements themselves may be anywhere from 20 to 100 percent pure phosphatidylcholine. For example, a 420-mg phosphatidylcholine supplement that is 90 percent pure phosphatidylcholine (378 mg) yields approximately 38 mg of choline.

Nutrient producers often combine choline with inositol and other nutrients, or include choline in B-complex and multivitamin supplements. Choline is also found in combination supplements, which go by names such as Choline Cocktail, Memory Boost, and Memory Fuel.

Some people experience fishy-smelling body odor and breath as a result of taking choline supplements. Dividing doses (consuming lesser amounts a number of times per day rather than a large dose all at once) or taking lecithin and phosphatidylcholine avoids this side effect. Most nutritional authorities say that, compared to choline, lecithin and phosphatidylcholine also tend to be more absorbable and less likely to cause minor side effects such as nausea, muscle stiffness and muscle-tension headaches, and digestive irritation. One of the drawbacks of lecithin supplements, on the other hand, is their tendency to become rancid.

According to the 1992 edition of the *Physicians' Desk Reference,* "No major side effects have been reported in connection with consumption of large quantities of phosphatidylcholine or commercially available (less pure) lecithin." Two Food and Drug Administration reports agree that taking up to 13.5 g of lecithin per day is safe.

A recent estimate of the average dietary intake of choline by Americans is 300 to 1,000 mg daily. An average daily supplemental dose is 100 to 200 mg of choline; 1,100 to 2,200 mg of phosphatidylcholine that is 90 percent pure; or 5 to 10 g, or 1 to 2 tablespoons of granules, of lecithin that is 20 percent phosphatidylcholine.

Coenzyme Q10

Coenzyme Q10 (coQ10) is a vitaminlike compound also known as ubiquinone, from the fact that it is naturally ubiquitous throughout the body. Discovered in 1957, the substance was unfortunately saddled with the misleading name of coenzyme Q10. Recent research indicates it could well have been termed a vitamin, since deficiency in it is possible and it is essential for well-being. Like many other vitamins, it acts as a coenzyme in the body to promote various chemical reactions. CoQ10 is needed to help the body's cells use oxygen and generate energy. In particular, it acts as a catalyst for the process by which the body produces adenosine triphosphate (ATP), necessary for energy at the cellular level. Coenzyme Q10 is also an antioxidant.

In humans coQ10 concentrates in certain organs, especially the liver and the heart, and it has been shown to help prevent or treat heart disease and hypertension (see Chapter 8). CoQ10 tends to stimulate the immune system and overall metabolism. It may be useful against diabetes, Alzheimer's disease, and obesity. Some people take coQ10 to boost energy levels (see Chapter 5), strengthen muscles and improve physical performance and endurance (see Chapter 4), and lose weight (see Chapter 17). It has also demonstrated excellent results in clinical trials on periodontal disease, speeding up healing time, reducing gum pockets, and improving other factors associated with gum disease.

CoQ10 is found in high amounts in organ meats and in cold-water fish such as sardines and tuna. Other food sources include polyunsaturated vegetable oils and spinach, though plant foods generally have only trace levels. The body does naturally produce coQ10; it needs sufficient B-complex vitamins and vitamin C for the process.

CoQ10 causes few side effects even when taken in amounts ten times higher than optimal recommended dosages.

There is no RDA for coQ10. An optimal intake level for adults is 15 to 30 mg daily.

Essential Fatty Acids

Essential fatty acids (EFAs) are fats that are needed by the body but are not manufactured by it and thus must be obtained through the diet. They are sometimes collectively referred to as vitamin F, though there is no established RDA. In the body EFAs act to strengthen cell membranes and promote the growth of muscles and nerves. They are used therapeutically to thin the blood and inhibit clotting, and to improve blood cholesterol and triglyceride profiles. They thus help prevent heart disease (see Chapter 8). EFAs also have natural anti-inflammatory effects, and so are potentially useful in the treatment of arthritis, allergies, asthma, and skin conditions (see Chapter 15). There is some evidence for a cancer-preventive effect (see Chapter 9).

Important EFAs include the omega-3's, such as eicosapentaenoic acid (EPA) and docosahexaenoic acid (DHA), and alpha linolenic acid, a plant-oil-derived EPA/DHA precursor. EPA and DHA are found primarily in the oil of cold-water fish. They usually occur together, and have similar effects on the body—reducing inflammation, lowering blood fat and cholesterol levels, and thinning the blood. Taken in excess they can reduce blood clotting capability to an unhealthful degree.

Other EFAs are the omega-6's, including linoleic acid and gamma linolenic acid (GLA). GLA is found in significant quantities only in oils derived from a few plants, especially evening primrose, borage, and black currant. Studies indicate GLA has potential therapeutic use in the prevention or treatment of heart disease, arthritis, skin problems, and PMS. GLA may also stimulate the growth of hair and nails. It has a soothing effect when applied topically to the skin.

The following substances are among the richest dietary sources of essential fatty acids. Supplements derived from these sources may need to be refrigerated. Many EFA supplements have vitamin E oil added in order to prevent rancidity. They are sold as liquids and capsules.

Concentrated fish oils. These are the fatty liquids expressed from certain cold-water fish, including salmon, mackerel, sardines, cod, blue-fish, herring, and tuna. The omega-3 fish oils are the most popular form of the essential fatty acid supplements. Most contain 1,000 to 1,250 mg of fish-oil concentrate, representing an EPA range of 180 to 360 mg and a DHA range of 120 to 240 mg. Look for products such as MaxEPA, SuperEPA, EPA Pure, Omega-3 EPA, Essential Fatty Acid Complex, and Balance Plus.

Cod liver oil. This is a fish oil rich in EPA and DHA. Unless the fat-soluble vitamins A and D have been removed, however, consuming too much cod liver oil may result in toxic levels of these vitamins building up in the body.

Borage oil. This is a vegetable oil derived from the seeds of a blue-flowering plant (*Borago officinalis*) that is also used as an herb in Europe, primarily to restore adrenal function and counter inflammation. The seed oil is taken as a supplement because it is one of the most concentrated natural sources of GLA—capsules providing 1,000 to 1,300 mg of borage oil usually have 240 to 300 mg of GLA.

Evening primrose oil. This fatty liquid is extracted from the seeds of a yellow-flowering willow-family plant (*Oenothera biennis*) that is a richly endowed source of the omega-6 essential fatty acid GLA. Evening primrose oil is produced primarily in Great Britain and is a popular remedy in Europe. Technically its use is still experimental in the United States, but few side effects have appeared. Since the late 1980s, evening primrose oil has been the subject of an ongoing regulatory dispute between the FDA and importers, who have had some shipments seized as an "unapproved food additive." Nevertheless, it is still available as a liquid or in capsules.

Black currant oil. The oil from this plant (*Ribes nigrum*) usually provides 50 to 100 mg of GLA per 1,000-mg capsules.

Rape seed oil. Rape seed (*Brassica napus*) is the source for canola oil, the popular cooking oil.

Flax seed oil. The flax plant (*Linum usitatissimum*) is used to make linen fiber as well as a seed oil rich in EFAs.

Hemp seed oil. This seed oil, derived from marijuana (*Cannabis sativa*), is a new one on the natural-foods market. It is pressed from sterilized seeds imported from Canada and has both omega-3's and some GLA. The seeds and the oil have no psychoactive property and are completely legal products in the United States (see "Resources" for the address of the producer).

"To a certain extent the omega-3's and omega-6's overlap," notes nutritional practitioner Shari Lieberman. "Both tend to enhance the body's ability to reduce inflammation and improve cholesterol profiles. Which one is best for an individual is often a matter of trial and error. Some studies have shown that the best results are achieved by using the omega-3's and omega-6's together."

An optimal supplement level of EFAs for adults is 250 to 500 mg daily.

Polyphenols and Flavonoids

Polyphenols are a large class of plant constituents with potent antioxidant (see Chapter 10) and disease-preventive properties. Among the most prominent polyphenols are the flavonoids, a group of often brightly colored compounds found in various fruits (especially citrus and berries), vegetables, grains, and herbs. They are also known collectively as vitamin P, the term applied to them by Szent-Györgyi, the vitamin C discoverer who also did pioneering research on the bioflavonoids. Flavonoids may help protect the body from viruses and allergens. They may also play an important role in preventing heart disease (see Chapter 8), cancer (see Chapter 9), and blood-sugar imbalances (see Chapter 13).

Some of the first flavonoids to be widely studied were hesperidin, quercetin, and rutin, which occur together in lemons, oranges, and other citrus fruits. They have been found to help protect capillaries and strengthen and stabilize cell membranes in the body. The convention has arisen (which we'll follow here) to refer to these as *bioflavonoids* (biologically active flavonoids) or *bioflavonoid complex,* though many other classes of flavonoids are also biologically active. Supplement manufacturers offer quercetin (as a single nutrient, typically derived from algae) and rutin (from buckwheat) in single supplements of 250 to 500 mg. More-popular products are the bioflavonoid complex and individual bioflavonoids in combination with other supplements, most often vitamin C (which protects quercetin, for example, from oxidation). These are usually found in sizes ranging from 500 to 1,000 mg. Look for products such as Citrus Bioflavonoid, Vital C Plex, and C Complex.

Some of the herbs rich in polyphenols and flavonoids include ginkgo, bilberry, European coastal pine, hawthorn, and milk thistle. Some popular beverages that are rich in polyphenols include green tea, red wine, and grape juice. Supplements based on the bioflavonoids and on compounds derived from these plants are now starting to appear in natural-food stores. Look for products such as C+ Herbal Polyflavonoids and C+ Super Polyflavonoids. These usually contain vitamin C, bioflavonoids such as quercetin and rutin, and herbs rich in various classes of polyphenols and flavonoids.

Ginkgo. Ginkgo contains bioflavonoids such as quercetin, the flavonoid-sugar derivative compounds known as flavone glycosides or simply flavoglycosides, and other flavonoids. Most supplement products are standardized for 24 percent flavoglycosides.

Bilberry. This is a blue-black berry, similar to the American huckleberry, that grows on a shrub (*Vaccinium myrtillus*) commonly found throughout Europe. Bilberry is rich in a class of reddish-blue flavonoid pigments known as anthocyanosides, which have a noted effect on vision (see Chapter 14). An Italian study of anthocyanosides also indicates that bilberry can lower blood cholesterol and triglyceride levels.

European or maritime coastal pine. The bark of this native French tree (*Pinus maritima*) is one of the few sources (along with grapes, cranberries, and a few other fruits and vegetables) to yield significant amounts of the flavonoids known as proanthocyanidins. A pine-bark extract rich in these powerful antioxidant plant constituents is sold as Pycnogenol, a registered trademark of the European-based company Horphag Research. Pycnogenol has been popular in Europe for a number of years and is increasingly catching on in North America. It is sold as Pycnogenol by various U.S. supplement companies and through multilevel marketing sources; most products are capsules containing 20 to 50 mg. Practitioners of natural medicine recommend it primarily as an antioxidant to reduce the risk of cancer and heart disease, but some also use it therapeutically to help strengthen blood vessels, boost circulation, or improve vision. It is safe and nontoxic.

Hawthorn. Hawthorn preparations are derived from the flowers, leaves, or berries of a thorny shrub (*Crataegus oxyacantha*) native to Europe. The plant is a rich source of polyphenols and flavonoids, including quercetin, vitexin, and catechin. Researchers have found that hawthorn can lower serum cholesterol, reduce blood pressure, and prevent palpitations and arrhythmias. Its many actions on the heart

have led most herbalists to recommend its use only with knowledgeable supervision.

Milk thistle. Herbal companies use flavonoid compounds found in
the seeds of this thorny, weedlike plant (*Silybum marianum*) to make the
standardized extract known as silymarin. The flavonoids in silymarin
appear to differ from other flavonoids by having special protective
effects on liver function (see Chapter 10). Milk thistle extract products
such as the popular Thisilyn are usually standardized for a flavonoid
content of 70 to 80 percent silymarin.

Red wine/grapes. Flavonoid compounds in red wine and red-grape
skins and seeds (or "pips") include the catechins, proanthocyanidins,
and anthocyanidins. Young red wines have higher flavonoid contents
than older wines; white wines have very low levels. A few producers
are now offering Pycnogenol-like supplements containing proantho-
cyanidin derived not from European coastal pine but from grape pip
extract. Look for single-source products such as Grape Seed Extract
and Grape Pips Proanthocyanidins and combination products with
names like Proanthanol (also containing ginkgo and bilberry),
Proflavanol, and OPC Plus (OPC is short for the technical term
oligomeric proanthocyanidins).

Green tea. The most popular beverage in the world, tea is derived
from a tropical and semitropical evergreen bush (*Camellia sinensis*) that
has been widely cultivated in Asia since ancient times. About three
quarters of the world's tea crop is used to make black tea, in which the
leaves are dried, rolled, fermented, and then fired. Flavor-generating
compounds in the leaves are allowed to oxidize, causing the leaves to
turn brown or black. A second type of tea, oolong, representing only
about 5 percent of world production, is a greenish-brown, semifer-
mented tea. The remaining 20 percent of the tea market is green tea,
the freshest and least processed form of tea. The tea leaves are green
because immediately after picking they are heated by steam or dry heat
to destroy the oxidizing enzymes and to prevent fermentation. This
lack of fermentation spares the compounds in tea that have now been
shown to have health-promoting properties.

Green tea can have appreciable levels of vitamin C, vitamin E, and
minerals, including tooth-decay-reducing fluoride. The most active
compounds, however, are polyphenols such as the flavonoids, which
may comprise 15 to 30 percent of the leaves' dry weight.

The principal flavonoid is the colorless plant constituent catechin,
technically epigallocatechin gallate (EGCG). Studies have shown that
EGCG can destroy harmful viruses and bacteria and boost overall

immunity. Catechins have also been shown to be powerful antioxidants that can reduce free radicals such as hydrogen peroxide. Researchers are now studying green tea extract for its potential to prevent dental caries, heart disease, and cancer.

Green tea comes in various grades, according to the age and form of the leaf. The finer grades include *gunpowder* (so named for the little balls of rolled-up leaves), *gyokuro, sencha, matcha,* and *extra choice.* When brewed, these yield a delicate drink that is a pale yellowish-green color and has a subtle flavor and aroma. *Fannings* and *dust* are lower-grade teas made from older leaves, twigs, stems, and leftovers. The Japanese teas termed *bancha* (literally "three tea," for its age in years at harvest) and *kukicha* ("twig tea") are considered low-grade tea. Green tea is sold in bulk and in tea bags; some manufacturers add flavors such as orange and lime.

The caffeine content of green tea is a matter of dispute, with some herbal companies claiming that green tea is naturally lower in caffeine than black tea. According to Richard J. Gilbert, Ph.D., author of *Caffeine: The Most Popular Stimulant,* green and black teas contain a similar amount of caffeine. It is possible to reduce the caffeine content of green tea by steeping the leaves or tea bags for only two to three minutes. This renders the flavor subtle and delicate, and keeps caffeine levels low (20 to 30 mg per cup). Note also that because caffeine is concentrated in the leaves, lower grades of green tea are naturally lower in caffeine content. Decaffeinated green teas are coming onto the market, though it is likely that the decaffeinating process also removes some of the healthful polyphenols.

Lengthy brewing of green tea can extract more of its unoxidized flavor compounds, yielding a bitter-tasting liquid. If you brew green tea, don't drink it scalding hot, which may reduce its benefits or even be harmful (possibly increasing the risk of cancer of the esophagus).

Green-tea extracts in capsule form are increasingly available from supplement manufacturers. Look for products such as Green Tea-Power and Preventin. Polyphenol content may range from 15 to 50 percent. For comparison, a cup of brewed green tea usually contains about 20 to 30 mg of polyphenols. So, for example, a 200-mg green-tea-extract capsule that has 25 percent polyphenols is equivalent to drinking about two cups of green tea. An average daily dose of green-tea polyphenols is 50 to 100 mg. Unless caffeine is added, most green-tea-extract capsules contain approximately 5 to 15 mg of caffeine.

As common food constituents, polyphenols and flavonoids are considered to be safe and nontoxic. The federal government has not set an

RDA for flavonoids. It is estimated that Americans consume approximately 1 g daily in fruits and other foods.

Beneficial Live Bacteria

The idea of eating live bacteria is counterintuitive, to say nothing of repulsive, to many people. Aren't bacteria the disease-causing agents that most of us try to avoid like the plague? (Bubonic plague was, in fact, caused by the bacterium *Pasteurella pestis*.)

Yet humanity has long been aware of the benefits available from certain lactobacilli, the bacteria that are used to ferment foods such as cheese, yogurt, kefir, and miso. In these foods, bacteria act as preservatives, nutritional enhancers, and digestion-promoting agents. Moreover, when these healthful bacteria reach your gut, they set up shop and work to balance intestinal acidity/alkalinity (pH) and intestinal flora—that is, the intestinal mix of the various useful and pathogenic bacteria, fungi, and other microorganisms.

Lactobacteria can also play a role in promoting a healthful balance of microorganisms in the vagina. A recent study of women with recurrent vaginal candida infections found that those who ate daily servings of yogurt considerably reduced their incidence of vaginitis.

The most prominent beneficial live bacteria are *Lactobacillus acidophilus* and *Bifidobacteria bifidum*. These are often referred to as simply acidophilus and bifidus, respectively.

Acidophilus. Acidophilus has become the generic term for various types of naturally occurring live bacteria that are increasingly popular as dietary supplements. Technically acidophilus is the strain *L. acidophilus,* though products sold as acidophilus may also contain *B. bifidus, L. bulgaricus,* and other strains of bacteria. *L. acidophilus* is the primary beneficial bacteria in the small intestine. Healthy colonies of *L. acidophilus* prevent food-borne pathogens—including species of salmonella, klebsiella, and staphylococcus, and fungi such as *Candida albicans* —from multiplying and impairing the function of the small intestine.

Bifidus. Bifidus is supplemental shorthand for *B. bifidum, B. breve, B. longum,* and other bifidobacteria, relatives of *L. acidophilus* and teammates in its efforts to maintain a healthy intestinal environment. Bifidobacteria are found in human breast milk, and quickly establish themselves in the previously sterile gut of a newborn. Unlike acidophilus, which is found in such common foods as cheese and yogurt, bifidobacteria are more difficult to obtain in large numbers through diet. They are the most prominent helpful bacteria of the large intestine, and should exist in greater quantities than any other intestinal microorganism. In proper balance with *L. acidophilus,* they help to inhibit harmful organisms, reduce blood-cholesterol levels, and create the environment necessary for synthesizing B vitamins.

Anyone who is taking oral doses of antibiotics (for which American doctors write over 110 million prescriptions annually) may benefit by supplementing the diet with acidophilus or bifidus. Broad-spectrum antibiotics such as tetracycline and ampicillin kill not only disease-causing bacteria but these friendly microorganisms, which the intestines need to function properly. When beneficial intestinal flora are missing, potentially harmful microorganisms more easily move in and take over. Supplementing the diet with acidophilus and bifidus helps to repopulate the intestines with beneficial bacteria and prevent toxic bacterial colonies from establishing themselves in the gut.

To distinguish beneficial bacteria from the harmful microorganisms that are targeted by antibiotics, foods such as yogurt and beneficial-live-bacteria products such as acidophilus and bifidus are now referred to as *probiotic.* At the same time, some nutritionists use the term *dysbiotic* for people suffering from the effects of an unbalanced colonic ecology, one characterized by a plethora of harmful bacteria, yeasts, and other microorganisms.

Live-bacteria supplements typically come in powders, tablets, gelatin capsules, and liquids. Some capsules are enteric-coated to help prevent stomach acids from destroying large numbers of the live organisms. Look for products that have labels providing information on how many live or "viable" bacteria are provided by each capsule or teaspoon of powder or liquid. Acidophilus products may be measured by colony-forming units (CFUs) per gram. Some capsules may provide 2 billion or more friendly organisms, while some liquids provide up to 5 billion per tablespoon. National Nutritional Foods Association guidelines call for beneficial-bacteria-product labels to state a specific minimum potency guarantee for each microorganism at the expiration date (some products offer only the number of viable organisms at the time of manufacture). Labels should also provide storage instructions and a listing of additional ingredients (avoid those preserved with BHT). Unless specially formulated, many live-bacteria products need to be kept refrigerated.

Live-bacteria products are nontoxic and safe (though expensive) to take indefinitely. A high-fiber, whole-foods diet can complement their positive effect on intestinal flora.

While you should avoid taking beneficial-live-bacteria products within two hours of taking antibiotics, many people take acidophilus and bifidus supplements both during and after a regimen of broad-spectrum antibiotics. Probiotic products can also help while taking birth control pills or following treatment with cortisone or chemo-therapy drugs. An average daily dose to replenish intestinal flora is 10 billion viable organisms daily. To maintain a healthy gastrointestinal tract, take $1/2$ to 1 teaspoon of powder or liquid daily, or capsules containing 2 to 3 billion viable organisms.

Melatonin

Melatonin is a bodily substance produced by a tiny endocrine organ, the pineal gland, in the center of brain. The pineal gland responds to a large variety of inputs, in the form of light and dark, temperature, and even magnetism, and sends messages to the brain that affect behavior. It does this by converting noradrenaline into melatonin, a hormone that is structurally related to serotonin. Scientists think that the pineal gland is linked to the eyes either by nerves or through the action of the part of the brain known as the hypothalamus. Thus melatonin secretion patterns are intimately affected by exposure of the eyes to sunlight.

Melatonin easily passes through the blood-brain barrier. Fluctuating levels in the body have been linked with changes in mood (see Chapter 6), performance, and fatigue. Since blood levels of melatonin tend to decrease progressively with advancing age, especially after age 70, some researchers into immunity and aging are now exploring melatonin's potential to extend longevity (see Chapter 10). Melatonin helps to stabilize the body's circadian (daily) rhythms and reset the body's biological clock, thus countering the effects of jet lag. Numerous well-controlled studies suggest that melatonin can be an effective remedy to regulate sleep and combat insomnia (see Chapter 12).

Unlike most remedies, for melatonin the time of day when you take it is crucial. You want to support the body's natural melatonin secretion pattern. Most people secrete their lowest levels of melatonin between 8 A.M. and 4 P.M. Secretion typically starts to rise in the early evening and peaks (at a level ten times higher than in the daytime) around 2 or 3 A.M. Consumed orally, melatonin is rapidly absorbed into the bloodstream. If you take melatonin during the day (assuming you're not a night-shift worker who sleeps during the day), you may experience unwanted effects, such as impaired memory, decreased alertness, and possibly even exaggerated symptoms of depression. You can avoid these side effects and enhance your body's natural biorhythms by taking melatonin in the evening, before you go to bed. Generally, healthy people should take it at the same time every night, within an hour of bedtime. If you suffer from insomnia, try taking it two to three hours before bedtime.

Studies indicate that melatonin is safe and causes relatively few side effects even when taken in doses much higher than recommended. Melatonin should not be taken by women who are pregnant or lactating, or by anyone suffering from kidney disease. Because it may affect growth-hormone levels, melatonin should also be avoided by anyone under the age of 20.

Synthetically derived melatonin supplements are available in natural-food stores and through mail order (see "Resources"). Melatonin typically comes in 750-mcg and 3-mg pills. Average doses range from 0.75 to 6 mg, depending upon the purpose for which it is being taken and the age of the consumer (elderly people usually need slightly higher doses to benefit from melatonin). See Chapters 6, 10, and 12 for recommendations on how to use melatonin. Most natural-health practitioners recommend starting with low dosages and increasing them if necessary. For best results melatonin should be stored in the refrigerator.

Amino Acids

Amino acids are the building blocks of protein molecules. The body makes proteins from twenty amino acids, eight of which are usually considered "essential amino acids"—those that must be obtained through diet or supplements. The essential ones are isoleucine, leucine, lysine, methionine, phenylalanine, threonine, tryptophan, and valine. A number of other amino acids that are produced by the body can nevertheless be taken in supplement form for their effects on the mind and body. These nonessential amino acids include tyrosine, arginine, and glutamine. In some circumstances nonessential amino acids may be required in the diet. For example, children may need arginine to help them grow. A few other amino acids found in the body, such as taurine and ornithine, have potential therapeutic effects but are not used by the body to build protein.

There are no RDAs or U.S. RDAs for amino acids.

In recent years researchers have determined that numerous amino acids can increase or decrease the body's supply of neurotransmitters. These important nerve chemicals have been shown to affect mood, sleeping patterns, sexual arousal, immunity, and other bodily functions.

Amino acid products come in single and branched-chain, or mixed, forms. Two of the most widely used single amino acids are phenylalanine and tyrosine.

Note that amino acids are technically referred to using the prefixes L- (for levorotatory or "left-handed") or D- (for dextrorotatory or "right-handed"), designating slight differences in molecular structure. Thus, for example, one sees the names L-tryptophan, L-tyrosine, and so forth. For most amino acids supplements, the naturally occurring L- forms are much more common than either the D- form or the mixed DL- form. Our practice throughout the book will be to drop the prefix L- except when it is necessary to distinguish specific forms, such as it sometimes is with phenylalanine.

Phenylalanine. The minor molecular differences between L-phenylalanine, D-phenylalanine, and DL-phenylalanine (also known as DLPA) account for their slightly different effects on the body. L-phenylalanine and DLPA act as nervous-system stimulants (see Chapter 5) and sexual stimulants (see Chapter 7), mood enhancers (see Chapter 6) and cognition enhancers (see Chapter 11), and appetite suppressants (see Chapter 17). While D-phenylalanine also apparently has antidepressant properties, it is taken primarily to control chronic pain (it seems to enhance the pain-relieving effects of acupuncture).

Phenylalanine is found in common protein foods, including poultry, meats, soybeans, fish, dairy products, nuts, and seeds, as well as the synthetic sweetener aspartame. Such sources supply the average person with an estimated 500 to 2,000 mg of phenylalanine from diet alone. In the body it is able to cross the blood-brain barrier. It stimulates production in the brain of the natural pain-killing and mood-boosting neurotransmitters dopamine, adrenaline, and noradrenaline. Some studies show a beneficial effect on people with Parkinson's disease.

Phenylalanine may cause stimulantlike side effects, including insomnia and anxiety. The L- form should be avoided by people with high blood pressure and those taking MAO-inhibitor antidepressants. Both L- and D- forms should be avoided by people with phenylketonuria, a genetic disorder of phenylalanine metabolism.

Average doses of phenylalanine depend upon the intended action; see specific chapters.

Tyrosine. Tyrosine is a nonessential amino acid that also helps the brain to produce dopamine, adrenaline, and noradrenaline. Tyrosine may play a role in relieving some forms of mild depression, according to studies (see Chapter 6). One placebo-controlled, double-blind study indicated that subjects respond to tyrosine at a rate similar to conventional antidepressants, though without their side effects. Like phenylalanine (from which it is derived in the body), tyrosine tends to increase energy levels and sexual desire (see Chapter 7). Some women take it to alleviate the lethargy and irritability of premenstrual syndrome. Tyrosine may also be a useful remedy to suppress appetite and to detoxify the body from cocaine and other drugs.

Tyrosine causes few side effects even at fairly high doses, according to Leon Chaitow, N.D., author of *Thorsons Guide to Amino Acids*. Nevertheless, most health practitioners agree that it is a good idea to consult with a knowledgeable nutritionist or naturopath before taking more than 2 to 3 g of tyrosine daily. Health practitioners may be able to determine, for example, whether you are more likely to have low brain levels of noradrenaline or of serotonin. The former may be helped by taking supplemental tyrosine and the latter by consuming tryptophan.

Like phenylalanine, tyrosine should be avoided by those who suffer from high blood pressure or who take MAO-inhibitor antidepressants —combining tyrosine and MAO inhibitors can also cause high blood pressure.

Also like phenylalanine, average doses of tyrosine depend upon the intended action.

Medicinal Mushrooms

Medicinal mushrooms are various types of fleshy fungi that have pronounced therapeutic properties when eaten. Mushrooms have long been treated much like herbs and used for medicinal purposes in China and Japan. Modern scientists have chemically analyzed some of these mushrooms and have determined that they contain compounds unlike those found in plants. Studies have also confirmed that certain mushrooms can lower blood-cholesterol levels, boost the immune system, and slow the growth of tumors. Most medicinal mushrooms can be consumed as either a food or a drug (in tablets and capsules, for instance).

Shiitake. Shiitake is the Japanese name for a dark, flavorful mushroom (*Lentinus edodes*) that has been prized in Asia for thousands of years for its medicinal properties, especially as a treatment for systemic conditions related to aging and sexual dysfunction. Studies indicate that shiitake extract can lower blood-cholesterol levels, shrink tumors, reduce blood pressure, and combat viruses and bacteria. Shiitake contains the polysaccharide lentinan, an immune booster (see Chapter 3) that may prove effective in the treatment of AIDS and in the prevention of cancer (see Chapter 9). Until recently shiitake was chiefly imported from Asia, but now is often American-grown. Herbal companies frequently combine it with other immune-boosting herbs. An average dose is 500 mg two or three times daily.

Reishi. One of the most potent medicinal mushrooms is the ganoderma. Several species grow in the United States, including *Ganoderma lucidum,* which is known by the Chinese as *ling zhi* and by the Japanese as *reishi.* (*Reishi* has also become the most widely recognized name for this mushroom in the United States.) The practitioners of the traditional medicines of China and Japan considered reishi to be among the most powerful adaptogenic and tonic herbs (see Chapter 13). Some ancient Chinese medical texts rank reishi among the "superior herbs," noted for its broad healing powers and lack of side effects. Asians used this "mushroom of immortality" for promoting longevity, boosting overall health, and speeding recovery from illness. It is still widely taken to balance the nervous and digestive systems, regulate blood sugar, and increase oxygenation of blood. People suffering from dizziness, nervous disorders, or poor sleep may benefit by supplementing their diet with reishi. Others who have reported positive results from using reishi include those suffering from chronic fatigue syndrome, asthma, and ulcers.

In addition to being an effective energizer, reishi is an antioxidant that protects the body from the harmful effects of radiation and free radicals. It contains polysaccharides and other compounds that may combat bacteria and viruses and boost the immune system (see Chapter 3). Because there is some evidence that reishi extract lowers cholesterol and blood pressure and reduces platelet stickiness, another cardiovascular risk factor, it is being studied for its potential in the treatment of heart disease. Finally, reishi may prevent cancer and even help reduce tumors (see Chapter 9).

A shelf fungus that grows on trees in heavily forested areas, reishi is an attractive mushroom characterized by an off-center cap with a deep, glossy, reddish-brown top and a white underside. In the West reishi is infrequently used as a food, since it is hard, bitter, and woodlike. Though a rare treasure when found in the wild, reishi is easily cultivated. Reishi supplements are widely available at natural-food stores in powders, capsules, teas, standardized extracts, and other preparations.

Supplement producers also sometimes include reishi in herbal and medicinal mushroom combination products. Look for products such as Mycelin3. Like shiitake, it is one of the more expensive natural substances. An average dose is 500 mg two to three times daily.

Beyond Herbs and Nutrients

Two important additional categories of natural remedies that are represented a number of times in upcoming chapters are the essential oils and the homeopathic remedies. Like herbs and nutritional supplements, the essential oils are used to treat some conditions, prevent ailments, and influence bodily functions ranging from sleep to sexual desire. For the most part, homeopathic remedies are taken to address specific illnesses and conditions, and rarely to increase athletic performance, boost brain power, or achieve most of the other goals that are the focus of this book. Yet some homeopathic remedies can aid relaxation, improve digestion, or otherwise benefit the basically healthy person.

Essential Oils

Aromatherapy remains popular in France, Great Britain, and Italy today, with over a thousand medical practitioners using essential oils in France alone. In the United States, interest is growing, and many natural-food stores carry diverse lines of essential oils. Although there are dozens of popular oils to choose from, you can benefit from aromatherapy after getting to know just a few. Some of the most popular ones mentioned more than once in this book include:

Lavender. This multipurpose essential oil is prepared from the leaves and blue flowers of a Mediterranean shrub (*Lavandula officinalis*). The Romans added lavender to their bath water, and herbal preparations of lavender have been used since ancient times for skin complaints and for scent in perfumes, soaps, and cosmetics. Lavender is grown mostly in the sunny regions around the Mediterranean. The true wild lavender is now more prized for its oil than the hybrid lavandin (*Lavandula* x *intermedia*) that colors southern France in the summer. As an herb, lavender has traditionally been used to treat coughs and the common cold. The oil is widely used in cosmetics and perfumes.

Aromatherapists and other practitioners of natural medicine recommend the essential oil for both internal (inhaled) and external applications. Applied to the skin, Lavender has mild pain-relieving and anti-inflammatory effects, and is used to heal burns, wounds, sprains, insect bites and stings, athlete's foot, and muscular aches and pains. The oil is mild enough to be applied full strength and is often recommended for use on children. It also helps kill germs—its name, from the Latin *lavare* "to wash," reflects a use that continues in some parts of the world: to wash and disinfect hospitals and sickrooms.

When inhaled, Lavender's fresh, flowery aroma stimulates a region of the brain in a way that has a sedating effect on the central nervous system. It is a mild soporific that can help induce sleep, alleviate stress, and reduce depression and nervous tension. It may also boost immunity and alleviate headaches.

Peppermint. Although herbalists in ancient Egypt and China first started using some mint species thousands of years ago, the familiar garden perennial peppermint (*Mentha piperita*) is a relative newcomer to the medical scene. Peppermint apparently began to be cultivated and used in England around the beginning of the eighteenth century. It was being grown commercially in western Massachusetts by the end of the eighteenth century, and being distilled into oil by 1812. The plant is native to Europe, and is still grown there and in the United States primarily for its essential oil, now widely used as a flavoring agent in foods, candies, chewing gum, and toothpastes. An estimated 1 percent of Peppermint oil is used medicinally.

Peppermint-leaf tea has long been popular as a digestive remedy, and some herbalists still prescribe it for indigestion, nausea, diarrhea, flatulence, and cramps. The essential oil contains azulenes, tannins, and menthol, a medicinally active alcohol that exhibits significant antimicrobial and anti-inflammatory powers. Like the tea, the essential oil helps to regulate digestion (see Chapter 16); it is also mildly stimulating (see Chapter 5). The essential oil is also applied externally for itchy skin, hemorrhoids, toothaches, muscle aches, and insect bites. The oil may irritate some people's skin if applied undiluted or in high doses.

Ylang-ylang. Pronounced *EE-lan EE-lan,* this is a tropical Asian tree (*Cananga odorata* var. *genuina*) whose freshly picked flowers are used to produce a pale yellow, sweet-smelling essential oil. It is a popular essential oil for use in cosmetics and perfumes. Therapeutically, Ylang-ylang is most commonly used for its calming effect. It helps to reduce blood pressure, regulate heartbeat and breathing, lower adrenaline levels, and quiet the nervous system. It can offer relief from anxiety, stress-related problems, and insomnia.

HOW TO USE ESSENTIAL OILS: Essential oils are extremely concentrated substances and are generally *not* taken orally. There are a number of other ways to take advantage of essential oils' healthful properties:

Vaporization. Mix 2 or 3 drops of essential oil with water in a small bowl. Put the bowl on a working radiator to allow the oil to be gradually dispersed into the room. Another option is to use a lightbulb ring or an essential oil vaporizer (most are clay bowls, heated by electricity or a candle, to which you add 8 to 10 drops of essential oil and a small amount of water). You can also put 8 to 10 drops of oil in a water-filled spray bottle or plant mister and spray a fine mist into the room.

Inhalation. Inhale an essential oil directly by placing a few drops on a tissue or clean cloth and inhaling deeply. You can also do steam inhalation by adding 5 to 7 drops of essential oil to a bowl of piping hot water. Drape a towel over your head and the bowl. Hold your face over the water for a few minutes, breathing deeply to capture the steam as it rises.

Massage. Mix 3 to 5 drops of essential oil per tablespoon of carrier oil. For a carrier oil, use a high-quality vegetable oil such as almond, safflower, sunflower, avocado, or jojoba. Wheat germ oil also works well and is naturally high in vitamin E, which acts as a preservative.

Bath. Add 6 to 8 drops of essential oil to a full tub of warm water (hot water will quickly evaporate the oils) and stroke the water a few times to disperse.

Compress. Put 3 to 4 drops of essential oil in a cup of warm water and soak a cotton cloth in the solution. Wring the cloth slightly and apply it to the skin.

Homeopathic Remedies

Some of the most popular single homeopathic remedies include:

Chamomilla. This is derived from the whole fresh chamomile plant (either German chamomile, *Matricaria recutita,* or Roman chamomile, *Chamaemelum nobile*). It is used to treat restlessness and insomnia, toothaches and childhood teething pains, earaches, fever, and joint pain. The *Chamomilla* patient is frequently irascible, stubborn, and inconsolable. *Chamomilla* is a common ingredient in combination remedies for teething, diarrhea, earache, insomnia, and menstrual problems.

Nux vomica. This is derived from the toxic, strychnine-containing seeds of the poison nut plant (*Strychnos nux vomica*). Homeopathically diluted, it is used principally to treat nausea and vomiting, especially from ailments due to overeating or drinking. The remedy may be beneficial for flatulence, constipation, or indigestion. It is also used to treat motion sickness and some types of coughs, backaches, fevers, headaches, and insomnia. *Nux vomica* is a common ingredient in combination remedies for cold and flu, back pain, constipation, fatigue, flatulence, headache, hemorrhoids, indigestion, and insomnia.

Pulsatilla. Pulsatilla is derived from the poisonous pasque flower (*Anemone patens*). In homeopathic dilutions, people take it internally for colds characterized by a profusely running nose and coughing. Homeopaths also recommend it for certain eye and ear ailments, skin eruptions, allergies, insomnia, fainting episodes, and gastric upsets, particularly when the patient is sensitive and prone to crying. *Pulsatilla* is a common ingredient in combination remedies for colds and the flu, earache, fever, indigestion, insomnia, menstrual problems, and sinusitis.

HOW TO USE HOMEOPATHIC REMEDIES: When you buy homeopathic remedies you will notice they are available in different strengths. For instance, the label may say "*Apis* 6X" or "*Apis* 30X." The 6X and 30X refer to the number of dilutions needed to produce the remedy. Dilutions are either decimal (and noted as 1X, 2X, etc.) or centesimal (1C, 2C, etc.) in scale. A 1X remedy is one that was made by adding one part pure mother tincture and 9 parts alcohol, and then succussing the solution. It is thus a 10-percent solution. To make a 2X (or 1C) remedy, homeopathic manufacturers add one part of a 10 percent solution to 9 parts alcohol. The resulting solution is now one part mother tincture and 99 parts dilution, or a 1-percent solution. The process is continued so that, for instance, a 6X (or 3C) remedy is essentially a one-part-in-a-million dilution, and a 12X (or 6C) remedy is a one-part-in-a-trillion dilution.

A few dilutions or "potencies" are more commonly used than others. Most natural-food stores and some pharmacies carry lines of homeopathic products that are labeled as either 6X, 12X, 24X, or 30X, or 6C, 12C, or 30C. Homeopaths consider these to be relatively low potencies that are best for self-care purposes. The higher potency remedies, such as 400X and 200C (up to and beyond 2,000,000X!) are usually reserved for use by professional homeopaths, since these remedies are thought to be more powerful and deeper-acting than lower potencies.

Homeopathic remedies are widely available in pellet and tablet form. A common dosage is 2 to 4 tablets up to four times per day. Follow directions on labels.

Working with Supplements

Though taking supplements is fast and easy, some people still find that the time and commitment necessary to take them is elusive. So before going any further, here are some tips for better integrating the stay-well herbs and nutrients into a healthy lifestyle.

• Spread your supplement-taking out over the day. Rather than trying to take a dozen pills at breakfast, bring some to work for taking at lunchtime, and get in the habit of setting aside some others for taking later in the day. Most supplements can be taken with meals to reduce the likelihood of digestive upset. Taking supplements in divided doses makes it less of a chore to choke down the supplements you want to take. It also reduces the risk that any one herb or nutritional substance will cause an adverse effect due to the size of the dose.

• Use supplements as motivating techniques for improving other aspects of your health. Rather than telling yourself, "I haven't got time to exercise today, I'll just take my chromium picolinate instead," get in the habit of telling yourself, "I'll take my chromium picolinate now and exercise too to boost its effectiveness."

• Learn how to take natural substances in safe and responsible ways that avoid addictive patterns of use. Natural substances that are most likely to lead to such abuse include the supplements that stimulate energy and aid in relaxation. If you find you have to take pills every day or regularly throughout the day for these purposes, you need to look for ways to improve your diet and lifestyle that will lessen the need for such supplements.

• Adjust your supplementation program depending upon how it is working for you. For example, the vast majority of people can take 1,500 mg of vitamin C in divided doses every day without experiencing loose bowels, an infrequent side effect that usually doesn't show up until daily doses of C exceed 2 to 5 g. However, if you do notice this or some other apparent side effect from taking vitamin C or any of the other natural substances discussed here, reduce the dosage accordingly or switch to another supplement with similar potential benefits.

• When you've determined what supplements you want to take on a daily basis (see below), adjust your daily routine in a way that makes the taking of them habitual. For example, some people keep important daily supplements in the medicine cabinet next to their toothbrush, so they're reminded to take the supplements every morning before brushing their teeth.

• Experiment with different forms of supplements. Many herbs and nutrients are now available in powders, tablets, capsules, and liquids. If you don't like swallowing large capsules, such as those that contain fiber or amino acids, try liquid forms or powder dissolved in a liquid. You can crush large tablets into a powder and ingest it, or add the powder to your favorite drink, to make them easier to take. An increasing number of supplements, including adult multivitamins, acidophilus, and antioxidant combinations, are available in pleasant-tasting chewable tablets, though usually at a premium price. A popular method for taking a capsule is to swallow it with a large mouthful of water. A number of health-product catalogs now offer handy devices for crushing pills and organizing or dispensing supplements; see "Resources."

• In general, it is best to take nutritional supplements with meals. Notable exceptions (such as melatonin, best taken before bedtime) are pointed out. Herbs are more flexible. "While most vitamins work best when taken with food, it is not necessary to take herbal formulas with food," notes naturopath Linda Rector-Page, Ph.D. "Unlike vitamins, herbs provide their own digestive enzymes for the body to take them in. In some cases, with herbs for mental acuity, for instance, the herbs are more effective if taken when body pathways are clear, instead of concerned with food digestion."

Every individual is unique. You need to determine what works for you and what doesn't.

Setting Your Supplement Priorities

Many people feel overwhelmed by the sheer volume of natural substances on the market today. Large health-food stores have aisle after aisle of herbs and nutritional supplements, representing hundreds and hundreds of individual substances, combinations, and formulas. The store may have a half-dozen or more complete lines of nutritional supplements, each with fifty or more distinct products, some overlapping with other lines' products and some apparently unique. The diversity can be bewildering even to veterans of natural health.

Compounding the problem are the restrictions placed by the federal government on both product-label information and on what store employees can legally tell you. Basically, there are only a very few health claims that manufacturers or sellers can explicitly associate with herbal and nutritional products. These are the health claims that most people are already well aware of—calcium can help prevent osteoporosis, for example. If you ask a store clerk, however, even a simple question such as "What do you recommend for a cold?" legally that clerk can only suggest places where you might look up that information.

So, to a great extent, you're on your own. The solution: Identify your needs before you go into the store. The information provided in this book and some of the others mentioned in "Resources" is meant to help you to set your priorities and develop a uniquely personal supplementation program.

For further help along these lines, the chart on pp. 64–65 reflects the top twenty supplements presented here and their various uses mentioned throughout subsequent chapters.

Use this summary to help you set your supplement priorities. Remember, you don't have to take anywhere near all of these healthful natural supplements to gain substantial benefits. If you're new to supplements, you'll probably want to start off by taking only a few of the most essential substances each day. That might include:

An insurance-level multivitamin-multimineral formula. An insurance-level supplement includes optimal amounts of the seven major vitamins and minerals in the chart plus any of the dozen or so of the others usually included in multinutrient formulas, but especially vitamin B complex and selenium. Many supplement companies offer insurance-level formulas that cover these and often a few more minerals, such as chromium. Keep in mind that because of the advantages of taking optimal levels of nutrients rather than merely the RDA, a good insurance-level multivitamin-multimineral formula will involve more than one tablet a day. An average formula may require taking four to six tablets or capsules per day.

Garlic. This is probably the safest and most multipurpose herb, with loads of scientific studies backing up its positive effects on health. It can't hurt to take it on a daily basis, and in all likelihood it will benefit your overall health immensely.

Coenzyme Q10. This is an essential vitamin in all but name, with important applications in heart and energy functions. It is required in only small doses, so even in capsule form it is tiny and easy to take.

An antioxidant formula. This might be in the form of an ACES (vitamins A/beta carotene, C, and E, and the mineral selenium) nutritional supplement or one of the flavonoid-rich herbal supplements, such as green tea, Pycnogenol, or ginkgo.

One of the medicinal mushrooms. Shiitake and reishi offer a diverse range of potential health benefits.

You can take all of these supplements in perhaps eight to ten pills or capsules daily. If you take just three or four of these natural supplements at breakfast and the same number later in the day, you will have substantially increased your energy levels, boosted your immune system, lowered your risk of heart disease and cancer, and strengthened and balanced your overall system. The total cost for all of these nutritional substances would probably not exceed a dollar or two per day, about what you may already spend for your first cup of takeout coffee. Taking these herbs and nutrients also serves as an excellent base program for using additional herbs and nutrients as needed, such as for temporary relaxation, sexual stimulation, or mood enhancement.

	Actions					
	Immunity	Strength/ endurance	Energy	Mood	Sex	Heart

Supplements

Herbs

	Immunity	Strength/ endurance	Energy	Mood	Sex	Heart
Garlic	•					•
Ginkgo			•	•	•	•
Ginseng		•	•		•	•
Siberian ginseng	•			•		

Vitamins/minerals

	Immunity	Strength/ endurance	Energy	Mood	Sex	Heart
A/beta carotene	•					
Vitamin C	•	•		•		•
Vitamin E	•	•			•	•
Calcium/magnesium		•	•	•		•
Chromium		•				•
Zinc	•				•	

Nutritional substances

	Immunity	Strength/ endurance	Energy	Mood	Sex	Heart
Choline				•	•	
Coenzyme Q10		•	•			•
Essential fatty acids						•
Polyphenols/flavonoids						•
Live bacteria						
Melatonin				•		

Amino acids

	Immunity	Strength/ endurance	Energy	Mood	Sex	Heart
Phenylalanine			•	•	•	
Tyrosine				•	•	

Medicinal mushrooms

	Immunity	Strength/ endurance	Energy	Mood	Sex	Heart
Shiitake	•					
Reishi	•					

Others

	Immunity	Strength/ endurance	Energy	Mood	Sex	Heart
Essential oils			•	•	•	
Homeopathic remedies			•	•		

Actions *(continued)*

Cancer	Longevity	Brain	Nerves	Tonics	Senses	Skin	Digestion	Weight loss
•	•			•			•	
	•	•			•			
	•	•		•				
				•				
•	•				•	•		
•	•	•			•	•		
•	•				•	•		
•		•	•			•		
				•	•			•
•		•		•	•	•		•
		•						•
								•
•						•		
•	•			•	•			
•							•	•
	•		•					
		•						•
•								
•				•				
		•	•			•	•	•
			•				•	•

TWO

Using Herbs
and Nutrients in
Your Everyday Life

3

Boost Your Immunity

The human body has a marvelously intricate and effective system for protecting it from harmful microorganisms, such as bacteria, viruses, parasites, and fungi, or invaders such as tumor cells. When your immune system is working well, it quickly and readily recognizes these potential threats, marshals a whole host of cells, hormones, and proteins that engulf or otherwise neutralize them, and in some cases even remembers relevant information in anticipation of future protection. The immune system thereby helps to protect you from the possible consequences of disease-causing agents, or pathogens, including such common conditions as colds (most people get two or three per year), flu, herpes, and candidiasis. Illnesses ranging from allergies to AIDS to cancer are also a function, in part, of the immune system not working as it should.

Keeping your immune system functioning well can be as important to your overall health as maintaining a strong heart or protecting your lungs from pollutants. In many ways, however, the immune system is harder to visualize and understand than the heart-based circulatory system or the lung-based respiratory system. Let's first take a look at the principal actors in the immune system before discussing the herbs and nutrients that you can take to keep it in top shape.

The organs and glands of the immune system include the following:

Skin and mucous membranes. These barriers are the first line of defense against many invading bacteria and viruses. The skin is the largest and most external organ, while mucous membranes line body cavities and organs of the alimentary canal and respiratory tract. Skin and mucous membranes can both physically block and chemically destroy microbes.

Thymus. This gland at the juncture of the neck and upper chest is sometimes referred to as the master gland of the immune system. White blood cells that enter the thymus become T lymphocytes or simply T cells, key agents in the cellular battle against viruses and possibly cancer cells. The thymus also secretes immune-active hormones.

Adrenals. Two small glands that sit atop each of the kidneys, the adrenals secrete a number of hormones that affect immune function and other bodily processes.

Bone marrow. This inner core of the bones produces the immune cells known as B lymphocytes, or B cells, which produce antibodies capable of attacking specific microorganisms.

Spleen. In addition to performing functions not related to the immune system, this fist-sized organ in the left side of the upper abdominal cavity produces antibodies and other immune cells that fight infection.

Lymphatic system. This is a system of nodes, tissues, and vessels throughout the body that collects, carries, or drains lymph, a body fluid containing white blood cells and other substances. The spleen, the tonsils (on the back of the throat), and the appendix (branching off the large intestine) are made up of lymphoid tissue. Only in recent years have scientists begun to identify subtle immune-related properties for the tonsils and appendix, sometimes still referred to as "vestigial" (having no current function) by conventional doctors.

Among the most active and important agents of the immune system are the white blood cells, also known as leukocytes. White blood cells help your body defend itself from pathogens and reduce your susceptibility to disease. White blood cells can be loosely classified by how they work. Some white blood cells are "eaters" capable of swallowing and digesting a bacterium, for instance. Actually, these phagocytes, or macrophages (big phagocytes), work by surrounding and engulfing foreign cells, and then releasing enzymes that break down the invader. The neutrophils made in the bone marrow are common phagocytic white blood cells.

Another category of white blood cells, the lymphocytes, are more subtle than the eaters in their attack. When a B lymphocyte encounters a bacterium, for example, it manages to multiply and then create an army of allies (the antibodies) that attach to the invader and mark it as prey for the phagocytes. A pair of T lymphocytes, the helper and killer cells, work as a team to latch onto a tumor cell or other abnormal cell and release chemicals deadly to the invader.

"All of these cells are influenced, in part, by the nutritional state of the body," says Jon D. Kaiser, M.D., author of *Immune Power*. "Their functioning is enhanced by the presence of certain vitamins and natural compounds and depressed by deficiencies of the same." Herbs, vitamins and minerals, nutritional substances such as organic germanium compounds and the amino acid arginine, and medicinal mushrooms are potential allies in your immune system's efforts to keep you well.

The Immune-Enhancing Herbs

Ask a conventional doctor, one with little or no training in nutrition (like most of them), what you can take to boost your overall immune system, and he or she will probably tell you that there are no generally used drugs to do that. (If you ask a doctor, on the other hand, about drugs to *suppress* the immune system—in order to prevent a transplanted organ from being rejected or to help treat an autoimmune disorder such as rheumatoid arthritis—he or she will be able to suggest a dozen potent drugs.) By training and inclination, practitioners of conventional Western medicine generally don't think in terms of boosting the body's innate immunity, with the exceptions of using vaccines to cause the body to produce specific antibodies or administering substances such as human immune globulin to temporarily boost immunity against certain infectious agents. Rather, the medical profession's focus is on identifying the disease-causing agents in the body and administering specific drugs to kill them.

Herbalists, nutritionists, and most practitioners of natural therapies also recognize the value of using remedies to destroy invasive microorganisms. Indeed, many natural substances have potent antibiotic, antiviral, and antifungal powers. Natural practitioners, however, also see boosting immunity as an important healing and disease-preventive function. From their perspective, nourishing the bone marrow, thymus, white blood cells, and other agents of the immune system to improve their efforts in the fight against illness is a safer, more economical, and more effective way to deal with disease than treating an already-existing condition. Indeed, in ancient times patients of some practitioners of traditional Eastern medicine paid their doctors only when well—illness was a sign of the doctor's failure. Many modern herbalists retain this ancient focus on maintaining wellness by recommending immune-boosting herbs.

Herbalist Christopher Hobbs, author of *Handbook for Herbal Healing,* makes the useful distinction between herbs that act as immune tonics and those that act as immune stimulants. He notes that this distinction corresponds to the two types of herbs that practitioners of traditional Chinese medicine and the traditional medicine of India used to treat "deep" and "surface" conditions. For example, Hobbs says that immune tonics, such as astragalus and the medicinal mushrooms, nourish and support the immune system at the deepest level. Immune tonics are typically taken for three to six months to help treat "deficient states" and long-term immune deficiencies such as cancer, AIDS, or chronic fatigue syndrome. On the other hand, the immune-stimulant herbs are useful for "illnesses that come and go and are not deeply seated or chronic." Immune stimulants, such as echinacea, are typically taken for a week or so to help treat or prevent colds, the flu, bronchitis, candidiasis, sore throats, and common infections.

Garlic. Garlic is a popular, multipurpose herb with a foot in both of the immune-tonic and immune-stimulant camps. You can take it at the first sign of a cold (see "An Immune-Boosting Remedy for the Common Cold," below, for dosage recommendations) or you can take somewhat lower doses on a daily basis indefinitely for its overall antiviral and immune-enhancing properties. Andrew Weil, M.D., says, "I recommend one or two cloves of garlic a day to people who suffer from chronic or recurrent infections, frequent yeast infections, or low resistance to infection." In supplement form, an average daily ongoing dose to boost immunity is 600 to 1,000 mg of garlic extract or concentrate; 1,800 to 3,000 mg of fresh garlic equivalent; or 1,800 to 3,600 mcg of allicin.

The Herbal Immune Tonics

The three following herbs—astragalus, ligustrum, and Siberian ginseng—are immune tonics and "adaptogens" (herbs that balance bodily functions; see Chapter 13). It is safe to take these herbs at the dosages suggested below on a daily basis for extended periods of time.

Astragalus

Astragalus, one of the most famous Chinese herbs, is derived from the root of a plant (*Astragalus membranaceus*) in the pea family. It is also known as milk vetch root (astragalus species grow in the United States; some are used to make the widely used food additive tragacanth gum) and, in China, *huang qi*. Astragalus is an antioxidant (possibly due to its being a good source of the essential trace mineral selenium) and an adaptogen. In addition, it is an overall bodily tonic used to treat fatigue and to strengthen (or "tonify") the body's overall vitality. Cancer patients in China take astragalus to support the spleen and boost immunity after chemotherapy or radiation treatment. Chinese researchers have shown that people taking astragalus get fewer and less severe colds.

Among the medicinally active compounds that researchers have identified in astragalus are certain complex carbohydrates known as polysaccharides, which stimulate the immune system. Polysaccharides are promising as immune stimulants because they help to produce more of certain immune agents or help to activate various white blood cells, including neutrophils, T cells, and interferon (a group of infection-fighting proteins that the body produces in response to a viral invasion). Human studies have confirmed astragalus's growing reputation as a white blood cell catalyst and an immune stimulant. For example, astragalus and another Chinese herb and immune stimulant, ligustrum, were recently tested on cancer patients and healthy persons by researchers in Houston. The scientists found that astragalus extracts were remarkably effective at restoring T-cell function in the cancer patients to normal levels. Another study found that astragalus helps protect the liver from some of the adverse effects of chemotherapy. Still others have found that astragalus increases production and secretion of interferon.

Astragalus is one of the most promising herbs for use in what the Chinese call *fu–zheng* therapy. *Fu* means "to fortify" and *zheng* means "constitution." According to herbalist Steven Foster and Chinese plant authority Yue Chongxi, authors of *Herbal Emissaries: Bringing Chinese Herbs to the West,* "Fu-zheng refers to treating disease by either enhancing or promoting the host defense mechanism or normalizing the central energy. . . . In the 1970s and early 1980s, Chinese scientists published a number of reports on the use of astragalus and other Chinese herbs as immune-system enhancers for patients undergoing chemotherapy for various cancers. The results showed that astragalus and other herbs acted as nonspecific immune system stimulants and helped to protect adrenal cortical function while patients are undergoing radiation or chemotherapy. . . . The end result was a significant increase in survival rates for the patients receiving fu-zheng therapy as an adjunct to western medical cancer treatments."

Astragalus is among the most nontoxic of herbs.

HOW TO USE ASTRAGALUS: Astragalus is sold fresh or dried and in capsules, concentrated drops, tinctures, and extracts. An average dosage to take two to three times daily is 250 to 500 mg of the powdered herb in capsules, or 1 dropperful of tincture or liquid concentrate.

Siberian Ginseng

In addition to being one of the premier adaptogens for balancing bodily functions, Siberian ginseng also has traditionally been used to enhance overall resistance to disease. A recent double-blind study by German researchers demonstrated the herb's potential to boost immunity. They administered an alcoholic extract of Siberian ginseng to 36 healthy volunteers three times daily for four weeks. While leading to no side effects, the extract caused a "drastic increase" in the number of T cells and other immune cells. The researchers concluded that Siberian ginseng "could be considered a nonspecific immunostimulant." Other studies have found that Siberian ginseng has a positive effect on interleukin and interferon. The exact mechanism by which it boosts immunity has not been determined.

Siberian ginseng has low toxicity and rarely causes side effects even in doses well beyond average ones.

HOW TO USE SIBERIAN GINSENG: Siberian ginseng comes in teas, tablets, capsules, extracts, tinctures, and concentrated drops. An average dosage is 250 to 500 mg once or twice daily, or 1 to 2 dropperfuls of the concentrated drops or tincture two or three times daily.

Ligustrum

Ligustrum is a principally Chinese herb (they refer to it as *nu zhen zi*) prepared from the dried and powdered fruits of an evergreen shrub (*Ligustrum lucidum*) also known in the United States as Chinese privet. It has traditionally been used in the East as a general strengthener for the liver and kidneys. Recent studies in China and the United States indicate ligustrum boosts immunity. Along with astragalus, it is being looked at as an agent for *fu-zheng* therapy to enhance white blood cell counts in cancer patients undergoing drug or radiation treatment. Herbalists also use ligustrum to help prevent respiratory-tract infections.

HOW TO USE LIGUSTRUM: Ligustrum is an ingredient in a number of herbal combination products sold in the United States. It is also sold as a powder, capsules, extracts, tinctures, and concentrated drops. An average dosage of the concentrated drops is 1 to 2 dropperfuls two or three times daily.

The Herbal Immune Stimulants

Take echinacea, goldenseal, and osha at the dosages suggested below for four to six days at a time if you feel a cold or respiratory infection coming on, have an injury, or otherwise need to boost the immune system. You can use these herbs for weeks or months at a time, but if you do it is best to dramatically reduce the dosages. For example, take 10 to 15 drops of echinacea, goldenseal, or osha in concentrated drop form.

Echinacea

Echinacea is derived from the roots and other parts of the purple coneflower (*Echinacea angustifolia, E. purpurea*). It is a versatile herb that is applied externally to a variety of injuries such as cuts, bites, and stings, and taken internally to fight bacterial and viral infections, lower fever, and calm allergic reactions.

Echinacea's reputation as a substance that activates white blood cells, boosts the immune system, and short-circuits colds and other respiratory infections has made it America's most popular healing herb. A recent survey of medical herbalists found that echinacea was by far the most important herb in their practices, outdistancing by a factor of two the runner-up, goldenseal. Echinacea is also among the most popular immune stimulants in Europe, especially in Germany, where pharmacies carry some 150 echinacea-based remedies. Germany has also been a leader in echinacea research. German scientists have conducted so many convincing studies on echinacea since the 1930s that medical claims for echinacea are now approved by the German government.

Echinacea is the ideal immune stimulant, according to Hobbs, author of *Echinacea: The Immune Herb!* He says, "Echinacea is probably one of the most promising immune strengtheners and modulators, with numerous scientific studies and rich clinical evidence in its favor." He notes that echinacea promotes healing and fights such common infectious conditions as influenza, herpes, and candidiasis. Researchers in Germany and elsewhere have found that echinacea shortens the duration of colds and flu and reduces the severity of their symptoms.

Studies have identified polysaccharides such as inulin and other compounds with immune-boosting and anti-inflammatory effects in echinacea. Herbal researchers have determined that it increases levels of the antiviral substance interferon as well as an immune-related blood protein known as properdin. The herb inhibits the bacterial enzyme hyaluronidase, thus helping to prevent pathogens from entering the body through the skin or mucous membranes. Echinacea prompts the thymus, bone marrow, and spleen to develop more of their various immune cells. Hobbs says that oral doses of echinacea juice, tincture, or drops may even stimulate immune tissue located under the tongue.

As a cold and flu remedy, echinacea is frequently combined with goldenseal, garlic, and other immune-stimulating herbs such as thuja (*Thuja occidentalis*). Look for products such as Insure Herbal, Cold-Sentry, Herbal Defense, and Vita Biotic.

HOW TO USE ECHINACEA: It is found freeze-dried and as fresh juice, tablets, capsules, concentrated drops, tinctures, and extracts. An average immune-stimulant dosage to take two or three times daily for four to six days at the first sign of illness is 1 to 2 dropperfuls of the tincture, juice, or concentrated drops; 750 mg of the dried root; or 300 to 400 mg of a dry extract.

Goldenseal

Goldenseal preparations are derived from the yellow root of a small perennial plant (*Hydrastis canadensis*) native to eastern North America. It is one of the most widely used herbs, with both internal and external applications. It is taken orally to alleviate colds, fevers, digestive ailments, and diarrhea caused by infectious agents. Numerous studies have proven that a number of goldenseal's alkaloid compounds, notably berberine, have pharmacological powers, including the ability to activate macrophages and other immune cells to counter bacteria. Goldenseal promotes the function of the spleen by increasing its blood supply and stimulating the organ's release of immune-boosting compounds.

Two additional berberine-containing plants are barberry (*Berberis vulgaris*) and its close relative Oregon grape (*Berberis aquifolium*).

Avoid taking goldenseal if you are pregnant or lactating or have high blood pressure.

HOW TO USE GOLDENSEAL: It is sold as a powder and in capsules, concentrated drops, and extracts. An average dosage is 500 mg of dried root, or 1 dropperful of tincture or concentrated drops two or three times daily.

Osha

Osha is a North American herb, prepared from the dried roots of a plant (*Ligusticum porteri*) in the carrot family, that Native Americans have traditionally used to treat sore throats, chest colds, and the flu. It is garnering increased attention from scientists for its ability to boost immunity and counter viral infections, though it has not been as well tested as other immune-boosting herbs. Especially in the western United States, herbalists are now using osha to help treat such conditions as bronchitis, herpes, and the flu.

Avoid osha during pregnancy and lactation.

HOW TO USE OSHA: It is available in capsules, extracts, tinctures, and concentrated drops. An average dosage of the tincture or concentrated drops is 1 dropperful two or three times daily.

Vitamins and Minerals for the Immune System

There is little doubt that taking optimal levels of certain nutrients can enhance the functioning of your immune system. A Canadian study published in *The Lancet* in 1992 suggested that taking even relatively low amounts of vitamins and minerals could cut in half the average number of days many older people are sick from colds, other infections, and immune-deficient conditions. Conducted by renowned immune researcher Ranjit Kumar Chandra, M.D., director of the World Health Organization's Center for Nutritional Immunology, the study looked at 96 people over age 65. One group took daily vitamin and mineral supplements, mostly at mere RDA levels (usually considered far short of optimal levels). The nutrient group experienced fewer than half as many days with infectious-disease episodes than the placebo group (23 days, compared to 48 days for the placebo group) over the course of a year. When they did get sick, those who took nutritional supplements recovered in about half the time it took the placebo group. Blood tests confirmed that the nutrient-takers had higher numbers of immune cells and that the cells were more active. The importance of this and similar studies is underscored by the fact that infections are a major cause of death among the elderly.

It is no accident that many of the vitamins and minerals that boost immunity are also potent antioxidants capable of scavenging excess free radicals. Free radicals can damage many important components of the immune system, including the thymus gland and cell membranes in the lungs and elsewhere. "When free radicals initiate damage to cell membranes, inflammatory substances such as prostaglandins are released," note the authors of *The Natural Health Guide to Antioxidants.* "This in turn can lead to immunosuppression, food and chemical sensitivities, lowered resistance to infection, and eventually degenerative inflammatory disease, autoimmune diseases, and cancer."

Vitamin A/Beta Carotene

Vitamin A and its precursor beta carotene are widely recognized as prominent infection-fighting nutrients, useful in the prevention or treatment of such conditions as respiratory infections, measles, candidiasis, and possibly AIDS. Nutritionally aware physicians recommend vitamin A/beta carotene to promote the healing of wounds and to prevent immune problems in patients undergoing surgery, radiation, or chemotherapy. There is good evidence that taking optimal levels of vitamin A/beta carotene can lower your risk of getting certain cancers.

Vitamin A/beta carotene boosts immunity by increasing both the number and the activity of antibodies such as T helper cells. Vitamin A/beta carotene also helps the thymus to grow and protects the gland from the harmful effects of stress. Vitamin A/beta carotene is necessary for healthy mucous membranes and thus helps protect the respiratory system from viral infections. More so than vitamin A, beta carotene is a potent antioxidant that defends the thymus gland from harmful free radicals. Some studies have found that beta carotene has an immune-enhancing effect separate from its vitamin A activity.

According to Shari Lieberman, a registered dietitian and the coauthor of *The Real Vitamin & Mineral Book,* "In my clinical experience, I have found that vitamin A supplementation is an excellent and safe immune system booster. Patients who get frequent sore throats, colds, flu, sinusitis, or bronchitis have shown a marked decrease in the frequency and severity of these respiratory infections."

Taking high doses of preformed A (such as 100,000 IU daily for months, or 500,000 to 1,000,000 IU daily for two to three weeks) can allow it to accumulate in the body and cause potentially serious adverse health effects. On the other hand, the body converts to vitamin A only as much beta carotene as it needs. Extra beta carotene is stored, but the only adverse effect of such storage is a slight orange tinge to the skin.

How to use vitamin a/beta carotene: It comes in a wide variety of tablets and capsules. An average daily immune-boosting dosage is 5,000 to 10,000 IU of vitamin A plus 25,000 to 50,000 IU (15 to 30 mg) of beta carotene or, even better, beta carotene plus mixed carotenoids.

Vitamin B₆

This B-complex micronutrient, found most commonly in supplements as pyridoxine, is well known for its ability to help protect against nervous disorders. Yet it is also the most important of the B vitamins for keeping your immune system working optimally. Animal studies indicate that optimal levels of B_6 may help prevent cancer and slow the growth of tumors. Studies done on elderly humans confirm a positive effect on the immune system. A B_6 deficiency can lead to immune-system dysfunctions by reducing the number of circulating antibodies and interfering with the proper functioning of lymphoid tissue and thymic hormone.

The adult RDA is 1.5 to 2.2 mg. Vitamin B_6 is extremely safe, though daily megadoses in excess of 500 to 1,000 mg may be toxic for some people, or induce a B_6 dependency. Many nutritionists recommend taking B vitamins as part of a B-complex supplement rather than individually, to avoid imbalances.

How to use vitamin B_6: It comes in tablets and capsules. An average daily dosage for increased immunity is 25 to 50 mg.

Vitamin C

This is the most popular supplement to boost the immune system and help the body resist infection by bacteria and viruses. Many people take high doses of vitamin C to reduce the symptoms of the common cold. Though the vitamin's effect on colds is still a matter of heated dispute among some scientific researchers, the consensus that has emerged is that at the very least C will shorten how long a cold stays with you and will often reduce its severity. Many people who take vitamin C on a daily basis also report getting fewer colds; the studies that have been done are more equivocal on this potential effect.

Vitamin C is important to the thymus gland and white blood cells such as lymphocytes. Without adequate levels of C, immune cells become sluggish and ineffective. High doses of C, on the other hand, stimulate the production of phagocytes and lymphocytes while also making them more mobile and active. It also increases interferon levels.

How to use vitamin C: Vitamin C comes in a wide variety of

powders, tablets, and capsules. An average dosage to boost immunity is 250 to 500 mg two or three times daily.

Vitamin E

Vitamin E enjoys a growing reputation as an immune stimulant that can boost the body's ability to resist various diseases, including lung and breast cancer and certain autoimmune diseases such as rheumatoid arthritis. Animal and human studies indicate that taking optimal levels of vitamin E improves antibody response and T-cell activity. Vitamin E deficiency, on the other hand, is characterized by lowered immunity and higher rates of some cancers.

Vitamin E's effect on the immune system is thought to be partially due to its role as an antioxidant that protects the thymus and lymphatic tissue. Vitamin E also helps to protect the integrity of cell membranes. Healthy cell membranes are necessary for warding off invading pathogens. Researchers say that E may also benefit the immune system by limiting the number of hormonelike substances known as prostaglandins, which tend to suppress the immune system.

How to use vitamin e: It is sold as a liquid and in dry and oil-filled capsules. An average daily dosage to boost immunity is 400 to 600 IU.

Zinc

This trace mineral is essential for various bodily functions, including proper functioning of the immune system. It has been shown to improve the healing of wounds and speed recovery from injuries and surgery. Zinc can check the spread of viruses such as herpes simplex in the body. Several studies also suggest that high concentrations of elemental zinc in the throat, from sucking on zinc lozenges, can counter the local viruses responsible for the common cold.

In one noted double-blind clinical trial, 37 subjects dissolved in their mouths two zinc gluconate lozenges (each containing 23 mg of elemental zinc) at the first sign of a cold. These subjects subsequently sucked on one additional lozenge every two waking hours. Another 28 subjects were given identical doses of a placebo. Zinc succeeded in eliminating cold symptoms, in some cases within hours and in about 20 percent of the subjects within a day. The average number of days before zinc-taking subjects became symptom-free was 4, while the placebo subjects took on average 11 days to become symptom-free.

Other human and animal studies confirm that taking zinc supplements can benefit overall immunity. An antioxidant, zinc protects immune organs such as the thymus from the adverse effects of free radicals. Zinc supports the body's efforts to produce thymic hormones and increases the number of T cells. People who suffer from zinc deficiencies often experience depressed immune function that can be reversed by taking zinc supplements.

Supplement manufacturers frequently combine zinc with copper, selenium, and other minerals and vitamins. Lozenges containing 23 to 25 mg of elemental zinc, and sometimes additional nutrients such as vitamin C and echinacea, are sold as Zinc Cold Care and Cold Season Plus. Flavored lozenges disguise zinc's metallic flavor.

Zinc is nontoxic at dosages many times the adult RDA of 12 to 19 mg. Most people experience no adverse effects from taking 100 to 150 mg daily for weeks, though this is more than is necessary for optimum health. Adverse effects such as gastrointestinal irritation and vomiting may result from single megadoses in the range of 1,000 to 2,000 mg.

How to use zinc: Zinc comes in liquids, lozenges, tablets, and capsules. An average daily dosage to boost immunity is 17 to 25 mg taken with a meal. For optimum effect, combine zinc with beta carotene or beta carotene plus mixed carotenoids (25,000 to 50,000 IU) and with copper (2 to 4 mg).

To short-circuit a cold, suck on a lozenge at the first sign of a throat tingle and then again every two hours, up to six times per day, until you are symptom-free. Avoid taking such high levels of zinc for more than about a week.

Selenium

This essential trace mineral has become increasingly popular in recent years for its well-established antioxidant effects. Studies have shown that selenium can help protect against such age-related diseases as heart disease, cancer, and arthritis. Selenium may also be beneficial in the treatment and prevention of immune-deficient conditions, including AIDS.

Researchers who have administered selenium supplements to animals report dramatic increases in both the number and the average activity of various immune cells, such as lymphocytes and phagocytes. Similarly, studies indicate that when a selenium deficiency exists, animals and humans experience decreased levels of antibodies and their activity is impaired. Numerous studies have also demonstrated that people who suffer from immune-suppressed conditions, such as AIDS, are often deficient in selenium.

Exactly how selenium boosts the immune system is unclear. Researchers speculate that the immune stimulation may be due to selenium's antioxidant activity and its ability to protect important immune-related tissues in the lymph system and the thymus against free-radical damage. Like vitamin E, selenium may also play an important immune-related role by protecting the integrity of cell membranes, thus improving their overall function.

The body requires only tiny amounts of selenium every day. Dietary sources of selenium, including fish, brewer's yeast, and plants that have been grown in selenium-rich soil, are often not sufficient to safeguard against a deficiency. Selenium is safe to take on a daily basis at levels three to four times the adult RDA, which is 50 to 75 mcg. Its potential toxicity does not appear to begin until dosages in excess of 1,000 mcg daily. Organic selenium is generally thought to be safer and more effective than inorganic sodium selenite.

HOW TO USE SELENIUM: Selenium is widely available in tablets and capsules ranging in size from 50 to 200 mcg. An average daily dose for boosting immunity is 100 to 200 mcg. Take selenium in combination with vitamin E for increased effect.

Other Nutritional Supplements to Increase Immunity

Some of the most popular nutritional supplements for boosting immunity are the bee products and green-food products. Bee products include:

Royal jelly. This is a light-colored, highly nutritious gelatinous substance secreted in the salivary glands of young worker honeybees. In the hive, royal jelly is used to feed all bee larvae for the first few days and then to stimulate the growth and development of larvae chosen to be queen bees, who feed on royal jelly exclusively.

Bee pollen. This is a powderlike nutrient collected from bee hives that are specially set up to gather flower pollen as it falls from the bees' legs. Similar products are sold as flower pollen and bee-free pollen (harvested without the bees).

Bee propolis. Propolis is a sticky substance derived from plant resins collected by bees along with pollen and spread around the hive, possibly for its antibacterial effects. Studies confirm that it contains a natural antibiotic. There is some evidence that it also boosts immunity and helps prevent the spread of infection in the throat. Allergic reactions to bee products are rare but possible. Experiment with tiny amounts before taking larger doses.

Natural-food stores sell two basic types of chlorophyll-rich green-food products, differentiated by source: algae products grown in water, and young grasses grown on land.

Spirulina. Among the most concentrated sources of chlorophyll and diverse carotenoids, spirulina is a whole-food supplement derived from certain primitive, spiral-shaped, blue-green microalgae commonly cultivated in tanks in California, Hawaii, and Asia. Some nutritional practitioners recommend spirulina therapeutically to lower cholesterol levels and boost immunity. It is sometimes sprinkled on foods as a condiment.

Chlorella. Chlorella is an easily digested green-food supplement derived from a single-celled microalgae. Most products are cultivated in tanks and imported from Japan or Taiwan.

Barley grass. This is the young, green barley plant harvested before the grain develops. Producers make supplements by juicing and then drying the plants. Barley-grass extract has shown antioxidant activity, and studies indicate barley grass may protect cells from damage by X rays and chemical pollutants. Products go by names such as Green Magma and Green Energy.

Wheat grass. Supplements are made from the dried juice of immature wheat plants harvested before the grain develops. A dose of 3 to 5 g is nutritionally equivalent to an average serving of spinach or other dark-green leafy vegetable.

In general, both bee products and green foods supply a varied concentration of easily assimilated and naturally balanced vitamins, minerals, enzymes, trace elements, essential fatty acids, and other nutrients. Although relatively few rigorous scientific studies have been done on these supplements, many people who take them swear by their ability to increase not only immunity but energy levels and physical performance. Because chlorophyll-rich supplements are concentrated foods rather than isolated nutrients, they are among the safest nutritional supplements on the market.

Bee products and green foods come in powders, tablets, capsules, juices, liquid concentrates, and extracts. In addition, new "whole-food concentrate" supplements combine herbs, nutrients, green foods, and bee products. With names such as Nutra Greens, Kyo-Green, Complete Greens, Green Magic, and From the Earth, such products bring together elements including spirulina, flower or bee-pollen extracts, barley, chlorella, wheat-grass juice, herbs, enzymes, and other phytonutrients. Many people are attracted to this shotgun approach to nutrition, and it has its advantages: no single nutrient is likely to be contained in levels high enough to be possibly harmful, and all sorts of as-yet-unidentified nutrients may well be present to some degree.

Check product labels for dosage recommendations for bee products and green foods.

Two supplements with more-established scientific track records for boosting immunity are arginine and organic germanium compounds.

Arginine

Arginine is found in chocolate, peanuts and other nuts, various seeds, and peas. An amino acid, it straddles the line between essential and nonessential. While nonessential for many adults, it is an essential amino acid for children, and possibly for some adults undergoing stress or recovering from injury. Along with the essential amino acid lysine, it is often thought of only in terms of how it affects the herpes virus. Though the evidence is not conclusive, arginine may promote herpes outbreaks, while lysine may inhibit them. These possible effects on herpes, however, are hardly the only actions these amino acids have on the body. Increasingly, research on arginine has focused on its well-demonstrated ability to stimulate certain glands, including the pituitary (which secretes growth hormone in the body, leading to muscle-building and fat-burning; see Chapter 4) and the thymus.

Since the thymus plays a central role in immune function by producing certain white blood cells, it is not surprising that arginine supplements show particular promise in boosting immunity and possibly speeding the healing of wounds. Recent test-tube, animal, and human studies confirm that arginine increases the number and activity of immune cells.

Pregnant women, anyone with kidney or liver diseases, and people under the age of 20 (whose bones are still growing) should not take supplemental arginine. Since it is possible that high levels of arginine can reactivate latent herpes viruses in some individuals, if you have herpes it is best to combine arginine with equal amounts of lysine (which may prevent herpes outbreaks) to avoid this side effect.

Arginine is frequently combined with such nutrients as ornithine, methionine, and B_6 in supplements aimed at the muscle-building market.

HOW TO USE ARGININE: It is available as a single ingredient in capsule and powder form. An average dose for immune enhancement is 250 to 500 mg daily.

Organic Germanium Compounds

Germanium is a trace mineral found in soil and some herbs and foods, including garlic and shiitake mushrooms. (It is not found, however, in the flowering plant with the similar name, geranium.) Although the mineral itself appears to have limited effects on human health, researchers have recently developed synthetic organic compounds with potentially dramatic medicinal effects. The most prominent of the new compounds was developed by Japanese researchers and dubbed Ge-132 or Ge-Oxy 132 (also known as organic germanium sesquioxide). Clinical studies in Japan indicate that this organic germanium compound improves oxygenation of tissues and restores the normal function of immune-boosting cells. In Japan and elsewhere Ge-132 is now being used to improve circulation, balance bodily functions, and help prevent cancer (see Chapter 9). Organic germanium compounds may also combat viral infections, AIDS, and chronic fatigue disorders, possibly by stimulating the activity of such immune agents as macrophages and interferon. "Studies regarding its immune-enhancing, anti-cancer and anti-viral activities seem promising and should be continued," comments Sheldon Saul Hendler, M.D., Ph.D., in *The Doctors' Vitamin and Mineral Encyclopedia.*

Organic germanium is relatively nontoxic. Adverse reactions are rare even among those who have taken several grams daily for a number of months, a much higher level of intake than is necessary or recommended. Skin rashes are the most common side effect at average doses. Expect to pay a premium for this supplement.

How to use organic germanium compounds: These come in powders, granules, and tablets, as well as capsules ranging in size from 25 to 250 mg. An average dosage for better immune function is 50 to 100 mg daily.

An Immune-Boosting Remedy for the Common Cold

At the first throat tingle or other sign of a cold, take the following combination of nutrients and herbs. Continue until your symptoms disappear, or up to one week.

• Vitamin C: 500 to 1,000 mg two or three times daily.

- Zinc: one 23-to-25-mg lozenge every two hours, up to six times daily
- Echinacea: 1 to 2 dropperfuls of the tincture, juice, or concentrated drops, or 750 mg of the dried root, or 300 to 400 mg of a dry extract two or three times daily
- Garlic: 1,000 to 1,500 mg of pure or concentrated garlic or garlic extract powder, or 2,400 to 3,600 mg of fresh garlic equivalent, or 3,600 to 4,800 mcg allicin per day

A number of companies now offer supplements that combine these and other immune-boosting herbs and nutrients. Look for products such as Quick Response and Under the Weather.

The Immune-Stimulating Medicinal Mushrooms

Taking mushrooms for their medicinal properties is still in its infancy in the United States. Yet worldwide annual sales of medicinal mushrooms recently passed one billion dollars, according to the First International Conference on Mushroom Biology and Mushroom Products, organized by UNESCO and the Chinese University of Hong Kong in late 1993. Continued growth in the field is likely to be spurred by ongoing studies into various mushrooms' abilities to reduce the risk of degenerative diseases.

According to natural-health advocate and mushroom authority Andrew Weil, M.D., one of the most promising aspects of medicinal mushrooms is their potential to change the function and activity of the immune system. In his recent article "Boost Immunity with Medicinal Mushrooms" in *Natural Health* magazine, Weil says that most of the hard, woody medicinal mushrooms from China and Japan contain polysaccharides like those found in echinacea, astragalus, and certain other plants. The antiviral, antitumor, and immune-stimulating properties of these polysaccharides suggest that medicinal mushrooms have been undeservedly overlooked as immune boosters. "It almost goes without saying," Weil notes, "that nontoxic compounds with these properties would be valuable, given the inability of conventional medicine to do much about viral infections and depressed immunity."

Japanese cancer researcher Dr. Goro Chihara notes that medicinal mushrooms such as shiitake can play an important role in augmenting "intrinsic host defense mechanisms"—boosting the body's inherent abilities to fight off invading agents. He says that such "host defense potentiators" should be a more important focus for cancer research than the current fascination with cell-killing substances.

Shiitake and reishi are the most common medicinal mushrooms in the United States today, though other varieties are beginning to become available either in fresh or packaged forms. Some of the new-to-the-market medicinal mushrooms most promising for their immune-stimulating properties include maitake, enokitake, and zhu ling.

Shiitake, reishi, maitake, and *enokitake* are Japanese names; *zhu ling* is Chinese. These medicinal mushrooms are also known by their English names, and most are either found wild or can be easily cultivated in North America. Since for the most part Asians have pioneered the medical research and the product development, and supplement makers in the United States typically use the Asian names, those are what is used here as well.

Shiitake

A Japanese scientist isolated the polysaccharide lentinan from shiitake in the early 1970s. Since then, researchers have used lentinan in numerous clinical trials and found it to have a beneficial effect on the number and activities of immune cells such as macrophages and T cells and on the production of interferon. Shiitake's immune-boosting effects are so well documented that in Japan lentinan is an approved drug for use in conjunction with cancer chemotherapy. Researchers have found that lentinan or shiitake extract can shrink tumors and combat viruses and bacteria. As an immune booster, shiitake may prove effective in the treatment of AIDS.

Until recently shiitake was chiefly imported from Asia, but now is often American-grown. In the United States it is sometimes known as Black Forest mushroom.

Reishi

Reishi is one of the most versatile medicinal mushrooms. It has long been used in Asia as an energy tonic to promote longevity and overall health. Studies indicate that reishi is an antioxidant and contains polysaccharides and other compounds that may boost the immune system. Reishi is taken to counter bacteria and viruses and has shown promise as an agent to help prevent or treat cancer, chronic fatigue syndrome, and other conditions. Russian researchers at the Cancer Research Center in Moscow have had positive results using reishi extracts to boost the immunity of cancer patients.

Maitake

Maitake (*Grifola frondosa* or *Polyporus frondosa*) may be the most promising new medicinal mushroom of the 1990s. Although scientists have not yet identified the relevant polysaccharide in this mushroom, it appears to be the most effective immune-boosting mushroom of all, says Weil. He notes in *Spontaneous Healing* that maitake belongs to a family of medicinal mushrooms that in the Far East is "highly esteemed as medicinal herbs, especially in the class of superior drugs, the tonics and panaceas that increase resistance and promote longevity." Studies in Japan tend to confirm that maitake increases immune function. Some animal and test-tube studies also indicate that maitake may shrink cancerous tumors and counteract HIV. In Asia maitake is also used as an adaptogen to help balance bodily functions.

While relatively rare in the wild in Japan, maitake (which translates as "dancing mushroom," as it caused such joy when found in the wild) is not an uncommon forest mushroom in eastern North America (where it is known as hen of the woods). Mushroom hunters still rejoice when they find one of its large clusters on a hardwood stump, as it is a delicious edible mushroom in addition to being wonderfully healthful.

Enokitake

Enokitake (*Flammulina velutipes*) is another medicinal mushroom that is widely cultivated in Japan. A closely related strain is sometimes found in the wild or cultivated for sale fresh in North America, where it is called winter mushroom or velvet-stemmed flammulina. Enokitake have small, pale caps on long stems. Though not as delicious as shiitake, enokitake contains a potent polysaccharide called flammulin. According to Weil, flammulin may be a more effective immune booster when taken orally than shiitake's lentinan.

Zhu Ling

Also known as polyporus and grifola, zhu ling is a maitakelike Chinese mushroom (*Polyporus umbellatus, Grifola umbellata*) that is rarely found wild in the United States. Animal and human studies indicate that it can boost immunity and slow the growth of cancerous tumors. The Chinese frequently use it as a short-term tonic. Zhu ling caps are pleasant-tasting, but the medicinal parts of the mushroom grow under-ground. Zhu ling is sometimes included as an ingredient in Chinese herbal formulas.

How to Use Medicinal Mushrooms

Shiitake and reishi are the only medicinal mushrooms that are rela-tively easy to find in North American natural-food stores. You can add fresh shiitake to soups and other dishes that call for edible mushrooms. Shiitake and reishi are more commonly available in supplement form, usually dried and in capsules, tinctures, and extracts. An average dose of either in capsules is 500 mg two or three times daily.

Maitake, enokitake, and zhu ling are still relatively new to the United States and can be hard to find, especially fresh or dried. Maitake is sold in caplet form (500 mg of powder) under the brand name Grifon (see "Resources"). The Eclectic Institute (see "Re-sources") sells a freeze-dried extract of zhu ling in capsules.

Medicinal mushrooms can be quite expensive. For example, Fungi Perfecti, a premier mail-order mushroom enterprise (see "Re-sources"), sells limited quantities of certified organic dried maitake for $300 per pound.

Mushrooms in tablets and capsules are usually dried powder or ex-tracts, though some may be the actual compressed whole mushroom. Herbal companies often combine various medicinal mushrooms, sometimes with immune-boosting herbs such as echinacea and astraga-lus. Look for products such as Mycelin3.

Where to Start

Here's an easy-to-follow daily supplemental regimen that can boost your overall immunity. Each day, take:

- An insurance-level multivitamin-multimineral supplement, to cover the important immune-boosting nutrients vitamin A/beta carotene, vitamin B complex, vitamin C, vitamin E, zinc, and selenium
- One of the immune tonic herbs, such as astragalus or Siberian ginseng
- Shiitake, reishi, or one of the other immune-stimulating medici-nal mushrooms

Beyond Herbs and Supplements

Some of the same healthful lifestyle and dietary habits that promote longevity and prevent degenerative diseases also help your body to protect itself from disease-causing agents. Here are eight of the most important areas to work on for developing a strong immune system.

- Learn to manage your mental stress and reduce your levels of anger, guilt, and hostility. Explore biofeedback, meditation, yoga, self-hypnosis, journal-writing, or other techniques, if necessary.
- Get regular exercise or physical activity.
- Get sufficient sleep.
- Reduce your consumption of fats, cholesterol, refined grains and sweeteners, and alcohol, since studies show that consuming large amounts of these foods and beverages inhibits various immune functions.
- Eat a balanced, whole-foods diet rich in nutrient-dense and high-fiber vegetables, fruits, grains, beans, and legumes.
- Reduce your exposure to environmental pollutants, including cigarette smoke, toxic household products, auto exhaust, and strong electromagnetic fields.
- Stay positive in your overall outlook and make the most of the humor in your daily life.
- Stay connected to family, friends, coworkers, and neighbors.

Enhance Your Strength and Endurance

The pressure to succeed in athletics can be intense, whether you are an international tennis superstar or a high-school football player in a small town in Texas. Society lavishes money, prestige, and acclaim on winners, but causes everyone else to question themselves. A win-at-any-cost attitude can often lead athletes to look for shortcuts to success, including the use of drugs that can speed muscle development during training or boost endurance during performance.

Admittedly, some aspects of physical fitness, such as flexibility and coordination, are not much influenced by either drugs or natural substances. Other important aspects are, however. These include how you build and repair muscle tissue and prevent its breakdown, how your body uses the energy available to it during exercise, and how you can encourage greater endurance or cardiovascular capacity.

From Coffee to Steroids

The three forms of conventional drugs most popular with athletes today are stimulants, anabolic steroids, and growth hormones.

Stimulants. These include synthetic drugs such as amphetamine as well as substances such as caffeine and ephedrine, which may be either derived from plants (coffee, tea, ephedra/ma huang) or synthetically derived. (See Chapter 5 for more on caffeine and ephedrine.) Stimulants are most commonly used for events that require endurance, which these drugs do enhance. Studies have confirmed, for example, that if you consume enough of it, caffeine permits you to exercise longer and more intensively. Most researchers consider an effective dose for an average-sized person to be at least 300 mg of caffeine, the amount found in 2 to 4 cups of coffee. In one study, subjects on stationary bicycles who took 330 mg of caffeine an hour before the test experienced a 20 percent improvement in endurance.

Caffeine's effects on endurance may be due to its increasing the rate at which fat is burned. This allows you to postpone using up your stores of glycogen, the principal fuel your body needs for energy and endurance. Caffeine may also help reduce the amount of lactic acid your muscles produce during vigorous exercise. Cells produce lactic acid when they break down glucose to generate energy; a buildup of lactic acid in muscles can cause cramping. Caffeine's effects may be due in part also to its psychoactive properties—it can increase alertness, self-confidence, and aggression.

Some of the potential side effects from too much caffeine include heart palpitations, abdominal pain, nausea, and diarrhea. Because caffeine is a diuretic that promotes fluid loss and frequent urination, it can increase the risk of dehydration. (Having to stop and pee every few miles during a marathon can present its own set of problems.) Caffeine's stimulating effects on the nerves may be counterproductive for some sports. Running takes minimal coordination, but if you're jittery while tossing up your tennis serve, your play may suffer. Too much caffeine may also impair your judgment and increase your risk of injury. The long-term effects of regular caffeine use should also be considered, including addiction, stomach and bladder irritations, and higher blood-cholesterol levels.

International athletic competitions prohibit amphetamine use and either restrict or ban the use of caffeine and ephedrine. Drinking a cup of coffee before an event may not yield bodily caffeine levels high enough for you to be disqualified, but consuming too much caffeine is usually considered to result in an unfair advantage. Ephedrine use is a more common cause of disqualification. Some disqualified athletes claim not to be aware that they took ephedrine, an ingredient in many over-the-counter cold and flu medications, but much ephedrine use is decidedly intended to boost performance. The Argentine soccer star Diego Maradona was kicked out of the competition in the latter rounds of the 1994 World Cup because in post-game urine tests he tested positive for five different ephedrine compounds.

Anabolic steroids. Anabolic steroids are synthetic prescription drugs that when injected into the body mimic the effects of natural anabolic (muscle-building) hormones, such as testosterone and growth hormone. Anabolic steroids promote muscle growth, increase lean body mass, and boost protein synthesis, leading to large, bulky, "cut and ripped" bodies. (Among bodybuilders, "cut and ripped" means losing surface fat to accentuate muscle separation and definition.) Though the use of anabolic steroids by competitive athletes has been banned for almost 20 years, an active black market exists for them among bodybuilders, wrestlers, track and field athletes, football players, and various other athletes and image-conscious males (and, increasingly, females) down to the high-school level (estimates are that 250,000 to 400,000 U.S. teens use them).

Anabolic steroids cause notorious side effects in many people. In young people they can stunt normal growth and cause adrenal-gland, liver, and kidney dysfunctions (including cancer later in life). Steroids may lead to irreversible heart disease, since they increase the total cholesterol level and decrease the level of HDL, the good cholesterol. In addition, steroids can cause acne and premature baldness. Effects on the personality are also noticeable. Steroids can cause increased aggression (the Nazis pioneered steroid use on military troops in World War II) and even psychosis in high doses. When male athletes inject themselves with large amounts of synthetic hormones, their bodies cut back production of the natural stuff. Thus, testicles begin to shrink and sperm production falls, leading to diminished sex drive, femalelike breasts, impotence, and sterility. Young women who use steroids, on the other hand, may experience irreversible decreases in breast size, deepening of the voice, development of male-pattern baldness, and growth of hair on the face.

In essence, men can become feminized, women masculinized, and young people smaller as adults than they would otherwise be. Clearly, anabolic steroids are not all they are pumped up to be, to use an appropriate metaphor.

Growth hormone. Produced naturally in the body by the pituitary gland, growth hormone stimulates normal bodily growth and possibly immune function. Growth hormone helps the body break down fat faster, releases more energy to the muscles, and stimulates the buildup of muscle tissue. In recent years these effects have made growth hormone a controversial substance in both the medical and athletic communities.

Until recently growth hormone was obtained from human corpses and was thus in short supply and exceedingly expensive. With recent advances in genetic engineering, growth hormone is now more readily available as a synthetic drug. Some doctors are advocating its use on short children, to promote growth to "normal" size. Whether that is ethically warranted is being debated. There is also a question as to whether short children who take growth hormone grow any larger than they would eventually, without the drug. Long-term side effects are still unknown, though one adverse effect from taking high levels of growth hormone is a gradual thickening of the bones, resulting in coarsened facial features or deformities of the hands and feet. In body-building and some other athletic circles, injectable growth hormone has supplanted anabolic steroids as the drug of choice, in part because growth hormone is much harder to detect than anabolic steroids.

Using high doses of stimulants, or any amount of anabolic hormones, gives an unfair advantage to the user. This often sets up a vicious cycle in which non-drug-using opponents feel they too need to take drugs to level the playing field. In the long run, the game or race is over, while the athletes' health may be compromised for a lifetime. Alternatives from the fields of herbs, vitamins and minerals, and nutritional substances offer a saner choice.

Herbs for the Athlete

Herbs can potentially improve athletic performance in a number of ways. Obviously, stimulant herbs such as coffee and ephedra have notable effects during exercise itself. There are also herbs that tend to balance the body's functions, increase its innate vitality, and boost its overall function (see Chapter 13). These "tonifying," "tonic," or "adaptogenic" herbs are usually taken not so much for their effects on an athlete during a specific game or race, but for the herbs' effects during the training and recovery phases. Some of the herbs that are most attractive to athletes, such as ginseng, schisandra, and cordyceps, seem to combine mild stimulation with this overall system-boosting effect.

Ginseng

This herb surpasses all others as an athletic performance booster. Ginseng seems to combine elements of the stimulants and the tonic herbs, improving performance as well as strengthening the system for training and recovery. This has generated a minor industry in ginseng products, from ginseng-flavored soft drinks to expensive standardized extracts, and the herb is now being used by professional athletes and weekend warriors.

Ginseng is often thought of as an exclusively Eastern herb, but that's not so. Some Native American tribes traditionally used American ginseng (*Panax quinquefolius*) for much the same reason that Asians have long taken Chinese or Korean ginseng (*Panax ginseng*): to increase strength, energy, fertility, and overall health. Ginseng is one of the best tonic herbs for increasing overall vitality. It is also stimulating (see Chapter 5), capable of increasing alertness and decreasing reaction time. Because it is so effective at reducing feelings of physical and mental fatigue and restoring and building overall energy levels, it is widely acclaimed as the single best herb for athletes.

A number of studies done in Europe and elsewhere have confirmed that ginseng has effects on such factors as alertness, strength, endurance, reflexes, lung capacity, visual and motor coordination, and reaction time. For example, a study at Uppsala University in Sweden found that people taking ginseng showed improved motor function and concentration. At the Institute of Biologically Active Substances, a research institute in Vladivostok, Russia, researchers found that runners taking ginseng significantly improved their speed. A 1981 study of athletes ages 18 to 23 given a ginseng extract found that ginseng-treated subjects experienced an increase in performance factors such as oxygen absorption capacity along with a decrease in fatigue factors such as lactic acid production in major leg muscles. Other researchers have found that ginseng boosts work efficiency, prevents fatigue, and reduces recovery time. Ginseng lessens the effects of stress, possibly by stimulating a part of the adrenals.

Ginseng is a popular constituent in herbal athletic formulations. It is also widely available as a single herb and in combination with other ginseng species. Potency in ginseng products may vary considerably. Products that are standardized for ginsenosides often offer the most predictable results.

HOW TO USE GINSENG: Ginseng comes in myriad forms, including the whole root, capsules, tablets, tea bags, tinctures, and extracts. An average dosage to boost athletic performance is 500 to 1,000 mg of extracts standardized for 5 to 9 percent ginsenoside. An average dosage of some concentrated extracts and ginseng products with higher standardized percentages may be as low as 200 to 400 mg; check labels.

Schisandra

Schisandra (also spelled *schizandra*) is a common Chinese herb derived from the dried red berrylike fruit of a hardy vine (*Schisandra chinensis*) of the magnolia family, native to East Asia. The Chinese refer to it as *wu wei zi*. Schisandra is a major system-strengthening herb in Chinese medicine, long prized for its ability to prevent fatigue, increase stamina, and prolong youth. Some hunting tribes of northern China would take supplies of the dried berries whenever they went on long hunting trips during cold weather. Eating the schisandra berries helped them to stoke their internal fires and renew their flagging strength. In parts of China people still make a mildly stimulating tea from schisandra berries. They consider it ideal for such conditions as fatigue, nervous exhaustion, and lack of energy. Schisandra may even boost mood and increase memory and mental acuity. Use of schisandra has recently spread to Russia (where it is a registered medicine for vision difficulties), Scandinavia, Europe, and the United States.

Recent animal studies by Chinese researchers and others indicate that schisandra may improve aerobic capacity. In one 1989 study researchers fed schisandra-berry extract to polo horses. The animals' heart rate during exercise did not rise as much, and upon stopping the workout their normal rate of breathing returned more quickly. Overall performance improved.

As an energy booster, schisandra's effects are mild compared to nervous-system stimulants such as ephedra, though herbalists say that, compared to healthy people, people suffering from exhaustion may feel a more pronounced rise.

How to use schisandra: Schisandra is most commonly found in capsules, though it also comes in concentrated drops, tinctures, and extracts. An average dosage in capsule form is 250 to 500 mg once or twice daily.

Cordyceps

Cordyceps is a Chinese herb native to the mountainous regions of China and Tibet. It is derived from a parasitic fungus (*Cordyceps sinensis*) that grows on the larvae of certain moths. Cordyceps exploded into the limelight in 1993 when Chinese coaches credited it with helping a number of Chinese women runners break various world records— some long-standing—at the Chinese National Games. Many Western skeptics were quick to charge that the athletes were using illegal drugs or steroids. The runners' coach said that the athletes' sudden and remarkable success was attributable to better training practices, terrapin soup, and cordyceps.

Whether the surprising performance of the Chinese runners can be attributed to cordyceps, anabolic steroids, or some other performance-enhancing drugs is an open question. In the runners' defense, they did not have the overdeveloped musculature typically seen on athletes taking steroids, nor did any of the runners fail the drug tests that were administered. On the other hand, no third-party track officials administered drug tests to the Chinese athletes during training, and steroid use can be difficult to detect with the tests administered at the time of competition. When another set of female Chinese athletes, this time swimmers with bulky arms and shoulders, swept aside more world records in 1994, new questions were raised about Chinese athletes' possible steroid use. Previous instances of female athletes suddenly outstripping their male compatriots have been associated with steroid use, and indeed a number of female Chinese athletes did test positive for illegal anabolic steroids in 1994.

Clearly, just taking cordyceps will not make you a world-class runner or swimmer. No substance can be expected to substitute for practice, dedication, and skill. Yet cordyceps may provide you with an added edge. Chinese people have been taking it as a mildly stimulating and body-strengthening tonic for thousands of years, both for occasional weakness or tiredness and on a regular basis to maintain health. It is said to increase endurance and to strengthen or enhance sexual, respiratory, and immune functions.

Cordyceps isn't found naturally in the United States and has not been as widely studied in the West as ginseng and other tonic herbs. Some related American species, however, have been used for their medicinal properties. For example, deer-fungus parasite (*Cordyceps ophioglossoides*), which grows on the underground trufflelike fungi *Elaphomyces,* is thought to be stimulating to the immune system.

The Chinese consider cordyceps to be safe and mild enough for any adult to use. It is an expensive herb.

HOW TO USE CORDYCEPS: Cordyceps supplements are still hard to find in natural-food stores (see "Resources" for how to obtain them through mail order). Cordyceps is most commonly found as a tincture (an average dose is 1 dropperful per day) and as a powder that is used to make a tea or added to soups.

Performance-Enhancing Vitamins and Minerals

Your body uses the nutrients you obtain from foods and supplements for energy, for building and repairing muscle and other tissue, and for regulating the oxygen use, fat-burning, and other processes that turn the fuel you consume into the energy you expend. Strenuous workouts, long road races, tough squash matches, and other intensive activities demand higher amounts of nutrients and fuel; they even increase your resting metabolic rate. It is possible to use up too much of your bodily stores of vitamins and minerals; the resulting vitamin and mineral deficiencies can detract from your overall health as well as limit your athletic potential. Taking optimal levels of certain vitamins and minerals helps you avoid these problems, and can also significantly boost your energy levels, muscle development, and stamina.

Antioxidants for Athletes

Athletes and others who work out regularly benefit from taking increased levels of antioxidants, such as vitamins A/beta carotene, C, and E, and the mineral selenium (see Chapter 10). That's because exercise is a double-edged sword: it improves fitness, but also results in muscles and other tissues breaking down, drawing increased amounts of oxygen, and thus producing more free radicals. Antioxidants help to neutralize some of the free radicals generated during exercise before they can combine with other molecules and cause harm to cells. As a result, these nutrients enhance your tolerance of exercise, allowing you more of the benefits at lower risk.

Vitamin C

Vitamin C's effects go beyond its powers as an antioxidant. It performs a number of functions important to overall fitness, chief among them an ability to improve endurance and aerobic capacity. Researchers recently determined that this effect may be due to an improvement in the heart's efficiency, allowing it to beat at a slower rate and maintain lower blood pressure during exercise. Vitamin C has also long been recognized as an important antistress nutrient, capable of reducing the secretion of stress hormones that are typically elevated by strenuous activity. Vitamin C is intimately involved in how fats are circulated and burned in the body. One study found that when researchers administered 1,000 mg of vitamin C to trained athletes, the athletes' muscles burned fat more efficiently, providing "beneficial effects in both cardiovascular and metabolic parameters during exercise." Finally, vitamin C also helps build collagen, the tough, fibrous protein found in tendons and connective tissue.

How to use vitamin c: Vitamin C is available in a wide variety of powders, tablets, and capsules. An average daily dose for boosting athletic performance is 500 to 1,500 mg.

Vitamin E

The value of antioxidants for fitness has been noted with nonhuman athletes: researchers at the University of California at Berkeley found that vitamin E improves the performance of racehorses. Horses given vitamin E experienced less tissue damage and muscle breakdown during and after intense aerobic workouts. Studies on humans have not always found immediate enhancement of physical performance from taking vitamin E, though its antioxidant benefits have been confirmed. For example, a recent study published in the *International Journal of Sports Nutrition* found that world-class cyclists who took vitamin E supplements for five months experienced no changes in performance. The athletes did have reduced blood levels of certain markers of oxidative stress, suggesting a long-term protective effect from vitamin E for those who engage in strenuous exercise.

How to use vitamin e: It is commonly found as a liquid and in liquid-filled capsules; an optimal daily dose is 400 to 600 IU.

More for Your Muscles

In addition to the antioxidants, the trace element chromium, the major mineral magnesium, and vitamin B complex have important performance-boosting effects.

Chromium

Through its effect on insulin activity, chromium plays an important role in regulating the metabolism of proteins, carbohydrates, and fats. Athletes often use chromium to help control hunger, lower body-fat percentage, and encourage muscle development. Chromium helps insulin work more effectively at providing cells with the energy-supplying glucose and muscle-building amino acids they need. Strenuous physical activity increases an individual's requirement for chromium.

Studies performed both on animals and humans over the past two decades have confirmed that taking chromium supplements can lead to leaner, stronger bodies.

One of the most prominent chromium researchers is Gary Evans, Ph.D., a chemistry professor at Bemidji State University in Minnesota. He found that athletes who supplemented their diets with chromium picolinate lost more body fat and gained more muscle tissue than athletes who did not supplement. Another study found that after six weeks on chromium picolinate, overweight volunteers had lost more than four pounds of fat while gaining nearly a pound and a half of muscle. According to Richard Anderson, Ph.D., at the USDA Human Nutrition Research Center in Beltsville, Maryland, "Chromium picolinate, more so than any other form of chromium, increases lean body tissue." An animal study done on young pigs also found increased muscle mass and a loss in body fat among those fed chromium supplements.

Unless you're a sumo wrestler or an ultra-long-distance swimmer, losses in body fat accompanied by gains in muscle tissue should translate into better athletic performance. Some bodybuilders now routinely take 1,000 mcg of chromium daily, though Evans notes that this is three to five times the level necessary for the average person to see benefits.

Chromium is one of the safest nutritional supplements known. It does not cause side effects in amounts up to 100 times greater than the average adult dose, and can be taken on a daily basis indefinitely. Diabetics taking insulin, however, should consult with a physician before starting chromium supplements.

Chromium is sold in a number of forms and under a variety of brand names, most commonly GTF and chromium picolinate (which was developed by Evans). Some chromium supplements combine GTF, chromium picolinate, and other nutrients. The supplements available on the market include Chromoplex, Chromium Complex, and Performance Picolinate.

How to use chromium: Chromium supplements are widely available in tablets (usually 100 to 200 mcg), capsules, and liquids. An optimal daily dose for adults is 200 to 400 mcg. Most people see results within four to six weeks, especially if they combine chromium supplementation with exercise and a low-fat diet.

Magnesium

Two recent studies suggest that magnesium is an up-and-coming star in the performance-enhancement field, capable of both building stronger muscles and improving aerobic endurance. One study of weight-training subjects found that those whose daily consumption of magnesium was 507 mg (from foods and supplements) experienced a 17 percent greater gain in muscle strength compared to subjects whose magnesium intake was 246 mg. In another recent study, researchers at Western Washington University in Bellingham looked at 32 active individuals who took magnesium before engaging in endurance exercise. The magnesium allowed subjects to exercise slightly longer and experience less body stress. Researchers say that magnesium may work by increasing protein synthesis in the muscles and elevating the body's metabolic rate.

HOW TO USE MAGNESIUM: An average daily dose for boosting athletic performance is 300 to 600 mg magnesium in combination with 600 to 1,200 mg calcium.

Vitamin B Complex

A number of the B vitamins have demonstrated positive effects on aspects of physical fitness. Nutritionists note that in general you need much higher amounts of the B vitamins when you are involved in regular strenuous activity. Increased amounts of thiamine are also required if you are eating larger portions of complex carbohydrates, as are many nutritionally aware athletes. Some of the B vitamins, particularly B_6, play a role in processing protein, rebuilding muscles, and increasing muscle stamina. The body requires other B vitamins, such as niacin, thiamine, riboflavin, and pantothenic acid, to metabolize fuel efficiently and maintain optimal aerobic capacity.

HOW TO USE VITAMIN B COMPLEX: It is sold in tablets, capsules, and liquids. An average daily dosage for boosting athletic performance is 50 to 100 mg.

Nutritional Supplements for That Competitive Edge

In general, nutritional supplements taken for their presumed body-building and performance-enhancing effects should be approached with some caution. The recommended dosages may be relatively high, causing profound druglike reactions in the body. For example, products containing 7.5 mg or more of the trace element vanadium or the related compound vanadyl sulfate are frequently promoted in muscle magazines and sold in health-food stores as muscle-builders. Vanadium is found naturally in minute amounts in buckwheat, soybeans, seafood, and some other foods. Whether vanadium is essential for human health (it may help burn fats and control blood sugar) is still being debated, but if it is essential, it is probably needed only in tiny amounts, such as 50 to 100 mcg. A number of recent studies indicate that in much higher dosages, such as those found in bodybuilding supplement products, vanadium may cause toxic side effects, including depression of the immune system and destruction of red blood cells.

Two supplements with more established safety records and better evidence for positive effects on strength and endurance are the vitaminlike substances coenzyme Q10 and carnitine. Bee products are also popular as performance aids, though the evidence that they work is still mostly anecdotal.

Coenzyme Q10

Nutritionists say that in spite of coenzyme Q10's ubiquity in the body, physical activity can deplete the body's stores. Bodily levels of coQ10 also tend to drop with advancing age. Thus many active older people are deficient in it. CoQ10 plays an important role in how the body's cells use oxygen and generate energy. Although most of the scientific studies to date have focused on its ability to help prevent or treat heart disease (see Chapter 8), there is some evidence that taking coQ10 supplements may speed the burning of fat, strengthen muscles, and improve physical performance and endurance. Researchers have found that skeletal muscles that have been weakened by muscular dystrophy are strengthened when subjects take coQ10 supplements.

CoQ10 causes few side effects even when taken at dosages ten times higher than those recommended.

HOW TO USE COENZYME Q10: It comes in capsules ranging from 10 to 100 mg. An average daily dosage for promoting greater strength and endurance is 30 to 50 mg.

Carnitine

Carnitine is a compound synthesized in the liver and kidneys from the amino acid lysine and other nutrients, including vitamin C. It is also a vitaminlike nutrient—some nutritionists classify it as a nonessential amino acid—found in foods. In the body carnitine plays a vital role in fat metabolism. Carnitine escorts fatty acids to their place of combustion, inside cells' mitochondria. Here, the burning of fats produces adenosine triphosphate (ATP). The body's principal energy-carrying compound, ATP is necessary for contracting muscles. Thus, muscle tissue, including the heart, ultimately depends upon carnitine for fuel. When insufficient carnitine is present, muscles weaken, and the heart can't function normally. Recent studies have shown carnitine to be potentially useful in the treatment of some forms of heart disease (see Chapter 8) and muscular dystrophy. Carnitine deficiencies may result from extreme exercise, illness, and insufficient dietary intake.

Athletes are now taking supplemental carnitine to maximize fat-burning and to boost strength and endurance. A number of studies on animals and humans have supported such use. Taking carnitine supplements does increase carnitine levels in muscles, thus improving exercise endurance and athletic performance. Research into carnitine, however, is in the early stages, and some scientists dispute claims that it enhances fitness.

There is no RDA for carnitine, and average dietary intake is unknown. Food sources of carnitine include meats and dairy foods.

A number of studies suggest that the active, L-form of this amino acid derivative is safer and more effective than inactive D-carnitine or the mixed form, DL-carnitine. Almost all supplemental carnitine is L-carnitine. Most nutritional authorities consider ongoing L-carnitine supplementation on the order of between 1.5 and 2 g daily to be safe and nontoxic. According to Elson Haas, M.D., author of *Staying Healthy with Nutrition,* "This is basically safe and can be taken over an extended period, although it probably should be stopped for one week each month, until its long-term safety as a supplement is more clearly established."

Carnitine is frequently combined with other nutrients, for example magnesium, in products such as Carni Fuel.

HOW TO USE CARNITINE: It typically comes in capsules and tablets of 250 to 500 mg, and in liquid form. An average daily dosage for improved athletic performance is 500 mg for continuous use, or 750 to 1,000 mg one or two times daily for up to three weeks out of every four.

Bee Products

Bee products include pollen (flower pollen mixed with nectar), propolis (a sticky substance derived from plant resins), and royal jelly (a gelatinous substance secreted by the salivary glands of young worker honeybees). In general, the bee products, which come in a wide variety of tablets, capsules, liquids, and jellies, are rich in protein, vitamins, minerals, enzymes, bioflavonoids, fatty acids, and an array of other nutrients with positive effects on overall health. Athletes and others frequently take pollen, propolis, and royal-jelly products to boost endurance and athletic performance.

Unfortunately, much of the evidence for these products' ability to affect physical fitness is anecdotal. Most of the scientific studies showing positive results are unavailable for critical review, having been done in Eastern Europe and in areas of the former Soviet Union. The few well-controlled studies done in the West with weightlifters, swimmers, and healthy nonathletes have tended to show that bee products have no greater benefit on stamina, strength, and performance than do placebos.

Allergic reactions to bee products are rare but possible. Experiment with tiny amounts before taking larger doses.

How to use bee products: An average dosage of pollen is 250 to 1,500 mg, or 1 to 2 teaspoons of the granules; of propolis, 250 to 500 mg; and of royal jelly, 500 to 1,000 mg.

The Bodybuilding Amino Acids

When you lift weights, play basketball, or jog, you're breaking down muscle tissue. Protein and the building blocks that make it up, the amino acids, are crucial for repairing those muscles. Amino acids can work in at least two ways to promote greater muscular strength: they can increase protein synthesis, and they can promote the body's secretion of muscle-building hormones. To take advantage of these effects, a wide variety of performance-related amino acid products are now being sold in various forms, including branched-chain amino acids (BCAAs, named for their branchlike molecular structure) and single amino acids that may be "peptide-bonded" or "predigested" (processed in a way that breaks them down as in digestion).

The BCAAs isoleucine, leucine, and valine are among the most popular of the protein-synthesizing amino acid supplements, since they are essential amino acids (that is, they must be obtained from diet)

and have a number of important effects relating to muscle tissue main-
tenance and repair. The BCAAs can increase protein synthesis. They
can also be used as fuel when muscles are being rigorously exercised,
thus substituting for the muscle's own protein and preventing muscular
breakdown. Studies have found that BCAAs can be used to restore
muscle that has atrophied due to liver disease, injury, or surgery. Studies of athletes who were given BCAAs have also shown that the supplements can promote development of muscle mass and reduce
exercise-related muscle loss.

BCAAs are found in varying amounts in such protein foods as poultry, beans, and seafood. In health-food stores, BCAA products typically state the relative amounts of each amino acid (isoleucine, leucine,
and valine), as in "BCAA 1:1:1." They are sold under names such as
Amino Athlete, Muscle Octane, Amino Strength, Anabolic Fuel, and
Amino Fuel. They come in a wide variety of tablets, capsules, liquids,
chewable wafers, and powders.

Many bodybuilders and competitive endurance athletes take 10 to
15 grams or more of single and branched-chain amino acid products
on a daily basis. The long-term effects of such supplementation are not
well known. Amino acids can have a pronounced effect on neurotransmitters, hormones, and other bodily substances that affect mood, level
of sexual desire, and wakefulness. Taking large amounts of protein
supplements for extended periods of time can cause metabolic imbalances, high blood pressure, and other side effects. Excess protein may
also tax the body's ability to process it, leading to liver damage.

If rigorous weight training is not on your agenda, you probably
won't gain any benefit from eating additional protein and taking amino
acid supplements. Most Americans get much more protein from their
diet than they need. Boosting your body's secretion of its natural
muscle-building hormones, however, is a secondary strategy that may
provide benefits for even the everyday athlete.

The Natural Growth-Hormone Promoters

An alternative to taking synthetic growth hormone is to take supplements that boost the body's secretion of its own natural growth
hormone. Most amino acids have a slight effect on growth-hormone
secretion, but studies suggest that two in particular—arginine and ornithine—can significantly increase bodily levels of the hormone.

While the average dosages suggested for the amino acid products
discussed below are relatively low compared to what many bodybuild-

ers take, you may want to consult with a professional nutritionist before taking bodybuilding amino acid products over extended periods of time.

Arginine

Researchers have discovered that this amino acid stimulates certain glands, particularly the thymus (see Chapter 3) and the pituitary. Because the pituitary secretes growth hormone, arginine supplements have become the rage for their muscle-building and fat-burning effects. A number of studies have confirmed that arginine helps to improve muscle mass both in athletes and in people recovering from injury or surgery.

Pregnant or lactating women, anyone with kidney or liver disease, and people under the age of 20 (whose bones are still growing) should not take supplements of this amino acid. Since it is possible that high levels of arginine can reactivate latent herpes viruses in some individuals, combining it with lysine (which may prevent herpes outbreaks) is a reasonable precaution for those with the virus. Even those who do not harbor the herpes virus may want to combine arginine with equal amounts of lysine, since one of the most noteworthy studies showing an increase in growth-hormone secretion was done with subjects given 1,200 mg of arginine and 1,200 mg of lysine.

Supplement producers often combine arginine and lysine with other fitness supplements such as ornithine and vitamin B_6. Look for products such as GH Releasers, OKG Fuel, and Anti-Catabolic Fuel.

HOW TO USE ARGININE: It comes in powders, tablets, and capsules. An average daily dose for muscle-building is 250 to 500 mg of arginine, along with an equal amount of lysine, two or three times daily, with meals.

Ornithine and OKG

Ornithine is formed in the body when arginine is altered by an enzyme. Like arginine, ornithine stimulates the release of growth hormone and thus encourages muscle-building. Ornithine alphaketoglutarate (OKG) is a compound that, in addition to increasing secretion of growth hormone, increases release of another musclebuilding hormone, insulin; it also reduces protein metabolism and ammonia buildup, thus preventing exercise-related muscle fatigue. Some studies that have examined OKG's therapeutic potential for helping people to rebuild injured muscle tissue have found it to have positive effects similar to arginine's.

Supplement producers are now adding OKG to many bodybuilding products. Some products combine OKG with arginine, or have additional nutrients such as vitamin B_6.

The same precautions should be followed as for arginine and lysine: avoid using ornithine and OKG if you are pregnant or lactating, have liver or kidney disease, or are under age 20.

HOW TO USE ORNITHINE AND OKG: These amino acid products come in powders, tablets, and capsules. An average daily dose is 1,000 to 1,500 mg.

Where to Start

The following combination can safely be used by everyone from dedicated triathletes to weekend warriors for added strength and endurance:

- An insurance-level multivitamin-multimineral supplement, formulated to provide optimal levels of vitamin B complex, vitamin C, and vitamin E, and the minerals chromium and magnesium
- Coenzyme Q10 (30 to 50 mg)
- Carnitine (for ongoing use, 500 mg per day)

Beyond Herbs and Supplements

No matter how much ginseng, chromium picolinate, and OKG you take, you're unlikely to reach your full physical potential unless you also pay close attention to your diet, exercise, and lifestyle habits. You also can't expect to be really physically fit if you engage in such debilitating activities as drinking to excess and smoking. For the best effect, combine natural performance-boosters with such commonsensical fitness factors as the following:

- Commit to a long-term fitness plan with goals that are realistic for your body, personality, and lifestyle. If you've neglected your body for years, don't expect optimum strength and endurance to return overnight. Avoid injuries and burnout by starting slowly and celebrating what progress you do make.
- Eat a mostly whole-foods diet rich in complex carbohydrates, fiber, and nutrients, and low in fat and refined foods. A high-carbohydrate diet helps replace muscle stores of glycogen.
- Drink plenty of water. Dehydration can significantly detract from

athletic performance. Thirst kicks in only after your water stores are depleted, so drink water before and during workouts regardless of whether you're thirsty. Unless your workouts are long and intensive, sugary sports drinks provide no advantage compared to water—loss of sodium and other electrolytes through perspiration is usually a concern only if you sweat profusely for a number of hours.

• Vary your activities and exercises to focus on the four main aspects of bodily fitness: endurance (jogging, swimming, or aerobics, for example), strength (using free weights or resistance machines, rowing), flexibility (stretching, yoga, dance), and balance and coordination (racket sports, martial arts, juggling).

• Get adequate rest for your muscles after every workout and sufficient sleep every day.

Increase Your Energy Levels

The most popular stimulants in the United States today are derived from herbs. Indeed, Americans probably use herbs more for their stimulating effects than for any other purpose. Does this surprise you? Then consider the following list of plants used primarily as stimulants: coffee, tea, kola (cola), tobacco, and coca (the source of cocaine). Cacao (the source of cocoa and chocolate) is also used by some as a stimulant, though it's most popularly used as a flavoring agent. Unfortunately, most of American society's use of herbal stimulants is addictive and destructive to overall health.

The Caffeine Culture

Americans' favorite beverages are herbal stimulants in the form of caffeinated drinks, including coffee, tea, and cola. Caffeine is an alkaloid that is a potent nervous-system stimulant. It was first isolated from coffee, a shrubby tree native to Ethiopia (*Coffea arabica*), Saudi Arabia (*C. robusta*), and elsewhere, in 1821. Americans drink an average of 28 gallons of coffee annually, or approximately 10 ounces per day. They also spend more money on cola than on breakfast cereal or any other grocery item, according to the Department of Labor. Caffeine from other sources, including a number of over-the-counter pain medications, boosts the average caffeine consumption in the United States to between 175 and 225 mg per day. Nor is caffeine the only potentially stimulating chemical in coffee and other caffeinated beverages.

Tea is derived from the dried leaves and stems of an evergreen plant

(*Camellia sinensis*) native to Asia. Americans drink more iced tea (an estimated 95 million glasses a day) than hot tea. In Britain and many of its former colonies, where the drinking of black tea is a national pastime, addictions to tea are not uncommon. Most green tea is drunk in China and Japan, though green tea is beginning to become more common in North America as its potential health benefits are recognized (see Chapter 2). A 5-oz. cup of tea contains less caffeine (an average of 50 to 75 mg) than coffee (which contains anywhere from 75 to 150 mg) but slightly more than a cola (which has 35 to 55 mg per 12 ounces). Note that actual caffeine content may vary considerably depending upon such factors as quality and amount of herb used, brewing time, and brewing method.

Cola-flavored soft drinks are something of a misnomer. Though some colas in their early formulations contained extracts from the kola nut, today most colas contain little of the bitter herb. The kola nut is a seed kernel from a tree (*Cola nitida, C. vera, C. acuminata,* and other species) that is native to tropical Africa and is cultivated also in the Caribbean, South America, and Indonesia. The plant is in the same family as the cacao tree and, like cacao, contains the stimulants caffeine (about 1 to 3 percent by weight) and theobromine. Theobromine is a chemical relative of caffeine that has similar (though less potent) effects on the body. People in some parts of the world chew the kola nut for its stimulant effect.

Most of the caffeine in colas is either synthetically derived caffeine or caffeine from coffee. Cola drinks also typically are extremely high in sugar, with some containing the equivalent of 10 teaspoons per 12 ounces.

Another common source of caffeine in the American diet is chocolate. Derived from seeds (called cacao or cocoa beans) of the tropical cacao tree (*Theobroma cacao*), chocolate is a bitter-tasting herb that is almost always combined with large amounts of fat and sugar to make it palatable. It contains a small amount of caffeine but a relatively large amount of theobromine. Americans each consume an average of nine pounds of chocolate per year.

Caffeine is undeniably an effective central nervous system stimulant. It stimulates the brain, increases the secretion of adrenaline (epinephrine), and boosts heart rate. Although relatively safe, long-term use in excess of 250 to 300 mg daily may cause numerous health problems. Caffeine has been known to raise blood-cholesterol levels, deplete B vitamins, irritate the stomach and bladder, exhaust the adrenals, and possibly lead to breast and prostate problems. In high doses caffeine can

cause heart palpitations, headaches, anxiety, panic disorders, and insomnia. In industrial societies, its use frequently results in dependence.
Andrew Weil, M.D., an authority on psychoactive substances and the
coauthor of *From Chocolate to Morphine,* says, "I estimate that 80 percent of coffee users are addicted to it. The addiction is physical, with a
prominent withdrawal reaction when use is suddenly discontinued."
Withdrawal symptoms such as headaches and irritability usually start
within 24 to 36 hours of one's last caffeine dose.

Nicotine Madness

Tobacco is one of the most powerful stimulant plants known, primarily because of its chemical constituent nicotine. The effects of
nicotine when it enters the bloodstream via the lungs are almost immediate. Nicotine reaches the brain within seconds and stimulates the
secretion of adrenaline, thus boosting heart rate, increasing blood pressure, and causing greater alertness. The body quickly builds up a tolerance to nicotine's most obvious stimulant effects, though by the time
this happens virtually every user is addicted to the substance.

The disadvantages of tobacco use are so well known that it is not
necessary to dwell on them. Suffice it to say that nicotine is one of the
most addictive and toxic drugs known. One British study showed that
a young person who smokes more than one cigarette has only a 15
percent chance of remaining a nonsmoker. And it is harder to stop
smoking than to stop shooting heroin. Tobacco addicts who stop
smoking can expect to experience withdrawal symptoms such as hunger and irritability within 24 hours; other physical symptoms may last
for weeks. Tobacco addiction is a leading cause of heart disease, lung
cancer, and premature death in the United States. In 1990 cigarette
smoking killed more than 400,000 Americans.

The recent fad among young people of chewing tobacco for nicotine's stimulating effects is only slightly less damaging to health than
smoking. Chewing yields higher overall doses of nicotine, because
much of the nicotine in cigarettes is burned before being inhaled in
smoke. Since the drug is absorbed into the bloodstream more slowly
when tobacco is chewed, chewing is somewhat less addictive than
smoking.

Surveys have shown that people who smoke are also more likely to
consume large amounts of caffeine.

Refined Stimulants: From Cocaine to Diet Pills

American society's fascination with stimulants is hardly limited to natural substances such as coffee and tobacco, of course. Drug companies produce various synthetic stimulants, primarily amphetamine and similar drugs, that physicians prescribe for conditions ranging from obesity to depression to childhood hyperactivity. Synthetic stimulants often make it onto the black market, where students, truck drivers, and others use them to stay awake. There's also a significant market for illegal stimulants, principally cocaine.

Coca, Coca-Cola, and Cocaine

Coca (*Erythroxylum coca*) is a shrub native to the eastern Andes in South America. The plant is legal in Peru and Bolivia, where for at least a thousand years many of the native peoples have chewed dried coca leaves for their stimulating effect. Scientists have identified over a dozen drugs in coca leaves, most prominently cocaine. The leaves, however, are an extremely dilute source of the drug; less than 1 percent of the leaf is cocaine. Chewing the dried leaves (along with an alkali, such as ash) allows small amounts of cocaine and other ingredients in the leaves, including nutrients, to enter the body slowly and to provide a gradual stimulant effect. Researchers have determined that most of the psychoactive effects of coca leaves can be attributed to cocaine, though other chemicals in the leaves also affect the body physically and possibly psychologically.

Use of coca leaves spread from South America to Europe in the early nineteenth century. Because the leaves provide a dilute dose and have a gradual effect, anthropologists and drug experts agree that chewing the leaves rarely results in the type of abuse common among users of purified cocaine. Abuse became more common after the 1860s, when scientists first developed potent coca extracts and then isolated and refined cocaine from coca leaves. By the 1870s, coca extract was being used in Europe in lozenges, teas, and tonic beverages for its stimulating effect. Europe's most popular stimulant and a widely prescribed medicinal remedy in the late nineteenth century was Vin Mariani, a wine whose principal active ingredient was coca extract. The wine's inventor, Corsican chemist Angelo Mariani, was hailed throughout Europe and even given a special medal of appreciation by the Pope.

It was the widespread success of Vin Mariani that inspired the Georgia pharmacist John Pemberton to develop his "French Wine of Coca" and then, in 1886, Coca-Cola, which in its earliest formulations was promoted both as a refreshing soft drink and as a "brain tonic and nerve stimulant." According to *Secret Formula,* Frederick Allen's recent history of Coca-Cola, the original formula for Coke syrup included water, sugar, kola extract, synthetic caffeine, caramel for coloring, lime juice, citric acid, and phosphoric acid. Flavorings included vanilla extract, elixir of orange, and oils from lemon, neroli, cassia, and other fruits and herbs.

According to Allen, "Pemberton added to this brew the fluid extract of coca leaves. Exactly how much cocaine went into the inaugural batch of Doc Pemberton's new soft drink syrup is impossible to calculate more than a century later, but even a touch of the drug, in combination with the sugar and caffeine—four times the amount in today's Coke, or about the same as a strong cup of coffee—made Pemberton's concoction quite a stimulating beverage." Though in its modern formulation Coca-Cola still makes use of tiny amounts of coca and kola extracts, since 1903 it has had all traces of the cocaine removed.

The late-nineteenth-century medical community was as eager as the general public to embrace coca leaves and cocaine. In addition to using cocaine as a local anesthetic and to cure alcohol addiction, doctors promoted cocaine as a drug for feeling better, the Prozac of its time. It was said to increase agility and muscular strength and create a pleasant feeling of general exultation and alertness. Among its early proponents (and users) was Sigmund Freud. In an 1884 article praising cocaine he said, "Coca is a far more potent and far less harmful stimulant than alcohol, and its widespread utilization is hindered at present only by its high cost." The publication of his article encouraged many physicians to prescribe cocaine for depression or even anxiety.

It didn't take long, however, for the downside of widespread cocaine use to become evident. Psychiatrists recognized cocaine as an addictive substance capable of inducing psychotic episodes. Though physically it is not overly toxic, a cocaine craving is psychologically powerful. Users eager for another experience of its intense rush become psychologically addicted. They soon care more for the drug than for family, friends, and job. Early proponents, including Freud, were denounced, and U.S. drug officials made cocaine a controlled substance. Its medicinal uses today are limited to some types of eye surgery, for which cocaine is an effective topically applied anesthetic.

Despite enormous public funds expended on attempts to curtail illegal use, an estimated four million Americans use cocaine at least once a month, according to the National Institute on Drug Abuse.

Amphetamine and Diet Pills

Freud was interested in cocaine for personal reasons: He suffered from fatigue, nervousness, mental distress, and various psychosomatic complaints. This constellation of symptoms was termed *neurasthenia,* and around the turn of the century it was one of the most frequent diagnoses in psychiatry. The term has since fallen out of favor and is rarely used by psychiatrists today, though some herbalists and natural practitioners still use it, because there are herbs that effectively address the condition. (There are also signs that the diagnosis of neurasthenia is making a comeback among conventional doctors—in 1992 an issue of *Psychiatric Annals* was dedicated to "Neurasthenia Revisited.")

After cocaine use was restricted, neurasthenia, mild depression, and many fatigue-related conditions were increasingly treated with the synthetic stimulant known as amphetamine. Amphetamine experienced its heyday from the 1920s to the 1950s. Like cocaine, it was lauded as safe and effective. One physician, writing in the *Journal of the American Medical Association* in 1938, defended amphetamine by saying, "There is no evidence in the entire literature of medicine that stimulants become habit-forming." The government of Germany distributed amphetamine freely to its armed forces during World War II, while Japan gave amphetamine not only to its soldiers but to civilians. An estimated 10 percent of American troops are thought to have used amphetamine regularly as well.

In the 1950s drug companies developed new synthetic stimulants, such as methylphenidate (Ritalin). Ritalin is an amphetaminelike drug widely prescribed for children who are so active that they can't sit still and learn in school. Ritalin works on attention-deficit disorder not because the drug is calming but because it stimulates the central nervous system, enhancing alertness and ability to concentrate. Potential adverse side effects from long-term use of Ritalin and forms of amphetamine (such as are used to make the prescription drugs Dexedrine, Obetrol, and Desoxyn) include addiction, decreases in normal growth among children, and weight loss. Though amphetamine provides a more gradual effect than cocaine and is thus less addictive, it is arguably more toxic than cocaine, and the liver more easily neutralizes cocaine than amphetamine.

The last few decades have also seen the spread of stimulants into over-the-counter drugs. Diet pills, pain relievers, cold remedies, and nasal decongestants often contain either caffeine or the synthetic stimulant phenylpropanolamine (PPA). At the same time medical use of amphetamine has been drastically curtailed.

Conventional Energy-Boosters at a Glance

Product	Type	Active ingredients	Effect	Average dose	Toxicity/addiction potential
Coffee	Herbal beverage	Caffeine	Nervous-system stimulant	6–8 oz	Medium
Black tea	Herbal beverage	Caffeine	Nervous-system stimulant	6–8 oz	Medium
Cola	Artificial beverage	Caffeine, theobromine	Nervous-system stimulant	12 oz	Medium
Chocolate	Food, beverage	Theobromine, caffeine	Nervous-system stimulant	1–4 oz	Low to medium
Tobacco	Herbal inhalant	Nicotine	Nervous-system stimulant	1 cigarette	High
Cocaine	Refined concentrate	Cocaine	Nervous-system stimulant	15–25 mg	High
Dexedrine	Synthetic drug	Dextro-amphetamine sulfate	Nervous-system stimulant	5–15 mg	High

The Chemistry of Energy

Natural substances can increase energy levels in a number of ways. Stimulants usually work through the nervous and circulatory systems to provide an immediate though short-lived increase in alertness. Stimulants may also temporarily elevate mood and boost brain function (see Chapters 6 and 11). Stimulants' quick action frequently leads to their abuse. System boosters, on the other hand (see Chapter 4), are herbs, vitamins and minerals, amino acids, and other nutrients that provide a more sustained and gradual release of energy. Some herbs, the so-called nervine tonics, can also act as overall nervous-system strengtheners.

How Nervous-System Stimulants Work

Though stimulants such as caffeine, cocaine, and amphetamine are chemically different, they have similar effects on the body. Stimulants speed up most physiological functions. They increase alertness and the ability to concentrate. They also suppress appetite and, at least subjectively, increase muscular strength. Some stimulants (cocaine and amphetamine more so than caffeine) elevate mood and cause euphoria.

Though the brain is complex and there is much still to be discovered, stimulants, like almost all psychoactive drugs, are thought to act via neurotransmitters, the substances that transmit nerve impulses from one nerve cell to another. These neurotransmitters include adrenaline, the hormone released by the adrenal glands when a person is confronted with a threatening situation, and the related stimulant neurotransmitter noradrenaline, also secreted by the adrenals. Adrenaline and noradrenaline increase heart rate, dilate pupils, and send more blood to muscles and the brain and less to digestive organs and the skin. They also increase sweating, expand airways in the lungs, raise blood pressure, and boost metabolic rate.

In the body, amphetamine molecules (which resemble adrenaline molecules in structure) are able to slip into the tiny neurotransmitter-receiving spaces in the nerve endings that would normally receive noradrenaline. Once attached to the nerve cell, the stimulant molecules cause a chain reaction with nearby cells, resulting in a release of more neurotransmitters at each nerve-cell gap (or synapse). If the nerve cells are stationed next to other nerve cells, the result is eventually an electric charge moving through the fiber of a nerve. If the nerve cells are next to muscle or gland cells, the chain reaction results in muscle contractions or the release of hormones from the gland.

All the nerve, muscle, and glandular activity caused by stimulants also quickly causes the body to assume "fight or flight" readiness. When the emergency (or stimulant use) is over, however, the body is left with fewer available energy resources, and the person may feel tired and depressed. Many people become addicted to stimulants when they don't let the body rebuild its natural energy reserves, but instead take further doses of the stimulant drug.

Beyond Coffee, Coke, and Speed

Some stimulant herbs are not much of an alternative to coffee and black tea, since their boost comes from caffeine also. Herbal producers who are less than scrupulous may claim on the package that a product is caffeine-free when in fact it is not. The first three herbs listed below are caffeine-containing stimulants, and thus share the relative advantages and disadvantages of coffee; the fourth, green tea, is a special case.

Guarana. This herb is derived from the seeds of a jungle shrub (*Paullinia cupana*) grown in Brazil, where is it often used to make sweet colalike drinks. Guarana actually has higher caffeine levels (up to 5 percent by weight) than does coffee or tea. It is a common ingredient in some combination herbal energy (or "upper") products. It is also sold whole, dried, and in capsules. An average stimulant dose is 500 to 1,000 mg of the dried herb.

Maté. Maté, also called yerba maté, is the leaves of a holly plant (*Ilex paraguariensis*) grown in Argentina. Caffeine content is up to 2 percent by weight. The popular herbal tea Morning Thunder, made by Celestial Seasonings, contains maté. Maté is sold dried and in capsules. An average dose is one cup of brewed tea.

Kola nut. As mentioned, this is the herb that lends its name (though little else) to cola drinks. Its caffeine content as a percentage of weight is similar to coffee's. In the United States it is more generally available in tincture, extract, and concentrated drop form than either guarana or maté. An average dose is $1/2$ to 1 dropperful.

Green tea. The level of caffeine in unfermented green tea is similar to that of black tea. Many people prefer, however, to brew green tea for only two or three minutes, thus avoiding a bitter taste and yielding a beverage with fairly low caffeine levels (20 to 30 mg per cup).

Stimulant herbs are hardly limited to caffeine-containing ones, of course. Three of the most potent noncaffeinated herbal stimulants are ephedra/ma huang, ginseng, and yohimbe.

Ephedra/Ma Huang

Ephedra encompasses some 40 related species of primitive stemlike desert bushes, such as the North American species Mormon tea (*Ephedra nevadensis*) and the Chinese species ma huang (*Ephedra sinica*). The Chinese have used ma huang for thousands of years to help relieve bronchial spasms and treat asthma. This traditional use played a role not only in ephedra's recognition by Western science but also in the development of amphetamine.

Around the turn of the century, physicians realized that one of the most effective treatments for asthma is adrenaline. In addition to increasing heart rate and muscular strength, adrenaline also dilates the bronchial tubes, allowing the person to take in more oxygen and breathe deeper and faster. This effect is important to asthma sufferers, in whom bronchial-tube constriction interferes with free breathing.

Adrenaline poses a problem as an asthma treatment, however. When taken orally, adrenaline is rapidly destroyed by the digestive system, and little gets absorbed into the bloodstream. Chemists working on this problem hoped to produce a synthetic adrenaline derivative that would be effective and absorbable. Success eluded them until the early 1920s, when K. K. Chen, a pharmacologist working for the Lilly Drug Company in Indianapolis, began to investigate ma huang. Chen was familiar with its reputation as one of humanity's oldest medicines and as an herb for relieving respiratory complaints such as bronchitis and asthma. Chen investigated the properties of one of ma huang's active ingredients, the alkaloid ephedrine, which had first been isolated in the late 1880s, and discovered that it was chemically similar to adrenaline.

Though a natural substance rather than a synthetic derivative, ephedrine was a breakthrough drug for asthma. It could be administered orally and was effective at dilating bronchial passages and relieving nasal congestion. Like adrenaline, ephedrine boosted heart rate, metabolism, and blood pressure. Researchers also found it to be an effective diuretic (an agent that increases the flow of urine).

Asthma sufferers benefited from ephedrine, but the search for a synthetic adrenaline substitute was not abandoned. Drug companies claimed that ma huang was scarce, and that, as an asthma medicine, ephedrine had a number of unwanted side effects, such as nervousness, restlessness, and increased blood pressure. Another factor may have been that ma huang and ephedrine, being natural substances (ephedrine can also be produced synthetically) could not be patented, and thus offered limited profits for any one company.

Finally, in the 1930s, a Los Angeles chemist synthesized an ephedrinelike compound that asthma sufferers could inhale directly into their lungs. He called the substance amphetamine. Under the brand name Benzedrine, amphetamine inhalers quickly displaced ephedrine as the asthma treatment of choice. Ephedrine use fell off after the 1940s, but to this day it, as well as the related alkaloid compound pseudoephedrine (also found in some ephedra species or produced synthetically), is used as an ingredient in certain cold remedies and oral decongestants such as Sudafed, as well as some weight-loss products (see Chapter 17).

Some species of ephedra contain more of the stimulating substance ephedrine than others. Ma huang has high levels, for instance, while

Mormon tea has little or none. Ma huang is thus a potent herb, more powerful even than caffeine (though less powerful than amphetamine) in its ability to stimulate the central nervous system. As noted in Chapter 4, don't use it if you're entered in an Olympic event—it could get you banned (as could high blood levels of caffeine). Ma huang is a common ingredient in herbal "uppers." In some herbal uppers it is combined with caffeine-containing herbs such as guarana, yielding a greater effect than either stimulant on its own. Such herbal upper products often go by names such as Rocket Blast, which give a fair approximation of their effect on the body.

The Food and Drug Administration takes a negative view of ephedra. A 1993 *Import Bulletin* stated that the "FDA has no information to support the GRAS [generally recognized as safe] status of ephedra or conditions of safe use." It also stated that "manufacturers should be aware of FDA's continuing interest in ephedra."

Responsible members of the natural-food industry also recognize the potential hazards of ephedra. Both the National Nutritional Foods Association and the American Herbal Products Association (see "Resources") have endorsed a label warning for over-the-counter products that contain ephedra/ma huang (though not Mormon tea). The recommended wording is as follows: "Seek advice from a health care practitioner prior to use if you are pregnant or nursing, or if you have high blood pressure, heart or thyroid disease, diabetes, difficulty in urination due to prostate enlargement, or if taking a MAO inhibitor or any other prescription drug. Reduce or discontinue use if nervousness, tremor, sleeplessness, loss of appetite, or nausea occur. Not for children under 13. *Keep out of reach of children.*"

As with other potent nervous-system stimulants, ephedrine-based stimulants are easily abused. Tolerance to ephedra's stimulant effect builds up quickly with continued use, necessitating larger and larger doses. Ephedra abuse may also weaken the adrenal glands.

How to use ephedra: Ephedra is sold dried and in capsules, concentrated drops, tinctures, and extracts. Extracts are often standardized for an alkaloid (mostly ephedrine) content of 5 to 10 percent. An average stimulant dosage of an extract with a 10 percent alkaloid content would be 125 to 250 mg. If you prefer to use a tincture or concentrated drops, $1/2$ to 1 dropperful provides a pronounced stimulant effect for an average of two to four hours.

Ginseng

The root of the ginseng plant is widely used to strengthen or normalize physical function. People also take it to boost energy levels, enhance alertness, and improve mental performance. One study found that test subjects who took a ginseng extract took less time to react to visual and auditory stimuli than they had before. Another study of men and women ages 40 to 60 found that taking a ginseng extract improved reaction time and subjective feelings of vitality and energeticness.

The chemistry of the root is exceedingly complex; ginsenosides, saponins, and glycosides are key active ingredients. Scientists have identified some chemical constituents that can raise blood pressure, increase hormone and enzyme secretion, normalize blood-sugar levels, and boost heart and metabolic rates. Some research indicates that ginseng's noted antifatigue action is due to stimulation of the central nervous system, though according to Michael Murray, N.D., author of *The Healing Power of Herbs,* ginseng's effect on the central nervous system "is essentially different from that of the usual stimulants. Although stimulants are active under most situations, ginseng reveals its stimulatory action only under the challenge of stress."

Ginseng may also increase noradrenaline levels. Compared to American ginseng, Chinese or Korean ginseng is richer in ginsenosides that affect the central nervous system and thus is a more powerful stimulant.

Ginseng is generally not as stimulating as herbal products containing caffeine or ephedrine. Some people may not find it stimulating at all, while for others it will be too strong and should be used in moderation. Its effects are sometimes cumulative and may become more apparent after it is used regularly for weeks or months. For regular use, start with half of the stimulant dose mentioned below. Ginseng should be used with caution by anyone with high blood pressure.

HOW TO USE GINSENG: It is sold as a whole root and as powders, capsules, tablets, tea bags, tinctures, and extracts. Commercial ginseng products vary tremendously in potency. An average stimulant dose of capsules standardized for 5 to 9 percent ginsenosides is 500 to 1,000 mg. An average dose of some concentrated extracts and ginseng products with higher standardized percentages may be as low as 200 to 400 mg.

Yohimbe

Yohimbe is a stimulant and aphrodisiac derived from the bark of the yohimbe tree (*Pausinystalia yohimbe*), an evergreen indigenous to tropical West Africa. Most of the scientific studies done on the plant have focused on its purported sex-enhancing effects (see Chapter 7). Its principal active ingredient, responsible for both its stimulant and aphrodisiac effects, is the alkaloid yohimbine. Yohimbine dilates peripheral blood vessels and lowers blood pressure. The herb also elevates mood in some people and may be a weight-loss aid.

Like ephedra, yohimbe is a potent herb with the potential for abuse. It shouldn't be used by people with heart disease or low blood pressure.

HOW TO USE YOHIMBE: Yohimbe is sold dried and in tablets, capsules, concentrated drops, and extracts. It is usually not stocked in natural-food stores, though it can be ordered from some herbal suppliers (see "Resources"). A 500-mg capsule is an average dosage.

Stimulant Use Guidelines

With the possible exception of ginseng, stimulant herbs should generally not be used on a daily basis. Andrew Weil, M.D., suggests the following guidelines for safe use of stimulants, including caffeine.

• Limit how frequently you take stimulants, using them purposefully rather than for ordinary, everyday functions.
• Use dilute rather than concentrated forms, and avoid taking a stimulant by any means other than orally.
• Maintain good habits of nutrition, rest, and exercise.
• Don't combine stimulants with depressants or other drugs.

Herbal Circulatory Stimulants

In the traditional herbalism of both East and West, herbs are often classified as either "heating" or "cooling." In general, heating herbs are those that increase blood flow throughout the body. The stronger heating herbs may also boost metabolic rate. The exact mechanism by which herbs increase blood flow to tissues is not fully understood, but many people report relief from tiredness and fatigue when taking circulatory stimulants. The effect may be due to the increased blood flow supplying greater amounts of oxygen and nutrients to body cells. So consider trying circulatory stimulants when you're feeling physically cold and mentally sluggish.

The herb ginkgo seems to boost circulation in the brain, while two herbs with noted stimulant effects on the overall circulatory system are cayenne and ginger.

Ginkgo

Derived from the leaves of one of the world's most ancient tree species, ginkgo has been used by the Chinese for thousands of years to treat asthma and allergies, and it is quickly gaining popularity in the West for its ability to improve brain function and boost memory and alertness. Researchers say that ginkgo may play a role in the prevention or treatment of dizziness, depression (see Chapter 6), and Alzheimer's disease. The effects its active constituents, such as the flavoglycosides, have on neurotransmitter levels has made it one of the premier "smart drug" herbs (see Chapter 11). As a circulatory stimulant, it is known to affect predominantly the brain and ears.

HOW TO USE GINKGO: Ginkgo comes in tablets, capsules, concentrated drops, tinctures, and extracts. An average stimulant dose is 40 to 60 mg of a standardized extract containing 24 percent flavoglycosides. Its stimulating, mind-boosting effects last for about three to six hours; some people won't notice a stimulant effect at this dosage, though they will notice a mind-boosting effect after taking 40 mg three times daily for at least seven to ten days. Ginkgo is safe to take indefinitely.

Cayenne

Also known as red pepper, cayenne is both an herb and a spice, obtained from the dried, ground fruit of various hot chili peppers (*Capsicum frutescens*) popular in Asia and Central America. Hot chili peppers contain the compound capsaicin, an alkaloid that reduces pain and inflammation when applied topically. When cayenne is taken orally, capsaicin and other alkaloids stimulate circulation, digestion, and sweating. (Since perspiration ultimately cools the body, cayenne is sometimes used to break a fever.) In Asia cayenne is a "crisis herb," popular for its stimulating effects on the kidneys, lungs, stomach, and heart.

HOW TO USE CAYENNE: Cayenne is sold in capsules, concentrated drops, and tinctures. An average dose is $1/4$ to $1/2$ dropperful of the tincture or concentrated drops.

Ginger

Ginger is derived from the rhizome (underground stem) of a tropical plant (*Zingiber officinale*) native to Asia. It has been used since ancient times by the Greeks, Chinese, and others as a medicine, spice, and flavoring. Ginger is the premier natural remedy for nausea and is widely taken today for its calming effect on the digestive system (see Chapter 16). It contains a number of volatile oils (ginger is also used to make a popular essential oil with medicinal properties) that are thought to be responsible for its mildly stimulating effect on circulation.

How to use ginger: Ginger comes fresh or dried and in tablets, capsules, concentrated drops, tinctures, and extracts. An average dose is 500 to 1,000 mg of the dried herb, or 1 to 2 dropperfuls of tincture or concentrated drops.

Tonic Herbs for the Nervous System

When most people suffer from fatigue they look for a quick energy boost from caffeine-containing herbs such as coffee. Even followers of natural-health practices may turn to caffeine-containing herbs such as kola nut or guarana, or to herbal "upper" products that contain ephedra. If used too frequently, however, such herbs can lead to chronic restlessness, insomnia, and possibly circulatory problems. A better long-term approach is to use what herbalists call nerve (or nervine) tonics, such as oats, damiana, or gotu kola, on a regular basis. You can also turn to such overall system boosters (see Chapter 13) as Siberian ginseng, schisandra, and astragalus.

Nerve tonics work to strengthen and feed the nervous system, thus helping to increase average daily energy levels. They do have an immediate stimulant effect, but it is less pronounced than that from caffeine or ephedrine. They have a deep, long-lasting effect and can safely be taken every day.

Oats

Oats is part healing herb and part nutritional supplement. It is prepared from the whole plant and seeds of the hearty, widely cultivated cereal grass (*Avena sativa*) whose edible grain is a popular breakfast food. As an herb, oats is traditionally used to help recover from exhaustion and depression. It is also used as an aphrodisiac. Studies confirm that the plant contains saponins and alkaloids that stimulate and restore the nervous system. Oats also provides a range of nutrients, including calcium, that feed a debilitated nervous system. It is widely recognized as an excellent nerve tonic, gently stimulating the system and providing nourishment. Oats is also now used to help break addictions. In high concentrations oats can make people (and horses) highly excitable. It is most effective when taken for long periods.

How TO USE OATS: The herb is sold dried and as capsules, concentrated drops, tinctures, and extracts. An average dosage is 1 to 2 dropperfuls of tincture or concentrated drops.

Damiana

Damiana is derived from the leaves and flowers of a plant (*Turnera diffusa, T. aphrodisiaca*) native to Mexico and the Southwest that is touted for its stimulating and aphrodisiacal effects. It has been used traditionally to treat fatigue as well as depression and anxiety. Scientific studies on damiana are lacking, though chemical analysis shows that damiana contains alkaloids with constituents similar to caffeine. In addition to stimulation, some people taking damiana may experience a mild euphoria that lasts for up to an hour or so.

How TO USE DAMIANA: Damiana comes in capsules, concentrated drops, and extracts. An average dosage for its tonic action on the nervous system is one or two 400-mg capsules.

Gotu Kola

Gotu kola is a traditional restorative for the nervous system in India and Pakistan. A principally Asian, weedy plant (*Centella asiatica*) of the parsley family, it should not be confused with the unrelated, caffeine-containing herb kola nut. In the West gotu kola is used mainly as a tonic to increase energy and endurance, improve memory and mental stamina, and alleviate depression and anxiety. Gotu kola also has a reputation for promoting longevity. Though gotu kola has been chemically analyzed and scientifically studied, at this point the evidence for these effects is primarily cultural and anecdotal. Indian researchers are investigating gotu kola for use against leprosy and tuberculosis, and studies have generally confirmed that it also has potential medical uses externally as a wound healer, burn remedy, and psoriasis treatment.

Large doses of gotu kola may have a calming rather than energizing effect.

HOW TO USE GOTU KOLA: The herb is sold dried and in capsules, concentrated drops, tinctures, and extracts. An average dosage of the concentrated drops or tincture is ¹/₂ to 1 dropperful two or three times daily.

Herbal Energy Boosters at a Glance

Product	Active ingredient	Effect	Average dose	Toxicity/ addiction potential
Guarana	Caffeine	Nervous-system stimulant	500–1,000 mg dried	Medium
Maté	Caffeine	Nervous-system stimulant	6–8 oz tea	Medium
Kola nut	Caffeine	Nervous-system stimulant	1 dropperful★	Medium
Green tea	Caffeine	Nervous-system stimulant	6–8 oz tea	Low
Ephedra	Ephedrine	Nervous-system stimulant	¹/₂–1 dropperful★	Medium
Ginseng	Ginsenosides	Nervous-system stimulant, system booster	150 mg standardized extract	Low
Yohimbe	Yohimbine	Nervous-system stimulant	500 mg dried	Medium
Cayenne	Capsaicin	Circulatory stimulant	¹/₄–¹/₂ dropperful★	Low
Ginger	Volatile oils	Circulatory stimulant	500–1,000 mg dried	Low
Ginkgo	Heterosides	Circulatory stimulant	40 mg standardized extract	Low
Oats	Alkaloids, nutrients	Nerve tonic	1–2 dropperfuls★	Low
Damiana	Alkaloids	Nerve tonic	400 mg dried	Low
Gotu kola	Triterpenoid compounds	Nerve tonic	1 dropperful★	Low

★Dropperful measurements refer to tincture or concentrated drops

Using Essential Oils to Boost Energy

Herbs for increasing energy can also be used in the form of essential oils, concentrated resinous extracts used in minute doses. Energy-boosting essential oils include Peppermint, which is mildly stimulating, and Rosemary, which is considered a nerve tonic.

Peppermint

Essential oil of Peppermint is derived from the leaves of a garden perennial (*Mentha piperita*) that has long been used to make natural remedies. The essential oil contains menthol, a medicinally active alcohol that exhibits significant antiseptic and anti-inflammatory powers on the skin and a mild stimulating effect on the nervous system. The oil is sometimes used for the same conditions as the dried herb (to relieve upset stomach, heartburn, and nausea), as well as for fainting and dizziness.

Rosemary

The essential oil of Rosemary is derived from a shrubby evergreen bush (*Rosmarinus officinalis*) native to the Mediterranean region. The essential oil as well as the herb have long been used to treat conditions characterized by a weakened nervous system, such as mental fatigue, depression, and neurasthenia.

Stimulants and nervines are usually inhaled or applied through massage or bathing (avoid using Peppermint in a bath). See "How to Use Essential Oils" in Chapter 2.

Essential Oils at a Glance

Product	Active ingredient	Effect	Average dose	Toxicity/ addiction potential
Peppermint	Menthol	Mild nervous system stimulant	2–8 drops	Medium★
Rosemary	Pinenes, others	Nerve tonic	2–8 drops	Medium★

★Essential oils are highly toxic before being diluted; they are not addictive.

Vitamins and Minerals That Boost Overall Energy Levels

Fatigue is a common symptom among people who are deficient in certain nutrients, especially iron, magnesium, and vitamin B complex. Some people experience an increase in average energy levels when taking additional nutrients even when they have no deficiency. An insurance-level daily multivitamin–multimineral supplement can often begin to show immediate energy benefits.

Iron

Iron is a trace element found in meat, poultry, fish, nuts, sunflower and pumpkin seeds, whole grains, and dark-green leafy vegetables. The adult RDA is 10 to 15 mg. In addition to aiding in energy production, iron is necessary for proper immune function. It is part of the hemoglobin that helps carry oxygen in the bloodstream to tissues throughout the body. It is used therapeutically to treat fatigue and depression due to both iron-deficiency anemia and other causes.

The body readily stores iron, and too much iron can be toxic or possibly contribute to cardiovascular disease. It can also be countereffective. For instance, high levels may actually cause fatigue or compromise the immune system. Most nutritionists now recommend that iron supplementation be undertaken only if an iron deficiency has been clinically demonstrated.

HOW TO USE IRON: Iron is available in liquid formulas, capsules, and tablets. An average daily dosage is 10 to 15 mg.

Magnesium

Magnesium is an essential major mineral found primarily in dark-green leafy vegetables, soybeans, and nuts and seeds. Along with calcium, magnesium regulates the body's energy levels and maintains normal heart function and neurotransmission. Magnesium works with enzymes in the body to create energy by breaking down sugar stored in the liver. Magnesium is also required for strong, healthy bones. Supplements are used to treat fatigue as well as premenstrual syndrome, high blood pressure, and osteoporosis. Magnesium is probably the safest mineral, with no record of toxicity from supplements.

HOW TO USE MAGNESIUM: Magnesium comes in tablets and capsules;

it is often combined in a 1:2 ratio with calcium. An average daily dosage is 450 to 650 mg.

Vitamin B Complex

The B-complex vitamins play a wide variety of roles that affect alertness and energy levels. For instance, vitamin B_6, included in supplements most frequently as pyridoxine, is an important vitamin for the healthy bioelectric functioning of the central nervous system and the metabolism of the neurotransmitters noradrenaline and acetylcholine. Vitamin B_{12}, or cobalamin, aids in energy production from fats and carbohydrates and in the production of amino acids. Supplementation with B_{12} (often injected) is a common step in the treatment of fatigue.

How to use vitamin b complex: Take 50 to 100 mg daily, in divided doses, of B complex. This is a better supplement strategy than taking large doses of any single B vitamin, which may cause imbalances in the other B vitamins.

Kicking the Coffee Habit

If you're trying to cut back on a five-cup-a-day coffee habit, try gradually switching to a combination of the circulatory stimulant herbs, vitamin and mineral nutrients, and perhaps even a reduced-level caffeine source. (Some health authorities suggest that toxic processing chemicals, roasted hydrocarbons, or other compounds in coffee may be more injurious to your health than the caffeine itself.) For example, try the following combination:

- Ginkgo (40 mg three times daily of a standardized extract containing 24 percent flavoglycosides)
- An insurance-level multivitamin-multimineral supplement with optimal amounts of magnesium, B-complex vitamins, and coQ10
- Green tea (3 to 5 cups per day of tea brewed only two to three minutes to keep caffeine levels at approximately 20 to 30 mg per cup)

Energy Supplements

Two increasingly popular nutritional supplements, organic germanium compounds and coenzyme Q10, can be taken regularly to increase daily energy levels. Both have a positive effect on the body's use of oxygen as a fuel. They are thus more similar to the system-boosting vitamins and minerals than to stimulants such as caffeine and ephedra.

Organic Germanium Compounds

Organic germanium compounds such as Ge-132 act much like hemoglobin, carrying oxygen to tissues throughout the body and improving cellular function. They thus help increase energy supplies as well as restore the normal function of immune-boosting cells (see Chapter 3).

HOW TO USE ORGANIC GERMANIUM: Organic germanium comes in powders, granules, and tablets, as well as capsules ranging in size from 25 to 250 mg. An average dosage for increased energy is 75 to 150 mg daily.

Coenzyme Q10

Coenzyme Q10 (coQ10) is a vitaminlike compound whose biological importance is tied to its role in energy production and how the body's cells use oxygen. CoQ10 is an essential component of the part of cells that manufacture adenosine triphosphate (ATP), the substance that is the immediate source of energy for muscular contractions. Studies have demonstrated that coQ10 enhances the pumping capacity of the heart and increases the production of energy in heart cells. It acts as a mild metabolic stimulant for many people.

HOW TO USE COENZYME Q10: Coenzyme Q10 comes in capsules ranging in size from 10 to 100 mg. An average dosage for maximizing energy efficiency is 30 to 50 mg daily.

Energy-Boosting Amino Acids

Since amino acids play a major role in brain chemistry and the production of neurotransmitters, and since some are capable of crossing the blood-brain barrier, it is no surprise that they can have dramatic effects on alertness and the ability to concentrate. Students, writers, and other people are now taking various amino acids—including phenylalanine, aspartic acid, and glutamine—for their stimulant effects. In general, these are taken as single amino acids (often with other nutrients such as B-complex vitamins and vitamin C) rather than as one of many components in a branched-chain amino acid combination product. This is because amino acids compete with each other for uptake by the brain, and other amino acids such as gamma-aminobutyric acid (GABA) have relaxing rather than stimulating effects.

As a rule it is best to avoid continual daily use of single amino acids for more than two or three weeks at a time.

Phenylalanine

This essential amino acid's stimulant effect is due to its ability to increase production in the brain of certain neurotransmitters, particularly adrenaline and noradrenaline. Taken as a supplement (in the form of L-phenylalanine or DL-phenylalanine), it commonly improves alertness and elevates mood. Phenylalanine is the precursor for tyrosine, which can also be used in supplement form as an energy booster.

Phenylalanine should be avoided by pregnant or lactating women, people with high blood pressure, and anyone taking MAO-inhibitor antidepressants. It should also be avoided by people with phenylketonuria, a genetic disorder of phenylalanine metabolism. As with most other stimulants, its potential side effects include insomnia and anxiety.

How to use phenylalanine: L-phenylalanine is more frequently taken for its stimulant effects than is D-phenylalanine. You can also take a mixture of the two forms, which is sold as DL-phenylalanine or DLPA. L-phenylalanine and DLPA typically come in capsules of 375, 500, or 750 mg. An average stimulant dosage is 375 to 500 mg of L-phenylalanine or 500 to 1,000 mg of DLPA, taken in the morning 30 minutes before breakfast.

Aspartic Acid

This nonessential amino acid, also known as potassium magnesium aspartate, plays a major role in the energy cycle of the body. It helps transport potassium and magnesium into cells and is found in high concentrations in the brain. Aspartic acid has an exciting effect on neurons in virtually every region of the central nervous system. Alternative practitioners often recommend it to increase stamina and endurance and relieve fatigue. Studies support its use as a fatigue remedy, including one study that showed that between 75 and 91 percent of some 3,000 patients treated with 1 g twice daily of aspartic acid reported pronounced relief from fatigue.

How to use aspartic acid: Aspartic acid comes in powders and capsules (usually 500 mg). An average stimulant dosage is 1,000 to

2,000 mg daily. Some people taking aspartic acid report positive results within a week, while others may not see a benefit for 5 or 6 weeks.

Glutamine

Glutamine is a brain fuel that increases mental alertness and clarity of thinking. It works in part by lowering levels of ammonia in the brain. Ammonia is created by the breaking-down of proteins necessary for brain metabolism. Glutamine in the brain produces the chemical glutamic acid, which neutralizes ammonia and improves brain function. Since glutamine is also a fuel used by cells for metabolic energy, it doesn't cause the type of letdown common with stimulants such as caffeine.

High doses of glutamine may cause headaches and other side effects in some people, especially those sensitive to monosodium glutamate (MSG), a glutamic acid compound added to some foods as a flavor enhancer.

How to use glutamine: Glutamine comes in powders, tablets, and capsules. An average stimulant dosage is 500 to 1,000 mg.

The Bee Boosters

Bee products such as pollen, propolis, and royal jelly are popular energy supplements in various cultures. Scientists have done fewer studies on these products compared to the research performed on herbs and nutritional supplements. Thus, most of the evidence for bee products' efficacy as energy boosters comes from anecdotal accounts. Most bee products are concentrated sources of vitamins and minerals, amino acids, enzymes, and other nutrients, which may explain in part their apparent energy-boosting effects. Bee products are generally taken on a daily basis as system boosters rather than as temporary stimulants.

Bee Pollen

Bee pollen is a dense source of protein, amino acids, and certain nutrients such as the B vitamin pantothenic acid, which is essential for many metabolic processes. In addition to its use to boost energy, it has long been a popular folk remedy to increase endurance, aid in weight loss, and improve immunity.

How to use bee pollen: Bee pollen comes in tablets and capsules ranging from 100 to 500 mg, and in liquids. An average dosage is 250 to 1,500 mg daily. Pollen causes allergic reactions in a small number of people (less than 1 percent of the population), so it's a good idea to start off by taking only half a tablet or capsule per day, gradually increasing the dose if you don't experience allergic symptoms such as wheezing or a skin rash.

Propolis

Propolis is a rich source of bioflavonoids, B vitamins, and minerals. It has traditionally been taken to increase energy and improve endurance.

Propolis products may contain pollen and thus can cause allergic reactions in some people, so the same warning as for bee pollen applies: Start with a low dose and increase it gradually if no ill effects are noted.

HOW TO USE PROPOLIS: Propolis comes in tablets, capsules, extracts, tinctures, and concentrated drops. An average dosage is 250 to 500 mg daily.

Royal Jelly

Royal jelly is rich in amino acids, certain fatty acids, minerals, enzymes, acetylcholine, and B vitamins, especially pantothenic acid. As a supplement, it is taken to boost energy levels and combat fatigue, as well as to prolong youth and increase longevity. Proponents also claim that it supports the adrenal glands and helps people lose weight. Producers of Chinese herbs often combine it with ginseng, astragalus, and other tonic herbs.

HOW TO USE ROYAL JELLY: Royal jelly comes in liquids and capsules ranging from 200 to 500 mg. An average dosage is 500 to 1,000 mg daily to promote energy.

A Homeopathic Remedy

Homeopathy offers a much broader range of substances with sedating effects than ones with stimulating effects (see Chapter 12). There is one remedy to consider for mild stimulation or relief from fatigue: *Nux vomica.*

Nux vomica

Strychnine is an alkaloid extracted as a white crystalline substance from the seeds of the poison nut plant (*Strychnos nux vomica*). In small doses strychnine is a heart stimulant. It was once taken to increase alertness and make perceptions more vivid, and it still has some minor medicinal uses. Unfortunately, strychnine is also an extremely poisonous substance, and the difference between a stimulant dose and a toxic dose is slight. The only safe way to use it is in the form of the homeopathic remedy known as *Nux vomica,* an extremely dilute preparation

Nutritional Substances at a Glance

Product	Type	Active ingredient	Effect	Average dose	Toxicity
Iron	Mineral		System booster	10–15 mg	High
Magnesium	Mineral		System booster	500 mg	Low
B complex	Vitamin		System booster	50–100 mg	Low
Organic germanium	Synthetic organic compound		System booster	75–150 mg	Low
Coenzyme Q10	Vitaminlike compound		System booster	30–50 mg	Low
Phenylala-nine	Amino acid		Stimulant, system booster	500–1,000 mg	Medium
Aspartic acid	Amino acid		Stimulant, system booster	1,000–2,000 mg	Medium
Glutamine	Amino acid		Stimulant, system booster	500–1,000 mg	Medium
Bee pollen	Flower substance	Amino acids, pantothenic acid	System booster	250–1,500 mg	Low
Bee propolis	Plant resin substance	Bioflavo-noids, B vitamins	System booster	250–500 mg	Low
Royal jelly	Bee secretion	B vitamins, pantothenic acid	System booster	500–1,000 mg	Low

of the poison nut plant. *Nux vomica* is most commonly used as a nausea and digestive remedy (see Chapter 16), but homeopaths also sometimes recommend it to boost energy and treat fatigue.

HOW TO USE NUX VOMICA: Homeopathic remedies come in tiny pellets or tablets; remedy "strength" (actually, the number of dilutions) is denoted with an *X* or *C*. An average dosage of *Nux vomica* is 2 to 4 tablets of 12X to 30X strength up to 4 times daily.

How to Choose

Stimulants are obviously a large and varied class of natural substances. What works best for you will depend upon such factors as your metabolism, your overall health, and how active you are. Keep the following considerations in mind as you make your choices.

• Ephedra and yohimbe are among the most potent stimulants, but are also the stimulants with the greatest likelihood of causing side effects. Regular use of such strong stimulants can be habit-forming.

• Single amino acids may also lead to unexpected health problems if used in high dosages for extended periods of time.

• Optimal doses of vitamins and minerals, nutritional substances such as organic germanium compounds and coQ10, and bee products enhance overall health and can safely be taken on a daily basis indefinitely.

• In the East, ginseng is sometimes used by taking it for two weeks and then abstaining for two weeks.

Beyond Herbs and Supplements

Stimulants and system boosters can help anyone to feel more alert and alive on a daily basis. No substance or remedy, however, should be expected to take the place of the everyday practices and habits necessary for health and happiness. For best results, combine energizing substances with daily physical activity, aerobic exercise for at least 20 to 30 minutes two or three times per week, a low-fat natural-foods diet, a positive outlook and emotional life, and regular relaxation or meditation.

6

Elevate Your Mood

Almost 40 million American adults frequently fall into negative moods, characterized by loneliness, boredom, and restlessness, according to a report from government health researchers Charlotte A. Schoenborn and John Horm of the National Center for Health Statistics. Another 10 million Americans suffer from clinical depression each year, they found. The NCHS study was based on an extensive survey of 43,782 adults done in 1991, in which respondents were asked if they had felt such negative moods in the previous two weeks. Schoenborn and Horm said that smokers and heavy drinkers were especially prone to depression.

The potential market for mood-elevating drugs is hardly lost on pharmaceutical companies. The drug giant Pfizer Pharmaceuticals takes out full-page ads in *The New Yorker,* for instance, to tout pharmaceutical answers to depression. "Depression. It can affect you in ways you would never suspect," the ad says, going on to list such possible indicators of depression as sleep disturbances, unusual irritability, difficulty in concentrating or remembering, and a loss of self-esteem or an attitude of indifference. Pfizer advises, "Do something for yourself and for those you love. See your doctor"—who will presumably write a prescription for the unmentioned Pfizer anxiety-and-tension drug Vistaril.

Since Dista Products, a division of Eli Lilly, introduced the antidepressant Prozac at the end of 1987, worldwide sales of this drug have skyrocketed to $1.2 billion annually. Prozac enjoyed the fastest acceptance of any psychotherapeutic medicine ever. By 1993 over four million Americans had taken it. Doctors and psychiatrists are now writing more than a million prescriptions a month.

Many of the people currently taking drugs such as Vistaril and Prozac are not clinically depressed. Doctors diagnose depression by at least eight criteria. In addition to those mentioned in the Pfizer ad just referred to, the criteria include loss of energy and feelings of fatigue, recurrent thoughts of death or suicide, appetite loss or overeating, and withdrawal from activity and involvement in life. Four or five of the eight criteria must be present for two to four weeks in order for a diagnosis of depression to be applied.

Though clinical depression—a very debilitating condition that typically affects work, relationships, and of course physical health—is widespread, millions more Americans experience elements of depression without deserving the diagnosis of a full-blown clinical depression. It is not at all unusual to feel temporarily sad, helpless, hopeless, irritable, worthless, guilty, withdrawn, lethargic, or unable to experience pleasure. Psychiatrists even have a name for chronic discontent or low-level unhappiness that falls short of clinical depression: *dysthymia*.

The dramatic success of Prozac and other mood-elevating drugs such as Zoloft and Paxil is due in part to a greater willingness to treat short periods of depressed mood, a deeper understanding of the chemistry of emotions, and a more sophisticated neurological mapping of the brain. Drug manufacturers and research scientists are working on developing new drugs that can target specific parts and functions of the brain, perhaps opening new avenues for understanding and treating depressed mood. The ultimate social value of this approach is the subject of controversy.

From Lithium to Prozac

Until the latter half of this century, drugs to improve mood were principally highly psychoactive or stimulating substances such as opium, cocaine, and amphetamine. For the most part, these went well beyond merely restoring energy and increasing one's sense of well-being. Their ability to induce outright euphoria made them ripe for abuse, and indeed these drugs are physically and psychologically addictive. Though each enjoyed a brief period of acceptance as medicinal substances, they are now highly controlled and rarely used therapeutically.

Today's conventional antidepressants go back only to the 1940s.

One of the oldest is lithium (Eskalith, Lithane), a chemical element that any drug manufacturer can use as the basis for a drug, since it cannot be patented. From the turn of the century until the 1940s, lithium was used mainly as a tranquilizer. In the late 1940s it was discovered to dampen the mood swings of manic-depression and is now used mainly in the long-term treatment of that condition. Among its possible side effects are blurred vision, nausea, and drowsiness. Its toxic dosage level (it is especially damaging to the nervous system, heart, and kidneys) is close to its therapeutic level.

The specific biochemical mechanism by which lithium affects manic-depression is not completely understood even today. By the late 1950s, however, pharmacological researchers began to realize that mood could be altered by drugs that affect the levels of certain brain chemicals, the biogenic amines. These are complex chemicals that regulate a number of functions, including heart rate and neurotransmission. The biogenic amines that are known to affect mood, such as serotonin, noradrenaline, acetylcholine, and dopamine, are also called neurotransmitters. They play an important function in the process by which neighboring nerve cells relay electrical impulses and so can directly influence mood. When neurotransmitters such as noradrenaline and serotonin in effect go on strike, and don't do their impulse-relaying job properly, brain chemistry is affected in a way that leads to lethargy, irritability, and other symptoms of depressed mood. Researchers have also determined that certain drugs can help neurotransmitters loiter around in the synapse—the gap between the outer terminals of two nerve cells—giving the neurotransmitters more time and opportunity to take effect. Other drugs can destroy the enzyme that inactivates neurotransmitters. The effect is the same: more mood-elevating neurotransmitters are present in the brain.

This biogenic amine model of action has resulted in a revolution in antidepressant drug therapy. It has inspired pharmaceutical companies to develop dozens of new prescription drugs, though most fall within three classes: the monoamine-oxidase (MAO) inhibitors, the tricyclics, and the serotonin uptake inhibitors.

Monoamine-oxidase inhibitors (MAOIs). The first of these, iproniazid, was developed in the early 1950s as a drug to fight tuberculosis. It enjoyed a short-lived success only when its usefulness as an antidepressant became apparent in the late 1950s. Patients reported that it made them feel more joyful and optimistic while increasing their energy level and appetite. The manufacturer quickly withdrew iproniazid from the market because of its side effects, but related MAOI drugs such as phenelzine (Nardil) and isocarboxazid (Marplan) remain in use today.

Biogenic amines such as serotonin, dopamine, and noradrenaline need time to accomplish their mood-boosting effects in the brain. Anything that shortens their effective lifespan can have the effect of causing depression. One of those potential life-shorteners is MAO, an enzyme found in nerve cells. MAO inactivates various biogenic amines in the brain by oxidizing them. Therefore, a drug that inhibits the action of MAO has the effect of limiting the enzyme's amine destruction. To simplify, less enzyme equals more amines, and more amines means better mood. Drugs such as phenelzine thus improve mood and restore a sense of well-being by inhibiting MAO.

The initial enthusiasm for MAOIs was soon tempered by reports of the drugs' potentially serious side effects. When MAOIs in the body encounter the chemical tyramine, the interaction can cause an extreme reaction, including high blood pressure, headaches, and even (occasionally) strokes. This means that some relatively common foods and drinks (certain cheeses, wine, coffee, yogurt, and chocolate, among others), nutrients (especially the amino acids tryptophan or tyrosine), and various drugs (including nasal decongestants) must be avoided due to their tyramine content.

Since doctors shudder at the thought of having a patient drop dead from a dinner-induced drug reaction, MAOIs have never become as popular as somewhat safer drugs, such as the tricyclics.

Tricyclics. This popular class of antidepressant drugs is so named because their chemical structure is characterized by three carbon rings. The first tricyclic, imipramine (Tofranil), was introduced in 1957 and was hailed for being a "normalizing," nonstimulating antidepressant. It is now widely used, along with other closely related tricyclics such as amitriptyline (Elavil) and desipramine (Norpramin).

Like the MAOIs, which affect noradrenaline, serotonin, and dopamine, imipramine and other tricyclics tend to affect a number of neurotransmitters. Imipramine promotes the release particularly of noradrenaline and serotonin, as well as other amines including acetylcholine and histamine. Tricyclics allow amines to remain active in the nerve synapse, rather than being grabbed back by the transmitting cell. This gives the amines more time to affect brain chemistry and improve mood.

Though tricyclics don't cause potentially fatal increases in blood pressure, they do have numerous unwanted side effects. These include drowsiness, dry mouth, sweating, and constipation. Instead of noticing a brightening of mood, some people may notice only that they've activated their stress-inducing fight-or-flight system.

Because of the drawbacks associated with use of the MAOIs and tricyclics, pharmaceutical scientists beginning in the early 1960s sought to develop antidepressants that were more specific in their actions. The ideal antidepressant, it was thought, would somehow promote serotonin without much affecting the other amines. Despite millions of dollars in research money and the backing of giant pharmaceutical firms, it wasn't until the late 1980s that a breakthrough class of drugs was created.

Serotonin uptake inhibitors. Prozac (fluoxetine hydrochloride) is the principal drug in this category. Prozac works by selectively blocking the reabsorption of serotonin back into nerve cells. Prozac does this without dramatically affecting other biogenic amines such as noradrenaline, histamine, and acetylcholine. Increased serotonin in the nerve synapses has been found to lead to various mood-enhancing effects, including greater feelings of assertiveness, self-worth, and flexibility.

Prozac is now widely used for anxiety, depression, panic attacks, eating disorders, premenstrual syndrome, attention-deficit disorder, and other conditions. It is the drug that prompted Harvard psychiatrist Robert Aranow to coin the term "mood brightener," referring to agents that can "brighten the episodically down moods of those who are not clinically depressed, without causing euphoria or the side effects that have accompanied the mood elevators of abuse" (such as cocaine or amphetamine).

Prozac does not provide pleasure per se but rather restores the capacity for pleasure, notes Peter D. Kramer, author of the best-selling *Listening to Prozac.* It is not a nervous-system stimulant like cocaine. Its effects are subtle and take time to manifest themselves. According to Kramer, "Prozac seemed to give social confidence to the habitually timid, to make the sensitive brash, to lend the introvert the social skills of a salesman." His Prozac-taking patients seemed to acquire extra energy and become more confident, vivacious, and upbeat. Kramer also noticed that Prozac has the potential to seemingly change a person's personality, raising troubling questions in Kramer's mind about the ultimate purpose of mind-altering drugs. Is shyness, introspection, or impulsiveness, for example, sufficient reason to medicate with Prozac?

Prozac's specificity of action on serotonin makes it a relatively safe drug, especially when compared to the MAOIs. Patients on Prozac typically don't feel high or euphoric, and it thus has low potential for abuse. Still, Prozac does have some unwanted side effects, and recent studies indicate these may be more pervasive than originally thought. For example, as many as one in three patients may experience a loss of libido or difficulty reaching orgasm. Other common side effects include nausea, poor appetite, anxiety, and insomnia. Prozac should not be used in conjunction with MAOIs. Furthermore, the long-term effects are still unknown, since experience with this drug goes back only a few years. Other drugs, including cocaine and nicotine, were also hailed as harmless or even beneficial to health until more was known about them.

According to naturopaths Joseph Pizzorno and Michael Murray, the authors of *A Textbook of Natural Medicine,* "The biogenic amine hypothesis has become the primary treatment approach for many practitioners—psychiatrists, allopaths, and naturopaths alike. Many of the psychotropic drugs used by the M.D.'s, and the nutritional treatments employed by the N.D.'s and progressive M.D.'s, are designed to correct or lessen suspected imbalances in the monoamines (serotonin, melatonin, dopamine, epinephrine, and norepinephrine)." Despite this widespread acceptance, it is necessary to note that the biogenic amine hypothesis is not an all-encompassing model for how the mind and body generate moods and emotions. Imbalances in brain chemistry are no doubt often a factor, yet it is impossible to ignore the many other elements, from childhood upbringing to current interpersonal relationships, that affect daily moods and overall outlook.

Herbal Uplifters

Herbs can play a number of positive roles in helping to improve mood. Some herbs can strengthen and support the nervous system, thus helping to counter the physical exhaustion and debility that often underlies depression. These "nervine tonic" herbs include oats, damiana, and gotu kola (see Chapter 5). The stimulant herbs, such as ginseng and those that contain caffeine or ephedrine (also see Chapter 5), can have a mood-brightening effect by increasing alertness and energy. Here we'll look at herbs most often used specifically to raise the spirits, including St.-John's-wort, ginkgo, and Siberian ginseng.

St.-John's-Wort

This herb is a common North American and European perennial (*Hypericum perforatum*) with a number of promising medicinal properties. Herbalists have used St.-John's-wort since antiquity as a topical wound treatment and as an oral remedy for diarrhea, pain, and high fever. It has also traditionally been used in a manner similar to the nervine tonics to restore emotional stability and nervous-system strength to those suffering from melancholy, hypochondriasis, and depression. According to Simon Mills, author of *Out of the Earth: The Essential Book of Herbal Medicine,* "This combination of restorative and relaxant effect is not contradictory, and underlies the plant's recommendation for the treatment of a number of such conditions where tension and exhaustion combine."

How the plant came to be named St.-John's-wort is unclear. One theory is that the name is derived from a distinctive red oil exuded by both the leaves and the yellow star-shaped flowers. "Early Christians named the plant in honor of John the Baptist," according to Michael Castleman, author of *The Healing Herbs,* "because they believed it released its blood-red oil on August 29, the anniversary of the saint's beheading. (*Wort* is Old English for plant.)" Another theory traces the name to its use as a charm against witchcraft and evil spirits. Some European peasants believed that the St.-John's-wort gathered on St. John's day (June 24) possessed magical and devil-thwarting properties.

Scientific interest in St.-John's-wort has increased in recent years with evidence that it has potential not only as a mood-boosting substance but as an antiviral agent possibly useful against AIDS. The herb contains high concentrations of flavonoids, tannins, and carotenoids. Its effect on both viruses and mood is thought to be due to the reddish pigment compound hypericin concentrated in the flowers' essential oil. Preliminary studies of hypericin's ability to reduce depression, anxiety, and insomnia have been promising, particularly a small German study from the early 1980s that involved 15 depressed women. After taking hypericin the subjects reported beneficial effects such as increased appetite, fewer sleep problems, less anxiety, and a more positive self-image. German regulators have approved hypericin products for improving mood.

A limited number of studies on humans and animals suggest that hypericin improves mood by affecting brain chemistry. Hypericin apparently inhibits the activity in the body of MAO, much like the conventional MAO inhibitors. A clinical trial done in 1984 on six depressive women confirmed hypericin's effect on biogenic amines. Researchers measured subjects' urine for major dopamine and noradrenaline breakdown products, considered to be reliable indicators of mood enhancement. The hypericin did significantly increase breakdown-product levels, indicating it raised dopamine and noradrenaline levels in the brain.

In early 1994 a larger, double-blind study of 105 male and female subjects, 20 to 64 years old, found that taking 300 mg of St.-John's-wort extract three times per day for four weeks helped alleviate two types of depressive symptoms: neurotic depression and temporary depressive mood. Sixty-seven percent of those who received the St.-John's-wort extract responded positively, compared to only 28 percent of those who received a placebo.

The authors of the study, published in *Phytomedicine,* commented, "The *Hypericum* preparations were found to have an antidepression effect in the treatment of mild and moderate depression which can be compared to the therapeutic effect of traditional antidepressants, and did not cause any undesirable side effects. Hence, according to the authors' point of view, *Hypericum* should be used as a remedy of choice in the treatment of such categories of depression which in practice are most widely spread."

St.-John's-wort is less potent than conventional, pharmaceutical MAO inhibitors. To the extent that it does work like an MAO inhibitor, however, it shares the same drawbacks: instant results are rare, and typically the herb must be taken on a daily basis for at least a month before effects are noticed. Most natural-health practitioners recommend working with a knowledgeable herbalist or naturopath if you intend to take St.-John's-wort for its antidepressant properties.

Another drawback to St.-John's-wort is its ability to sensitize some people's skin to the sun. Fair-skinned people in particular may be prone to sunburns and allergylike phototoxic reactions after taking St.-John's-wort internally and then sunning themselves. Avoiding the sun after ingestion prevents this side effect. St.-John's-wort also should not be taken by pregnant women.

HOW TO USE ST.-JOHN'S-WORT: It is usually sold dried and in concentrated drops, tinctures, and extracts. A typical dosage of St.-John's-wort is 125 to 250 mg one or two times daily of a standardized extract containing 0.125 to 0.150 percent hypericin, or 1 dropperful twice daily of tincture or concentrated drops.

Ginkgo

An increasing number of people are turning to ginkgo to elevate mood and relieve depression. Ginkgo's ability to improve mood is thought to be tied to its effect on circulation to the brain. According to naturopath Michael Murray, author of *Natural Alternatives to Over-the-Counter and Prescription Drugs,* by increasing blood flow ginkgo boosts the amount of oxygen and other nutrients available to the brain. Researchers who have tested ginkgo extracts on subjects with less-than-optimal brain circulation have found that the herb can help reverse symptoms such as short-term memory loss, headache, lethargy, and depression.

Like St.-John's-wort, ginkgo may need to be taken for a number of months before its full effects are felt, though some people report benefits within two or three weeks. Says ginkgo researcher D. M. Warburton, "It seems that the longer the treatment is continued, the more obvious and lasting the result. Even at the end of a year, it was found that improvement was continuing and adherence to the treatment was good."

Ginkgo is safe and nontoxic even at doses well beyond average.

How to use ginkgo: Ginkgo comes in tablets, capsules, concentrated drops, tinctures, and extracts. An average dosage is 40 mg three times daily of a standardized extract containing a minimum of 24 percent flavoglycosides.

Siberian Ginseng

This versatile herb is among the premier adaptogens, herbs that help to strengthen and balance bodily functions (see Chapter 13). Studies indicate that Siberian ginseng's adaptogenic ability may also extend to balancing the relative levels in the brain of biogenic amines such as serotonin and dopamine. This has the effect of enhancing mood and increasing the person's overall sense of well-being. Herbal researchers have found that various manifestations of depression and mood disturbances, from hypochondriasis to insomnia, have been improved when subjects take Siberian ginseng.

One rat study found that a Siberian ginseng extract increased the biogenic amine content in the animals' brains, adrenals, and urine.

Siberian ginseng is safe and nontoxic at dosage levels well beyond the average.

How to use siberian ginseng: Herbal producers often combine Siberian ginseng with other herbs, such as schisandra. Siberian ginseng is also available dried and in capsules, tinctures, and extracts. An average dosage is 250 to 500 mg once or twice daily, or 1 to 2 dropperfuls of the concentrated drops or tincture two or three times daily.

Nutritional Supplements to Dispel SAD and Bad Moods

Many vitamins and minerals are involved in the complex interplay between the nervous system and the brain. Certain nutrients are crucial for hormone secretion, neurotransmitter production, and nerve-impulse transmission. A long-term deficiency in one or more of these nutrients thus can contribute to imbalances in brain chemicals such as noradrenaline, serotonin, and dopamine, possibly leading to mood disorders. Such symptoms as confusion, loss of energy and sex drive, fatigue, restlessness, and sadness can, on occasion, be alleviated by simple nutritional supplementation.

Some of the most important nutrients for preventing deficiency-induced depressive symptoms include:

Iron. Anemia from too little iron can lead to fatigue, lethargy, and other symptoms that are characteristic of depression also. Most nutritionists recommend taking supplemental iron only after a lab test has documented an iron deficiency.

Vitamin C. Depressed mood is an early symptom of scurvy, the vitamin C deficiency condition. A number of studies in which emotionally disturbed subjects were given vitamin C suggested that supplements can help elevate mood. For example, one random study of 40 psychiatric patients with chronic illness found that after three weeks, patients given vitamin C were less depressed than those given a placebo. Researchers have also found that, in general, patients in mental hospitals tend to have low blood levels of C. An average dosage of vitamin C is 250 to 500 mg two or three times daily.

Magnesium. A deficiency in this mineral has been known to lead to irritability and depression. An optimal daily dosage of magnesium is 450 to 650 mg; calcium supplements are usually taken in conjunction with magnesium at a 2:1 ratio.

Vitamin B Complex

While iron, vitamin C, and magnesium are important, the vitamin that is the most crucial to proper nerve function and neurotransmitter levels is vitamin B complex. Among the B vitamins with the most dramatic mood-elevating effects are thiamine (B_1), niacin (B_3), B_{12}, and folic acid. Researchers say that folic acid and B_{12} may help stimulate the formation of a compound necessary for the first step in synthesizing neurotransmitters, especially serotonin. People who suffer from

B-vitamin deficiencies often show symptoms of mild depression. Numerous studies have also found that deficiencies or low blood levels in these B vitamins are common among psychiatric patients suffering from irritability, apathy, anxiety, fatigue, and other symptoms related to depression. When depressive persons are supplemented with B vitamins, they often improve faster than those who are not. In some cases the person recovers completely from nothing more than supplementing the diet with the missing nutrient.

The B vitamin with perhaps the most dramatic mood-elevating effects is B_6, which is usually taken in supplemental form as pyridoxine. According to nutritional authority Alan Gaby, M.D., author of *B_6: The Natural Healer,* "Brain metabolism can go awry in countless ways, any number of which might trigger depression. Some of these abnormalities, and the depression they produce, can be corrected by vitamin B_6." Gaby notes that pyridoxine is the cofactor for enzymes that convert the dietary amino acids tryptophan and tyrosine to serotonin and noradrenaline, respectively. Pyridoxine is also necessary to convert the amino acid phenylalanine to the compound phenylethylamine (PEA), a neurotransmitter with stimulant effects. A pyridoxine deficiency is common among depressed patients, many of whom find that taking supplemental pyridoxine provides an emotional boost. Because oral contraceptives can interfere with the tryptophan-serotonin cycle, women who take birth control pills are particularly likely to benefit from taking extra pyridoxine.

How to use vitamin b complex: It comes in tablets, capsules, and liquids. An average dosage is 50 to 100 mg daily.

Choline/Phosphatidylcholine/Lecithin

If you suffer from some forms of depressed mood, in addition to making sure you are getting adequate levels of the basic micronutrients, you may want to consider using choline/phosphatidylcholine/lecithin to lift your spirits. The vitaminlike compound choline is intimately involved in the synthesis or release of certain neurotransmitters, particularly acetylcholine. When some types of neurons are deprived of adequate acetylcholine, the result may be memory loss or mood disorders. Choline has shown promise as a way to control mood swings. Increases in acetylcholine in the brain seem to elevate mood and improve alertness and mental energy, while low levels have been tied to depression and lack of concentration. Many people who use choline as a "smart drug" (see Chapter 11) notice an improvement in overall disposition. Studies have confirmed that choline boosts the mood of some Alzheimer's patients who take it.

Choline, phosphatidylcholine, and lecithin are safe and nontoxic at the dosages suggested below. Though megadoses of these nutrients (for example, 15 to 20 times the average dose) may have a role in the treatment of manic-depression and other serious psychiatric disorders, it is a bad idea to try to self-treat for these conditions. Such high doses of choline can be countereffective and actually cause depression in some people. You should also avoid taking choline supplements if you have gastric ulcers or Parkinson's disease, or if you are taking prescription drugs meant to block the effects of acetylcholine (atropine, diphenhydramine).

HOW TO USE CHOLINE/PHOSPHATIDYLCHOLINE/LECITHIN: Choline is available in powders, tablets, capsules, and liquids. An average daily dosage for boosting mood is 100 to 200 mg. Phosphatidylcholine typically comes in capsules; an average daily dosage of phosphatidylcholine that is 90 percent pure is 1,100 to 2,200 mg. Lecithin comes in granules, oil-filled capsules, and liquids; an average daily dosage of lecithin that is 20 percent phosphatidylcholine is 5 to 10 g, or 1 to 2 tablespoons of granules.

Melatonin

Just within the past few years researchers have begun to link melatonin levels with certain mood disturbances. One study that used psychological profiles found that melatonin benefited a half-dozen mood-scale categories, including tension/anxiety, depression/dejection, and fatigue/inertia. When manic-depressive patients are in the depressive phase they tend to have lower levels of melatonin than they do during the manic phase; they also experience lower levels of melatonin during episodes of suicidal behavior, according to studies. Scientists are now exploring a link between schizophrenia and melatonin dysfunction.

If you suffer from lousy moods primarily during the winter months, you may be a victim of Seasonal Affective Disorder (SAD). This form of "winter blues" is not uncommon in climes that get little sunshine during the winter, such as much of Scandinavia and northern North America. An estimated one in 20 people (four times as many women as men) who live in these sunlight-deprived areas experience some form of depression. During the winter months they tend to be tired, irritable, and lethargic. They gain weight, lose their ability to concentrate, and show no interest in having sex. While scientists are not sure that they understand the exact mechanism of SAD, it is thought to be linked with a malfunction in melatonin secretion. The lack of daytime light apparently diminishes the release of melatonin during the night. Researchers who have exposed SAD sufferers to especially bright, full-spectrum lights have found they can help these people become happier and more energetic. The SAD-busting lights, however, are expensive, and sufferers usually need to be exposed to them for many hours per day. Melatonin supplements show promise as an easier, more direct way to stimulate the pineal gland, regulate the sleep cycle, and enhance mood.

Studies indicate that melatonin is safe and causes relatively few side effects even when taken in doses much higher than recommended. Though many people are now taking melatonin to alleviate SAD and improve mood, a medical professional should evaluate and monitor any attempt to use melatonin for serious emotional illnesses such as manic-depression and schizophrenia. Melatonin should not be taken by women who are pregnant or lactating, or by anyone suffering from kidney disease. Because it may affect growth-hormone levels, melatonin should also be avoided by anyone under the age of 20.

Unless you're a shift worker who sleeps during the day, melatonin should always be taken at night, to support the body's natural melatonin secretion pattern and enhance your body's natural biorhythms. To improve mood or alleviate mild seasonal depression, most people find that melatonin works best when taken at the same time each night, within an hour of bedtime. You will probably sleep more soundly and be in a better mood the next day.

How to use melatonin: Melatonin comes in pills ranging in size from 750 mcg (0.75 mg) to 3 mg. An average daily dosage to elevate mood is 0.75 to 1.5 mg; elderly people may need to take 2 to 3 mg daily for a similar effect. Start with the lower dosage and increase if necessary.

Amino Acids to Elevate Mood

As we saw in the previous chapter on energy boosters, amino acids play a major role in brain chemistry. Some amino acids are precursors for the same neurotransmitters, such as serotonin, dopamine, and nor-adrenaline, that are affected by the conventional antidepressant drugs. The principal amino acids taken for their mood-elevating effects are tyrosine and phenylalanine. Tryptophan can also improve mood, though it is currently unavailable in supplement form in the United States.

Phenylalanine

Researchers have identified a number of possible mechanisms that may account for the mood-elevating properties of L-phenylalanine, D-phenylalanine, or DL-phenylalanine (DLPA). For example, scientists know that consuming supplemental phenylalanine affects bodily levels of other amino acids, including tyrosine and tryptophan, that in turn have been shown to influence directly neurotransmitters linked to mood. Phenylalanine, in fact, is a precursor of tyrosine, which can raise brain levels of the neurotransmitters dopamine and noradrenaline. In addition, D-phenylalanine acts to discourage the breakdown of endorphins, the body's natural opiates that reduce pain and encourage mild euphoria.

If the body has sufficient levels of vitamin B_6, it can also use L-phenylalanine to make PEA. Abundant in chocolate (which may account for chocolate's reputation as a love- and romance-inducer; see Chapter 7), PEA in the brain acts as a neurotransmitter with stimulant and mood-boosting effects. In one study, scientists noted that depressed subjects who had low levels of a PEA-related compound in their urine enjoyed improved moods after supplementing their diet with L-phenylalanine and vitamin B_6. In an uncontrolled study of 23 depressed patients, phenylalanine caused a positive response in 17 patients previously unresponsive to conventional tricyclic or MAOI antidepressants.

The major side effects associated with supplemental L-phenylalanine are those related to its stimulant properties, including insomnia and anxiety. You shouldn't take phenylalanine if you're already taking MAO-inhibiting antidepressants. Pregnant or lactating women, people with high blood pressure, and those suffering from the disorder known as phenylketonuria should also avoid taking phenylalanine supplements.

HOW TO USE PHENYLALANINE: It typically comes in powders and capsules. The usual recommendation for boosting mood is to take 375 to 500 mg of L-phenylalanine or 500 to 1,000 mg of DLPA supplements twice daily in the morning or at noon, half an hour before a meal. For maximum mood elevation, combine phenylalanine supplementation with 25 to 50 mg of B_6 or vitamin B complex. It may take a day or two to brighten mood; some depressed subjects in the studies didn't respond for a week.

Tyrosine

Tyrosine is a nonessential amino acid that helps the brain to produce the natural pain-killing and mood-boosting chemicals dopamine and noradrenaline. Tyrosine may play a role in relieving some forms of mild depression, according to studies. One placebo-controlled, double-blind study indicated that subjects respond to tyrosine at a rate similar to conventional antidepressants, though without the other drugs' side effects. Like phenylalanine (from which it is derived in the body), tyrosine tends to increase energy levels and alertness. Some women take it to alleviate the lethargy and irritability of premenstrual syndrome.

Tyrosine should be avoided by those who suffer from high blood pressure or take MAO-inhibitor antidepressants—combining tyrosine and MAO inhibitors can also cause high blood pressure.

HOW TO USE TYROSINE: It comes in capsules and powders. For mild lethargy and depression, take 500 to 1,000 mg twice a day with high-carbohydrate meals (in order to lower levels of competing amino acids). Take with 25 to 50 mg of vitamin B_6 or B complex.

Tryptophan

Tryptophan is an essential amino acid that, until it was banned as a food supplement by the FDA in 1989, was a popular natural sleep aid (see Chapter 12). Prior to 1989, tryptophan was also recognized as a relatively safe and effective treatment for some forms of anxiety and depression, even being included as an ingredient in two British antidepressants (tryptophan was withdrawn from the U.K. market also in 1989). If you've ever felt anxious, moody, and tense, eaten a snack rich in tryptophan and carbohydrates, and then begun to feel much better, you've probably experienced the subtle mood-brightening effects of tryptophan. Along with some B vitamins, these nutrients helped to increase your brain's supply of natural feel-good chemicals.

The calming and uplifting brain chemicals that tryptophan promotes in the body include serotonin and melatonin. When blood levels of tryptophan are low, synthesis of these neurotransmitters is reduced, and there may be adverse impacts on mood. In the years before tryptophan was banned, a number of scientific studies confirmed a connection between tryptophan consumption and emotional complaints. One researcher even found that countries with low average tryptophan intakes had higher rates of suicide than countries where average tryptophan consumption was higher.

One of the most dramatic demonstrations of tryptophan's effect on serotonin levels is done by feeding test subjects a diet almost totally lacking in tryptophan. When these subjects are then given an amino acid drink, again lacking in tryptophan, they experience a rapid depletion of serotonin in the brain. For some people this causes only relatively minor effects, while for others it results in fatigue, irritableness, and sadness, sometimes within hours. These feelings often lift when a normal diet that includes tryptophan is resumed. British researchers recently reported on a similar double-blind study in the *Archives of General Psychiatry*. They tested 24 males who were usually more aggressive than most men. The subjects who were given an amino acid mixture lacking in tryptophan experienced marked increases in anger, aggression, annoyance, quarrelsome tendencies, and hostility. The researchers warned that people who are prone to depression and who take amino acid supplements lacking in tryptophan may experience serious mood changes.

Recently a British psychiatrist reported on his experience with a 44-year-old male patient suffering from recurrent depression. Because the patient could not tolerate conventional antidepressants, the doctor recommended tryptophan supplements. On those occasions when the patient felt his depression returning, he took daily doses of 1.5 g of tryptophan for a few days at a time to help control his depression. When tryptophan supplements were no longer available, the man found that eating large amounts of pumpkin seeds for their tryptophan content was an effective mood elevator. Within 24 hours after eating the seeds, the psychiatrist commented, the patient "felt quite transformed. He was no longer anergic [lacking energy] or depressed and happily returned to work the following day."

In some studies of depressed patients tryptophan has worked as well as conventional antidepressants. For example, one study found a 65 percent improvement in 32 depressive patients after four weeks of daily supplementation with 4 g of tryptophan. Other medical studies, however, have not found tryptophan to be an effective treatment for depression. According to naturopaths Pizzorno and Murray, "The inconsistent results from studies utilizing tryptophan appear to be due to failure to address important considerations related to the nature of the depression and the factors affecting brain uptake."

The FDA recalled all tryptophan supplements from stores and banned future sales in the United States when they were tied to a rare illness called eosinophilia-myalgia syndrome that caused some 39 deaths. During the next two years, medical investigators determined that these ill effects were almost certainly caused by contaminated products and not by tryptophan itself. Whether tryptophan supplements are safe and deserve to be returned to the market remains controversial. Should the safety questions about tryptophan be resolved and supplements again become available, keep in mind that pregnant women should not take tryptophan supplements, nor should anyone who is taking MAO-inhibiting drugs.

HOW TO USE TRYPTOPHAN: When tryptophan was available in supplement form, it was frequently combined with 25 to 50 mg of vitamin B_6 and 250 to 500 mg of magnesium to promote its conversion into brain chemicals and enhance its effects.

Since supplemental tryptophan is currently not available in the United States, the only way that Americans can take advantage of its calming powers is through diet. The most effective strategy is to eat foods with high levels of tryptophan relative to other amino acids. Eggs, poultry (especially turkey), meat, and many other protein foods are rich in tryptophan, but they also contain large amounts of other amino acids that compete with tryptophan for uptake in the brain. Among the foods with the best ratios of tryptophan to other amino acids are roasted pumpkin seeds, dried sunflower seeds, bananas, milk, peanuts, and lentils. Still, you must eat relatively large amounts of these foods to approach the levels of tryptophan once widely available in supplements. For example, eating 100 grams, about 3.5 ounces, of pumpkin seeds, or drinking four cups of milk, provides a dose of about 500 mg of tryptophan. To boost mood, eat some of these tryptophan-specific foods while avoiding other sources of protein. Tryptophan can cause relaxation and even drowsiness in many people when used at night.

Another way to use tryptophan-rich foods is to consume them along with foods rich in complex carbohydrates, such as potatoes, bread, cereal, or pasta. The carbohydrates promote the secretion of insulin, which helps amino acids cross from the blood into cells. Insulin has less effect, however, on tryptophan than on the other amino acids. This leaves more tryptophan in the blood to cause a gradual rise in serotonin levels in the brain and affect behavior.

How to Choose

Consider the following questions as you evaluate the best choices for natural mood-brighteners. See "Where to Start" for a suggested mood-boosting daily program.

• Is your low mood an occasional problem? If your mood is a once-in-a-blue-moon problem, consider trying when necessary a quick-acting, stimulating mood-brightener such as phenylalanine or tyrosine.

• Is your sadness a more frequent and deeply ingrained problem? If so, you may be a good candidate for professional help, and for St.-John's-wort. Because of the safety considerations of long-term use, however, get appropriate supervision while using this herb.

• Do your low moods seem to be worse during the winter? You may suffer from SAD and respond to melatonin.

• Are you normally aware of and responsive to the odors that surround you? If so, you may be a good candidate for one of the essential oils, listed in the following section.

"Inhalable Prozac" and Other Uplifting Essential Oils

Many herbalists and aromatherapists recommend essential oils to uplift the spirits. Essential oils are concentrated aromatic liquids. They're usually steam-distilled from roots, leaves, flowers, or other plant material. Essential oils are volatile and can readily be evaporated or dispersed into the air, where they are inhaled and quickly affect parts of the brain that control mood and behavior.

A number of essential-oil producers now offer combination products, including massage and bath oils, that blend commonly used mood-enhancing essential oils such as Sandalwood, Ylang-ylang, Bergamot, Rosemary, and Jasmine. Look for products with names such as Euphoria and Depression. Two of the most popular single essential oils for enhancing mood are Rose and Thyme.

Rose

Thousands of species of rose exist, mainly modern hybrids developed for their dramatic size and colors. Only a few of the ancient, traditional cultivars, however, are widely grown nowadays for their exquisitely scented essential oil. Chief among these are damask rose (*Rosa damascena*) and cabbage rose (*R. centifolia;* also known as Provence rose), both probably native to the Middle East but now grown in Europe, China, and elsewhere.

People have been growing roses for use in perfumes since ancient times, and roses are still among the most popular perfume constituents, though many perfume producers now use synthetic rose oil. Until the Middle Ages, herbalists used roses for their medicinal properties, recommending the tea to treat nervous tension and other conditions. As an herb, rose is not in general use today, but the soothing qualities of the natural, pale yellow-green essential oil is much sought after to uplift the mood and spirit. Many aromatherapists recommend essential oil of Rose for depression and loss of appetite, as well as for such conditions as headache, lack of circulation, and menstrual problems.

"Rose essential oil is good for people with a very nervous disposition," says aromatherapist Daniele Ryman, a trained biochemist and the author of *Aromatherapy: The Encyclopedia of Plants and Oils and How They Help You.* "It seems to work on the nervous system, calming the patient, and is better received by women than men. Massage an oil into the solar plexus; apply a dilute oil after a bath, and drink rose petal infusions. Rose also helps insomnia." Ryman says that in a manufacturing plant such as those in southern France, where rose petals are steam-distilled to make essential oil, "one can get high on it, the nose is so completely saturated with the perfume."

The late French aromatherapist Marguerite Maury said that "the rose procures us one thing above all: a feeling of well-being, even of happiness, and the individual under its influence will develop an amiable tolerance." Think of it as inhalable Prozac.

Because more than three hundred pounds of rose petals are needed to make just an ounce of high-quality essential oil, rose is one of the most expensive essential oils. If it is not expensive, it is probably adulterated or mislabeled. (It does not necessarily follow, of course, that all expensive rose oil is therefore genuine.) For example, expect to pay at least $20 to 25 for a 1-ml bottle, $40 to 45 for 2 ml (^{1}/16th oz.). Essential oil of Rose is well worth the price if it works for you.

Thyme

This mood-enhancing essential oil is less expensive and more readily available than Rose. It is obtained through water or steam distillation of the leaves and flowering tops of a low-lying, perennial evergreen plant (*Thymus vulgaris*) of the mint family. Thyme is native to the Mediterranean but is now found worldwide. It was a popular medicinal herb of the Egyptians, Greeks, and other ancient peoples, principally for headaches, digestive problems, and respiratory complaints. As an antiseptic, it was strewn about or worn on clothes to ward off everything from plague to lice. Today it is widely known as a seasoning for meats and other dishes.

In addition to its medicinal use, thyme has also long been a favorite mood-enhancing herb. The Romans used it to treat melancholy; other herbalists have also favored it for nervous conditions and insomnia. The influential seventeenth-century English herbalist Nicholas Culpeper claimed thyme "helps to revive and strengthen both body and mind." In the late nineteenth century it was used to promote recovery in convalescing patients. Aromatherapists often recommend the essential oil for people suffering from mental stress, premenstrual tension, fatigue, and low spirits.

The highest-quality essential oil of thyme is clear or white rather than reddish in color. Look for products labeled Lemon Thyme (*T. citriodorus*), Sweet Thyme, or "linalol." These are less likely to irritate the skin than red thyme, but it is still a good idea to dilute essential oil in a carrier oil before applying to the skin.

Essential oils are extremely concentrated substances and are generally *not* taken orally. There are a number of other ways to take advantage of essential oils' relaxing properties; see "How to Use Essential Oils" in Chapter 2.

Homeopathic Remedies for the Blues

An experienced homeopath might recommend any of dozens of homeopathic remedies to someone complaining of depression, overall discontent, or despair. To find just the right remedy, he or she would need to consider many factors specific to the individual's unique situation and personality: Is the person's condition made worse by criticism? Does he dislike being in the company of other people? Does he have a tendency to brood? If the condition is serious and long-standing, it is definitely worth seeing a trained homeopath to work through these questions. For many people, though, a quicker and less expensive path is sufficient. Such people may prefer to take a homeopathic combination formula that contains many of the most commonly recommended remedies to lift a person's spirits. Although few homeopathic companies have developed combination remedies specifically for depression, many people may benefit by trying those labeled for fatigue, insomnia, or anxiety. Another option is to try two of the most commonly used single remedies for low spirits, *Arsenicum* and *Pulsatilla*.

Arsenicum

Arsenicum is prepared from arsenic trioxide, a compound of the poisonous chemical element arsenic. In microdilute homeopathic dosages *Arsenicum* is used to treat various physical symptoms ranging from certain skin rashes to food-poisoning-induced stomach upsets. It is also taken for types of depression, especially when the patient is exhausted, restless, pale, fearful, and anxious. This is the right remedy if you get obsessively neat and tidy when you're feeling down.

Pulsatilla

Pulsatilla is derived from the poisonous pasque flower (*Anemone patens*). In homeopathic dilutions people take it for runny nose, certain eye and ear ailments, and allergies. It may also help to boost the spirits of the person who suffers from insomnia, is oversensitive, tends to start crying at the slightest provocation, and constantly needs reassurance and attention.

See "How to Use Homeopathic Remedies" in Chapter 2.

Where to Start

The following three substances are profitably combined in an ongoing, daily program for improving too-frequent moodiness, loneliness, and boredom.

• Ginkgo (40 mg three times daily of a standardized extract containing a minimum of 24 percent flavoglycosides) is a better choice for most people than is St.-John's-wort. Ginkgo is somewhat safer than St.-John's-wort and has more varied positive effects on the body.

• An insurance-level multivitamin-multimineral supplement, with optimal daily levels of vitamin B complex, vitamin C, and magnesium, is a good idea.

• Choline (100 to 200 mg; or 1,100 to 2,200 mg phosphatidylcholine that is 90 percent pure; or 5 to 10 g, or 1 to 2 tablespoons of granules, of lecithin that is 20 percent phosphatidylcholine) not only brightens mood but can enhance overall mental function.

Beyond Herbs and Supplements

Just as it is a mistake to think that any drug, whether it is Valium or Prozac, is a magic bullet for the mind and emotions, so it is unwise to think that any herb or nutrient by itself can banish from your life all feelings of anxiety, irritability, and depression. Mood swings are a natural response to the challenges and the changes inherent in daily life. Accept them when you can; when you need help, recognize that natural substances should be only a part of the answer.

Whether you suffer from only occasional grumpiness or long-term manic-depression, it is likely that many causative factors come into play, from environmental influences to lifestyle decisions. Many such factors, such as one's love relationships or one's job satisfaction, are not addressed by the presence or absence of certain brain chemicals and neurotransmitters. Rather than relying on a drug or remedy, keep in mind the following suggestions.

• Take steps to discover the underlying causes of long-term depressed mood, through psychological counseling, dream work, hypnosis, or other mind/body techniques.

• Exercise or be physically active on a regular basis. Being physically fit improves your overall outlook and can help relieve depression, reduce anxiety, and decrease levels of anger and hostility.

• Be open to the possibilities for humor in everyday life. Laughing is an infectious, healthful way to spread positive feelings and good will.

• Avoid overuse of stimulants, including caffeine. Nervousness, depression, and anxiety are common side effects of prolonged stimulant abuse.

• Reduce your exposure to high levels of mental and emotional stress, or learn how to change your body's routine reaction to such stress, through biofeedback, meditation, or other techniques. Stress causes the adrenal gland to release higher amounts of hormones that may contribute to depression.

Stimulate Your Sexuality

What do oil of peppermint, cucumbers, marijuana, mandrake, oysters, and honey have in common? They have all been widely used at one time or another as aphrodisiacs, substances to increase libido (sexual desire) and boost sexual performance. They have also all been dismissed by most scientists as having no possible direct effect on sexuality. Indeed, some medical authorities say that *any* presumed aphrodisiac effect is merely psychological. For example, according to the *American Medical Association Encyclopedia of Medicine,* "No substance has a proven aphrodisiac effect, although virtually anything may produce the desired results if the person taking it believes strongly enough that it will work."

This dismissive attitude is due in part to the sheer number of purported aphrodisiacs. The *Dictionary of Aphrodisiacs,* written in the early 1960s, included 250 pages of entries. A large number of traditional aphrodisiacs in various cultures are foods that are associated with male fertility because they resemble the shape of a penis or are associated with female fertility because they are eggs. Clearly, what aphrodisiac effects these do have are essentially suggestive (though highly suggestive: the placebo effect is as high as 50 percent for aphrodisiac properties). Some purported aphrodisiacs work by diminishing sexual inhibition while intensifying sensory feelings (marijuana, for example). On the other hand, some foods, herbs, and nutritional substances have very definite physical effects on the body that could account for increases in sexual desire and performance. Natural substances can affect bodily levels of male and female sex hormones (androgens and estrogens), cause increases or decreases in brain levels of neurotransmitters associated with sexual desire, and even improve blood supply to erectile tissue such as the penis. Natural substances not only can increase short-term sexual desire but also can nourish and support the sex glands and the entire hormonal and reproductive systems, thereby increasing overall sexual vigor and, frequently, fertility.

The Body's Own Aphrodisiac

One of the key bodily agents in the expression of sex drive is the hormone testosterone. Most people think of testosterone as an exclusively male hormone, but women's bodies also naturally produce small amounts of it. Men produce testosterone in the testes, and women produce it, in tiny amounts, in the ovaries. When men or women lack sufficient testosterone, they may experience reduced sexual drive and performance, a condition that can be reversed by taking synthetic testosterone.

Testosterone is not found in the plant world; a popular synthetic form is the anabolic steroids. These and other synthetic testosterones, however, are not recommended as libido-increasing agents for most people. After an initial boost in sexual drive, men taking anabolic steroids may experience increased aggression and a higher risk of heart or liver disease. Synthetic testosterone can also actually reduce sex drive and sperm production in normal men. Women may experience the development of facial hair and a deepened voice.

A minority of women, however, do suffer from what Susan Rako, M.D., of Newton, Massachusetts, calls "female androgen deficiency syndrome." Compared to women who produce normal levels of testosterone, these low-testosterone women tend to make love less often and enjoy it less, experience difficulty in reaching orgasm, and have lower levels of vital energy. Rako has conducted workshops with women "suffering from a decrease in the normal, essential levels of this hormone," often due to menopause (when the ovaries naturally curtail production of testosterone), unnecessary removal of ovaries with hysterectomy, or from the effects of chemotherapy for cancer. Rako says, "No woman considers the prospect of using supplementary testosterone without concern about potential side effects." But restoring a normal level of testosterone to women with deficiencies can be beneficial to millions of women, she contends.

Sexual desire is a complex human function affected by both physical and psychological factors. Herbs or other natural substances should not be expected to provide a permanent answer for a flagging of sexual desire caused by such physical conditions as depression, fatigue, or regular drug use (including sleeping pills, birth control pills, and antidepressants). Nor can any substance substitute for treatment of reduced libido that is due to sexual abuse or sexual trauma.

Herbal Aphrodisiacs: Myth and Reality

Some of the classic herbal aphrodisiacs are best experienced secondhand—read about them if you like, but definitely don't take them. Though you can find many references to the following herbs in discussions of aphrodisiacs, in reality these present considerable disadvantages and relatively little proof that they enhance sex. These herbs are not found in herbal supplements and are not sold in natural-food stores. The plants are found in the wild, however, and occasionally are still used by the unwary. Do not use them.

Mandrake. This is a toxic plant (*Mandragora officianarum*) in the nightshade family. What studies that have been done on its purported aphrodisiac properties have not confirmed this traditional use.

Jimson weed. Also known as thorn apple, this plant was recently responsible for the death of two Texas teenagers. They ate plant parts harvested from the wild, presumably for their ability to cause intoxication or a hypnotic state. In addition, in 1994 more than a dozen other young people in New York and Connecticut were hospitalized after experimenting with jimson weed. In the nineteenth century jimson weed was sometimes used for its narcotic and pain-relieving effects, and, as noted in Chapter 1, alkaloids found in it are used in some modern drugs. Nevertheless, jimson weed is highly toxic. Fatalities are not uncommon; recorded poisonings go back to 1676 in colonial Jamestown, Virginia (*jimson* is an alteration of *Jamestown*). Even collecting the plant can cause swollen eyelids.

Poison nut. This aptly named plant is a small Asian tree whose seeds are the source of the poisonous alkaloid strychnine. At one time strychnine was an aphrodisiac for the adventurous—those who didn't mind that the toxic dose and the therapeutic one were dangerously close. The plant does have some excitatory and stimulant properties, but you should avoid it and, if so inclined, try instead the safe and nontoxic homeopathic remedy *Nux vomica.*

Two additional herbs, wild lettuce and hop, are not toxic like mandrake, jimson weed, and poison nut, but are similarly dubious as aphrodisiacs. Also known as lettuce opium, wild lettuce (*Lactuca virosa*) may have very mild sedative powers but some herbalists say that it is anaphrodisiac—that is, it decreases sexual desire.

The ability to reduce rather than increase sexual desire is also a trait of the bitter herb hop (*Humulus lupulus*). That's right, fellas, one of the primary ingredients in beer, that popular alcoholic beverage promoted in TV commercials as an instant, woman-attracting party-creator, may have an adverse effect on libido. Of course, the alcohol in beer, which has contradictory effects, is probably more potent than the small amount of hop used. As Shakespeare was among the first to note, alcohol increases the desire but detracts from the performance. Over time, excessive alcohol consumption lowers a man's sperm count and decreases his production of testosterone.

Sexual Stimulants

Yohimbe, damiana, and muira puama are among the few herbs that may truly deserve to be called aphrodisiacs, in that they increase sexual desire, enhance sexual pleasure, and stimulate sexual performance. Typically these herbs are taken on an occasional basis prior to lovemaking, rather than regularly, as are ginseng and other sexual-system balancers.

Herbal producers often combine yohimbe, damiana, and muira puama with other herbs that are either sexually stimulating or balancing, such as ginseng, sarsaparilla (*Smilax officinalis*), and saw palmetto (*Serenoa repens, S. serrulata*). Some of the products aimed at either men or women include Aphro, Hot Stuff, Romantic Mood, and Love Tea. Products aimed at men, often including nutrients such as zinc, go by names such as Super Male Plex and For Men Only.

Most herbal aphrodisiac products refrain from making any explicit claims about increasing libido on the label or in product literature. That's because the Food and Drug Administration bars from interstate commerce "any product that bears labeling claims that it will arouse or increase sexual desire, or that it will improve sexual performance, because there is a lack of adequate data to establish general recognition of the safety and effectiveness of any of these ingredients, or any other ingredient for OTC use as an aphrodisiac."

Yohimbe

Yohimbe is arguably the most potent herb with true powers of aphrodisia. For centuries some native peoples of West Africa have drunk a tea made from the bark shavings to treat impotence and to encourage sexual activity on special occasions. Scientific studies on yohimbe conducted since the 1930s have confirmed that the herb has definite effects on men's sexual organs—though at a price, as we'll see.

Researchers have identified and isolated the sex-active ingredient in yohimbe bark. It is an alkaloid called yohimbine. Today yohimbine is the only medicine approved by the FDA for treatment of certain types of male impotence. A number of pharmaceutical companies have for-mulated prescription drugs (Yocon, Actibine, Aphrodyne, Yohimex) using the compound yohimbine hydrochloride. Studies have shown that approximately one in three impotent men can get erections by taking yohimbine hydrochloride. (Clinical researchers always use yo-himbine hydrochloride, not the whole herb.) Nonimpotent males with normal libidos are also affected by yohimbine. One noted animal study, conducted by Dr. Julian Davidson and colleagues from the de-partment of physiology at Stanford University and published in *Science* in 1984, found that yohimbine-treated rats began to engage in a frenzy of sexual activity. Even males with apparently low libidos joined in the fun.

Studies show that yohimbine works by blocking the release of cer-tain neurotransmitters and thus causing small arteries to dilate. Yohim-bine also increases blood flow to erectile tissue and peripheral parts of the body, including the penis. At the same time veins in the penis are compressed, preventing blood from flowing out of the organ. Yohim-bine's actions are complex; its ability to increase libido has not been fully explained.

Though yohimbine does not affect testosterone levels, its effects on blood flow are enough to cause some men to experience powerful, rigid, and long-lasting erections. Frequency of erection is also in-creased. Yohimbine's downside is what you get along with the porno-movie performance. As Davidson has noted, "Yohimbine does help men get an erection, but they don't know what to do with it because they feel so lousy." Among the alkaloid's toxic side effects are nausea, tension, irritability, sweating, anxiety, panic attacks, elevated heart rate, hallucinations, dizziness, headache, and high blood pressure. You should avoid using yohimbine if you have high blood pressure, heart, kidney, or liver disease, are taking MAO inhibitors, are psychologically disturbed, or are pregnant.

Herbal preparations are also potent, depending upon the exact alka-loid content (often not provided on labels and thus difficult to deter-mine). Herbalists agree that yohimbe has the potential for abuse, and you shouldn't use it on a daily or even regular basis. The FDA classifies it as an unsafe herb. According to naturopath Michael Murray, author of *Male Sexual Vitality,* "I think there is some validity to this classification. I have used yohimbine in my practice and have found that, because of side effects, it is very difficult to work with." He says it is not an herb for self-medication, and recommends that it be used only under the supervision of a physician.

Individual reactions to the herb vary, and some yohimbe users do manage to have positive experiences with the herb. They take it occasionally as an aphrodisiac and for its stimulating or mood-elevating effects. Women generally avoid it, though some take it as a weight-loss aid. Some people say that it is a mild hallucinogenic that can heighten sensory effects.

Yohimbe is used as an ingredient in some aphrodisiac combination products, a form that some herbalists recommend over individual use. These products cannot be promoted as aphrodisiacs, according to FDA regulations, but product names like Man Power often suggest their intended use.

How to use yohimbe: Yohimbe is sometimes difficult to find in natural-food stores. Those with extensive selections of herbs may carry the dried bark, tablets, capsules, or liquids. (See "Resources" for mail-order sources that sell it.) If you do decide to experiment with yohimbe, start with low doses to avoid side effects. For example, take a single 500-mg capsule of the powdered herb, or drink a cup of the tea. You can make a mild tea by boiling an ounce of bark in two cups of water for 2 to 3 minutes and then lowering the heat and simmering for 10 to 15 minutes.

The safest way to use yohimbe is in its diluted homeopathic form, available by mail-order from some homeopathic suppliers.

Damiana

Damiana has long been a popular Mexican herbal aphrodisiac, and in recent years it has begun to make inroads north of the border. Herbalists formulate products from the leaves and flowers of a plant native to Mexico and the U.S. Southwest. Chemists have determined that damiana contains a volatile oil that is mildly irritating and gently stimulating to the genito-urinary tract when excreted. The plant also contains some alkaloids that may boost circulation, stimulate the nerves, and increase the sensitivity of the clitoris and penis. Some people experience a mild euphoria that lasts for an hour or so after taking damiana.

Folk use of damiana as an aphrodisiac was limited mainly to women, but today the herb is taken by both sexes. Some herbalists contend that damiana can help to increase sperm count, build testosterone levels, and strengthen the prostate and male sex organs. Unfortunately, damiana has not attracted the interest of researchers, and there are no clinical studies to back up the anecdotal and folk evidence for its powers as an aphrodisiac.

Damiana is a much milder, safer herb than yohimbe. Native Mexicans have long used it not only as an aphrodisiac but also to treat constipation, fatigue, depression, and anxiety.

Like yohimbe, damiana is also used in herbal combination products. If you're in Mexico, you might look for a damiana liqueur produced there. Small doses are recommended because of the alcohol's effects on sex.

HOW TO USE DAMIANA: Native Mexican women have traditionally used damiana by drinking a cup of tea about an hour before planned lovemaking. In the United States damiana is sold primarily in capsules, concentrated drops, tincture, and extracts. An average dosage is one or two 400-mg capsules of the powdered herb, or 1 dropperful of concentrated drops or tincture.

Muira Puama

Potency wood, the English name for this folk herb of Brazil, emphasizes its reputation as an aphrodisiac. Muira puama is derived from the wood, stem, or root of two Brazilian shrubs (*Ptychopetalum olacoides, P. uncinatum*). Native peoples in the areas surrounding the Amazon and Orinoco river basins have long used muira puama to enhance sex, stimulate or tonify nerves, and treat impotence.

Though muira puama has not been extensively studied, the herb's effects on sexuality have recently begun to be validated by scientists. For example, a clinical study at the Institute of Sexology in Paris looked at 262 patients with erection problems and a lack of sexual desire. Over half of the subjects given a daily dose of between 1 and 1.5 g of muira puama extract over two weeks experienced positive benefits to their sex lives. Researchers are, however, unsure about why muira puama works. Among its chemical constituents are a resin that may stimulate the central nervous system, as well as such compounds as lupeol, campestrol, and beta-sitosterol. How these constituents affect sexual stimulation is unknown.

Like yohimbe, muira puama is a somewhat uncommon herb in natural-food stores. It is found in combination herbals such as Cobra from PEP Products.

How to use muira puama: Shortly before planned sex, drink a cup of tea or take a dropperful of tincture of muira puama. Some people have also applied concentrated drops directly to the genitals.

Choosing Among the Herbal Aphrodisiacs

Yohimbe, damiana, and muira puama are among the few likely, though still not totally proven, classical aphrodisiacs. That is, they stimulate the desire for sexual activity within hours of consumption. Most of the rest of the natural substances reputed to be aphrodisiacs are more correctly sexual fortifiers. They nourish the sexual glands and promote overall sexual health, leading ultimately to increased desire for sex, but you wouldn't necessarily expect them to show immediate effect. So if you're the adventuresome type and really want to experience an aphrodisiac, yohimbe is it. Just keep in mind that you may not like it. Damiana and muira puama are less potent as sexual stimulants but also are much less likely to cause you to swear never to take another herbal product as long as you live. Of these, damiana is more readily available in easy-to-use capsule form.

Sexual System Balancers

The following are tonic herbs for the sexual system. These herbs can be taken on a daily basis by men or women to increase sexual energy and support the functioning of the reproductive organs.

Oats

Oats (also known as oat straw and wild oats) is the familiar, widely cultivated cereal grass (*Avena sativa*) whose edible grain is a hearty breakfast food. Herbal companies make oats products from the young, whole plant and unripe grain. Oats combines some of the properties of a healing herb and those of a nutritional supplement, being rich in alkaloids and other potentially medicinal compounds as well as nutrients such as calcium. It has traditionally been used as a remedy to support and nourish a debilitated nervous system. People take it to help recover from exhaustion and depression, to help break addictions, and to gently stimulate the nervous system. It has also long been recommended as a sexual tonifier and mild aphrodisiac that can help in the treatment of impotence. Scientific proof for oats' effects on sex drive is generally lacking, though one recent study of forty men and women given an oats-and-nettle product found higher levels of sexual desire and performance.

A popular oats-and-nettle product is Exsativa caplets from Scandinavian Natural.

How to use oats: It is sold dried and as capsules, concentrated drops, tinctures, and extracts. An average dosage of tincture or concentrated drops is $^1/_2$ to 1 dropperful two or three times daily.

Ashwagandha

Ashwagandha, also known as winter cherry, is a prominent tonic herb in Ayurvedic medicine, the traditional healing practice of India. Ashwagandha preparations are derived from the roots of a small branching shrub (*Withania somnifera*) of the nightshade family that grows abundantly in India. Herbalists recommend it to calm nervous tension and promote restful sleep. It is also sometimes used as an aphrodisiac by both men and women, and as a treatment for impotence.

Ashwagandha is safe to take on a daily basis for extended periods of time.

How to use ashwagandha: Ashwagandha is still a relatively new herb on the U.S. market. Most products are capsules standardized for 2 to 5 mg withanolides, as are the preparations preferred in clinical studies. An average daily dosage of these capsules is 150 to 300 mg.

Fo-ti

One of the most widely used Chinese tonic herbs, fo-ti is derived from the roots of a weedy, twining vine (*Polygonum multiforum*) in the buckwheat family. The name *fo-ti* sounds ancient but is a recent American coinage. In China the herb has long been known as *he shou wu* (also *ho shou wu*). Fo-ti is famous as a rejuvenating and longevity tonic in China, where it is taken to prevent premature aging. It is also said to increase fertility, strengthen sexual function, and boost a low libido.

Legend has it that the plant was named *he shou wu* over a thousand years ago after an elderly Chinese man. Childless and seemingly impotent at the age of 58, he tried the weed out of curiosity. His virility restored, he went on to father numerous children and live to the age of 130.

HOW TO USE FO-TI: It is sold dried and as a powder, tablets, capsules, concentrated drops, tinctures, and extracts. An average recommended dosage of the concentrated drops is ¹/₂ to 1 dropperful two or three times daily.

Ginkgo

Derived from one of the world's most ancient tree species, ginkgo is a traditional Chinese herb that is now catching on in the West for its ability to strengthen arterial tone and to increase blood circulation in parts of the body, including the brain and ears, without raising overall blood pressure. A few studies have also focused on ginkgo's effects on circulation to the genitals. For example, a clinical study done in 1989 by R. Sikora and colleagues and reported in the *Journal of Urology* indicated that a ginkgo extract can help relieve impotence due to insufficient blood flow to the erect penis. The researchers administered 60 mg of ginkgo daily for 12 to 18 months to 60 patients with erectile dysfunction. Even though this is a relatively small dose of ginkgo (most herbalists recommend 120 mg daily), sonograms showed that the patients began to experience increased blood flow to the penis after six to eight weeks and that after six months half of the patients had regained potency.

HOW TO USE GINKGO: Ginkgo is widely available in natural-food stores in capsules, concentrated drops, and tinctures. An average recommended dosage is 40 mg three times daily of an extract standardized for 24 percent ginkgo heterosides.

Ginseng

This sometimes phallic-shaped root has a varied résumé, including long use as an herb to increase virility and revitalize the sex organs. Ginseng-based love potions are part of the herbal traditions in China and India and among Native Americans. While human studies have yet to confirm ginseng's reputation as a mild sexual stimulant, a number of animal studies do indicate ginseng has a positive effect on aspects of sexuality. For example, a study published in the *American Journal of Clinical Medicine* showed that ginseng-treated animals are more sexually active than animals not given ginseng. Studies of rabbits, bulls, and rats to which ginseng was administered indicate that the herb encourages growth of the gonads and, in males, increases sperm quality or quantity. A ginseng compound was shown to protect mice against lowered sex drive due to induced stress. Ginseng has also been shown to stimulate egg-laying in hens.

Various chemical constituents isolated from ginseng have been shown to increase endocrine and metabolic activity and stimulate the heart and brain.

HOW TO USE GINSENG: Ginseng comes in a wide variety of forms, from the whole root to teas to standardized-extract capsules, and is one of the most popular herbs in natural-food stores. An average dosage for use as a sexual stimulant is 500 to 1,000 mg of capsules standardized for 5 to 9 percent ginsenosides. An average dosage of some concentrated extracts and ginseng products with higher standardized percentages may be as low as 200 to 400 mg.

Aphrodisiacs of the East

The diverse herbal traditions of Asia incorporate many plants used for their effects on sexual desire and performance. Some of these, including ginseng, fo-ti, and ginkgo, have begun to make considerable inroads into Western herbal practice. Less well known in the West are the so-called Chinese patent or prepared medicines, formulas that may contain a few or dozens of herbs. Practitioners of traditional Chinese medicine often combine herbs to take advantage of each herb's distinct properties, and also to reduce potential adverse effects. Chinese herbal formulas to boost sexual drive are often described by the Chinese in terms of their ability to correct "deficient *qi*" or "a lack of *yang*," concepts that don't readily translate into Western terms but basically mean lack of virile or vital energy.

From the Chinese perspective, sexual tonics also attempt to strengthen the internal organs necessary to support normal sexual activity. Daniel P. Reid, author of *Chinese Herbal Medicine* and other books on Chinese health practices, says, "Herbal aphrodisiacs, like all herbal medicines, have their own specific 'natural affinities' for certain organs and glands in the body. In the case of aphrodisiac potions, herbalists select ingredients with known affinities for the sexual organs, blood, and vital glands, especially the sexually all-important suprarenal glands. The herbs tonify these tissues, stimulate secretions from glands, and promote circulation to the minute capillaries of the sexual organs. The net result is an overall stimulation of vitality (energy) and hormones (essence); the enhanced sexual potency that follows is largely a *side effect* of this general tonification of essence and energy."

Two of the Chinese herbs most often found in traditional Eastern aphrodisiac formulas are the following:

Eucommia bark. Known in Chinese as *du zhong,* eucommia bark is derived from a hardy, rubber-producing tree (*Eucommia ulmoides*) with somewhat elmlike leaves. Widely cultivated in China, this species is the only one left in a tree family that once included representatives in Europe and North America. Eucommia bark is one of the earliest Chinese herbs, traditionally used as a system strengthener that, as Chinese herbal authorities Steven Foster and Yue Chongxi put it, "invigorates the liver and kidney, strengthens bones and muscles, [and] enhances vital essence and vital energy." Chinese herbalists use it to treat high blood pressure and other conditions, as well as impotence and general sexual dysfunctions. Research by Western scientists in the past few decades indicates it has pain-relieving and sedative properties; studies also confirm its promise as a treatment for high blood pressure.

Horny goat weed. This somewhat obscure Chinese herb, also known as lusty goatherb and epimedium (*Epimedium sagittatum*), is said to make goats fornicate after they eat it. It lives up to its name, according to Reid. He says, "Recent studies have shown that sperm count and semen density increase substantially in men during the first few hours after ingestion of this herb. Besides stimulating hormone production in the suprarenal glands, which in turn stimulates other related glands, this drug has a salutary effect on circulation of blood. When it enters blood vessels, especially the finer capillaries, its presence there causes them to dilate, thereby greatly enhancing circulation in tissues fed mainly by small capillaries, such as a man's penis."

Aphrodisiacs to Avoid from the Animal Kingdom

In the past the traditional pharmacopoeia of China and a number of other cultures around the world have made use of various animal parts for their presumed aphrodisiac effects. Perhaps the most notorious of the animal-derived aphrodisiacs is a Western product, the infamous Spanish fly. This purported aphrodisiac is made by drying and crushing into powder the green blister beetle (*Cantharis vesicatoria*) native to the Mediterranean and Near East. The active ingredient in the powder is a rapid-acting compound known as cantharidin that is one of the most potent blistering agents and urinary tract irritators known to medicine. As cantharidin passes through the urinary tract, it irritates and inflames the lining of the bladder and urethra. True, this action can prolong an erection and engorge the clitoris. But sexual ardor is usually overwhelmed by the excruciating abdominal pain, urinary burning, nausea, diarrhea, and urge to urinate.

The federal government classifies Spanish fly as a Class 1 poison and restricts its legal possession. A few milligrams of cantharidin is considered a toxic dose, with the potential to cause kidney damage or even kidney failure. Some 30 mg or so may be fatal, and Spanish fly has caused numerous comas and deaths. Cantharidin-based prescription drugs are primarily topical preparations—applied only by a doctor—to treat warts. The homeopathic remedy *Cantharis* is used to treat extreme suffering and excessive desire for sex.

Another notorious class of animal-derived aphrodisiacs is based on the presumed benefits of consuming parts of animals' genitals. Nowadays, obtaining some of these animal parts, such as the penises, testicles, or blood of tigers and lions, causes the destruction of rare or even endangered species. No amount of human sexual pleasure should justify the killing of animals, much less endangered ones, for their body parts. Only the morally depraved would defy the various governmental restrictions in place to prevent such animal abuse. Rhino horn, which is considered an aphrodisiac in some parts of Asia and the Middle East, is another example in which an animal's very existence is threatened as a result of the immoral demand for one of its body parts.

Other Animal-Based Aphrodisiacs

There are, however, a few animal-based aphrodisiacs that present no legal restrictions and, unlike tiger penises, may have more than symbolic reason for their use. Admittedly, environmentalists, animal-rights activists, vegans, and some others will nevertheless choose not to use the following.

Deer antler. Deer antler (*lu rong* in Chinese) products enhance male virility and reinforce overall *qi* or vital energy, according to practitioners of traditional Chinese medicine. Deer antler is also used to build athletic endurance, prevent the harmful effects of stress, and improve overall strength and performance. While Chinese herbalists contend that chemical analysis shows that deer antler contains certain sterols with potential testosteronelike effects, and that animal studies indicate deer antler extracts can cause the testes to secrete more testosterone and produce more sperm, herbal skeptics are unconvinced. Plant drug expert Varro E. Tyler, Ph.D., Sc.D., for example, says that deer antler has "never been proven to contain any constituent that stimulates libido or cures impotence."

Deer antler products are typically imported from China. Reputable producers do not harm or kill deer to obtain deer antler extract, relying instead on antlers that mature deer have naturally shed or on the soft, fresh tips of young deer's antlers, removed in a way that allows the deer to grow new ones. Obviously, if abuses in these procedures do occur, American consumers are unlikely to know.

Sea horse. The Chinese have long used the whole bodies of these small marine fishes with horselike heads to treat male infertility. From the Asian perspective, sea horse is a good tonic for anyone suffering from a deficiency of *yang*. Chinese herbalists say that recent studies of sea horses have identified certain proteins and amino acids that may help men to produce higher amounts of semen.

How to Use Chinese Prepared Medicines

There are a limited number of mail-order suppliers of Chinese herbs and prepared medicines (see "Resources"). You can also find Chinese herbs and prepared medicines in Asian pharmacies located in major cities' Chinatowns.

Herbs such as eucommia bark and horny goat weed usually come in bulk or powder form, which you can use to brew into a traditional tea.

Deer antler is usually available in pieces at Asian pharmacies; it is expensive. You can use these to brew a tea, or soak them in alcohol for several weeks to make a powerful tincture. Tablets (such as Alrodeer Pills; take four pills three times daily) and extracts (Pantocrin; use 10 to 20 drops in warm water) are also available. Deer antler is an ingredient in combination products such as Kidney Yang Qi.

Sea horse is usually sold in bulk, powder, or tablets. Prepared medicines such as Sea Horse Genital Tonic Pills are also available; an average dose of these small pills is 10 twice a day.

Especially for Women

Two of the following herbs, vitex and dong quai, are both ancient remedies long known as women's herbs for their positive effects on the female reproductive system, if not sexual desire per se. Vitex is a favorite European herb, while dong quai is a respected Chinese herb. Today women around the world are using these, as well as a third herb, wild yam, to help balance hormones and maintain optimal sexual function.

Supplement makers often include these herbs with nutrients in products specially formulated for women. Look for products with names such as Vita Gyn, For Women Only, Woman's Select, and Formula for Her.

Vitex

Vitex is derived from the small fruits of a shrub (*Vitex agnus-castus*) native to western Asia but now found throughout Europe and in the southern United States. Vitex is also known as chaste tree, chasteberry, and agnus castus (*castus* is Greek for "chaste"), reflecting some traditional people's ancient belief that this plant lowered sex drive rather than increased it. This belief was not universally accepted, though it persisted into the Middle Ages and was the reason why priests and nuns used a specially formulated vitex syrup to maintain chastity. Women have also long used vitex to treat various gynecological problems, including irregular monthly periods and the discomforts of menopause.

Vitex is still used today to treat "female complaints" such as PMS, fibroids, and excessive menstrual bleeding. Recent studies done on vitex have cast doubt on its anaphrodisiac effects while confirming that it can help to strengthen the sexual organs and glands by balancing production of the sexual hormones. "The truth is," says herbalist Rosemary Gladstar, "that vitex neither suppresses nor increases libido. It is a normalizing herb for the reproductive system."

Vitex apparently stimulates the pituitary gland in the brain to secrete luteinizing hormone, which helps control the function of the male and female sex organs. In women this leads to increased levels of the hormone progesterone, necessary for the healthy operation of the female reproductive system. Vitex can also play an important role during and after pregnancy. For example, studies suggest that it stimulates the flow of breast milk.

Vitex is safe for use over an extended period of time. Many women take it for six months or longer to effect a change in their hormonal cycle. Vitex should not be used, however, in conjunction with birth control pills.

HOW TO USE VITEX: It comes in tablets, capsules, concentrated drops, tinctures, and extracts. An average daily dosage is 500 to 1,000 mg of the dried herb in capsules or tablets, or 1 to 2 dropperfuls of the liquid extract or tincture.

Dong Quai

Also known as dang qui and tang kuei, dong quai is derived from the root of Chinese angelica (*Angelica sinensis*). It is used similarly to American and European angelica, and has long been prescribed by traditional Chinese and Indian herbalists to "harmonize vital energy," strengthen the blood, and maintain gynecological health. Dong quai has been extensively studied in China and found to nourish the reproductive system, enhance immunity, lower blood pressure, reduce pain, and improve circulation. It is often taken as a daily tonic when entering menopause or before menstruation. Dong quai's popularity has now spread to the West, where women take it to relieve gynecological problems, regulate hormones and uterine function, and alleviate menstrual cramps, PMS distress, and menopausal complaints. Herbal researchers say that dong quai encourages production of red blood cells and stimulates secretion of the natural sex hormone estrogen in the body.

Women with high blood pressure should avoid using dong quai. It is usually used during pregnancy only when clinically indicated.

How to use dong quai: It comes dried and as tablets, capsules, concentrated drops, tinctures, and extracts. An average daily dosage of the dried herb in capsules or tablets is 500 mg.

Wild Yam

This herb is derived from the long, twisting roots of various perennial species (*Dioscorea villosa, D. mexicana, D. paniculata, D. spiculiflora*) also known as rheumatism root, barbasco, and Mexican yam. The true yams are unrelated to sweet potatoes, and in North American supermarkets you'll only rarely find any yams—as a food, that is. Wild yam species are the plant source for sex hormones used in the manufacture of certain steroid products, including birth control pills and other medicines, making it one of the most widely used herbs in the world.

The Chinese have used wild yam as an herb for thousands of years. They recommend it as a liver tonic, digestive aid, and muscle relaxant. Ayurvedic practitioners also use related species of wild yam as a remedy for impotence and infertility.

The plant's ability to regulate hormone production and thus alleviate such complaints as uterine pain and menopausal discomfort has been confirmed by scientists in recent decades. In 1940 an American scientist in Mexico found that a species of wild yam was an unexpected source of sex steroids. Until then, sex steroids had been laboriously derived only from animal sources, keeping the price high and supply low. Plant chemists discovered that various other species of wild yam could be used to isolate certain saponin compounds such as diosgenin, a potent steroid chemical that could be converted in the lab into synthetic sex hormones, including testosterone and progesterone. This discovery spurred a boom in the market for synthetic hormone products that today includes such products as birth control pills and Progest, a progesterone cream.

As an herb, wild yam provides both men and women with compounds that their livers need to produce sex hormones. It has come to be more of woman's herb than a man's, however. This is because wild yam primarily produces progesterone, and it also balances the body's levels of progesterone to estrogen. Women who suffer from PMS, menopausal symptoms, and other gynecological conditions especially benefit from taking wild yam.

Wild yam is a generally safe and nontoxic herb. Many women take it on a regular basis to regulate hormone production.

HOW TO USE WILD YAM: It comes in powders, tablets, capsules, liquid drops, and extracts. An average dosage of the powdered herb is 250 to 500 mg.

Especially for Men

A number of herbs seem to have an affinity for the male sexual system, including damiana, ginseng, and ashwagandha. Siberian ginseng may help to balance hormone production. Saw palmetto, however, is the one herb most widely taken for its nourishing effects on the male reproductive and genitourinary systems.

Saw Palmetto

Saw palmetto herbal products are derived from the dark berries of a small, shrubby palm tree with swordlike, fan-shaped leaves. The plant is native to Florida, other regions of the southeastern United States, and parts of the Caribbean, where traditionally it has been used as a mild aphrodisiac and sexual rejuvenator. Saw palmetto is also known as a nutrient and tonic for the male reproductive system and the prostate gland in particular. Studies confirm that it reduces symptoms of benign prostate enlargement and has an effect on male sex hormones.

Saw palmetto has a reputation as a safe herb with few known side effects. Along with damiana, sarsaparilla, ginseng, and certain vitamins and minerals, it is also a common ingredient in herbal formulas for male sexuality. Look for products such as Male Change, Virility Two, and Maxi Pros Plus.

HOW TO USE SAW PALMETTO: It is sold as tablets, concentrated drops, extracts, and tinctures. An average dosage of the standardized berry extract is 100 to 200 mg twice daily.

Nutritional Supplements for Better Sex

Many of the vitamins and minerals play at least a minor role in some aspect of sexual function, whether it is hormone production or protection from harmful free radicals. Make sure you take adequate levels of the major nutrients and extra antioxidants (see Chapter 10). A few nutrients, such as choline and the amino acids phenylalanine, tyrosine, and histidine, can be taken on an occasional basis to temporarily boost a dormant sex drive. Others, such as vitamin E and zinc, are especially crucial to male reproduction and sexual performance.

Choline/Phosphatidylcholine/Lecithin

The vitaminlike nutrient choline, and the choline-rich substances phosphatidylcholine and lecithin, stimulate the brain to synthesize or release various neurotransmitters, particularly acetylcholine, noradrenaline, and dopamine. These neurotransmitters help to regulate bodily functions such as mood, immunity, and sex drive. Scientists say that acetylcholine, for example, can help maintain an erect penis by allowing the muscles in the arteries to relax.

High doses of choline may cause depression. You should also avoid taking choline supplements if you have gastric ulcers or Parkinson's disease, or if you are taking prescription drugs meant to block the effects of acetylcholine (atropine, diphenhydramine).

Choline is an ingredient in combination supplements such as Choline Cocktail from Twinlab. Choline Cocktail is promoted as an energy drink, but its ingredients, including 1,500 mg of choline, the compound DMAE (see Chapter 11), the herb ginkgo, vitamins E and B_{12}, and carnitine (a vitaminlike compound found in high concentrations in sperm), can also help increase sexual performance. Take it half an hour before lovemaking—though perhaps not at night, since it also contains a hefty 165 mg of caffeine, from guarana extract.

HOW TO USE CHOLINE/PHOSPHATIDYLCHOLINE/LECITHIN: Choline is available in powders, tablets, capsules, and liquids. An average daily dosage for increasing sex drive is 100 to 200 mg. Phosphatidylcholine typically comes in capsules; an average daily dosage that is 90 percent pure phosphatidylcholine is 1,100 to 2,200 mg. Lecithin comes in granules, oil-filled capsules, and liquids; an average daily dosage of lecithin that is 20 percent phosphatidylcholine is 5 to 10 g, or 1 to 2 tablespoons of granules.

Phenylalanine and Tyrosine

These amino acids serve as precursors for the neurotransmitters dopamine and noradrenaline, which play a central role in sexual performance and arousal.

Phenylalanine comes in L-, D-, and mixed (DLPA) forms. Taking L-phenylalanine also increases brain levels of the neuropeptide phenylethylamine (PEA), the chemical (also found in chocolate) that seems to be associated with feelings of romance and love. Indeed, studies have found that people who have lost interest in sex tend to have low levels of PEA. Some researchers have speculated that the well-known habit of gorging on chocolate after splitting from one's lover may be an attempt to reestablish high levels of PEA.

Phenylalanine and tyrosine may cause stimulantlike side effects, including insomnia and anxiety. They should be avoided by people with high blood pressure or phenylketonuria, a genetic disorder of phenylalanine metabolism. They should also be avoided by those who take MAO-inhibitor antidepressants.

HOW TO USE PHENYLALANINE AND TYROSINE: These amino acids typically come in capsules and powders. To boost a flagging libido, take 500 mg of L-phenylalanine or tyrosine once or twice daily for up to two to three weeks. Take with 25 to 50 mg of B-complex vitamins and 500 mg of vitamin C.

Histidine

Histidine is an amino acid that is the precursor of the neurotransmitter histamine, which is stored in nerve endings, brain cells, and elsewhere. Histamines are best known for the central role they play in allergies and immune response, causing the familiar symptoms of runny nose and sneezing. Histamines also dilate blood vessels and are released by both sexes during sexual arousal and the flush of orgasm. Since it is possible that low bodily stores of histamine can thwart sexual response, taking histidine supplements, along with niacin and vitamin

B$_6$ to promote histidine's conversion to histamine, may improve sexual function for some people.

Histidine should be avoided by anyone taking antihistamines or suffering from manic-depression. Men who take high levels of histidine may experience premature ejaculation.

This is not one of the more widely available amino acids in supplement form. If your local health-food store doesn't carry it, you can mail-order it from one of the large vitamin discounters with extensive product lines (see "Resources").

HOW TO USE HISTIDINE: An average dosage to improve sexual function is 500 mg before meals two or three times daily for two to three weeks, along with 25 to 50 mg of vitamin B complex, for the niacin and B$_6$.

Vitamin E

Vitamin E is sometimes called the virility or sex vitamin. As an antioxidant, it protects cell membranes and unsaturated fatty acids, including those found in sperm, from the harmful effects of free radicals. Vitamin E also plays an important role in the production of hormones and the formation of sperm. Some test-tube studies have demonstrated that vitamin E improves sperm's ability to fertilize eggs. Other studies have indicated that 600 to 800 IU of vitamin E daily may increase the number and motility (spontaneous motion) of sperm.

HOW TO USE VITAMIN E: Vitamin E is widely available in liquid-filled capsules. An average optimal level of supplementation to support the sexual system is 400 to 600 IU daily.

Zinc

This trace mineral is a key actor in numerous bodily functions, including male reproduction, virility, and sexual response. For various reasons, zinc is much more important to males' sexual response than to females'. Adequate zinc is necessary for hormone metabolism, sperm formation and motility, and the makeup of semen. The body requires zinc to produce testosterone; the prostate, which is normally rich in zinc, needs it to help metabolize testosterone. Semen is rich in zinc, and frequent ejaculation can deplete levels of zinc in the body. When this happens, sex drive is naturally diminished, thus allowing the body to replenish its supplies of zinc. Inadequate zinc can lead to impotence or infertility, low sperm count, and reduced libido.

Some of the foods that, according to folklore, are effective aphrodisiacs or enhance virility, such as oysters, are particularly high in zinc.

HOW TO USE ZINC: Zinc is a component in most multivitamin-multimineral tablets and is frequently combined with copper (also important for the prostate), selenium, and other minerals to prevent a deficiency in them. You can also take it in tablets, lozenges, and other forms. The adult RDA is 12 to 19 mg, and an average optimal daily intake is 17 to 25 mg.

The Love Drug

A new "smart drug," longevity aid, and antidepressant also seems to have the pleasant side effect of markedly increasing sex drive. In the United States today, it is a prescription drug, not an herb or nutrient such as the substances that make up the bulk of this book. The drug does, however, seem to be safe and to act in the body in a manner similar to the neurotransmitter-affecting amino acids, so it's included here.

Deprenyl

Also known as selegiline (Eldepryl, Jumex), deprenyl was approved for sale in the United States in 1989 after establishing itself as a remarkably effective drug for treatment of Parkinson's disease. It has since largely replaced the drug L-dopa to manage this degenerative disease of later life. Deprenyl can not only delay the onset of Parkinson's symptoms, but it can also cause marked improvements in Parkinson's patients' memory, attention span, and energy levels. Deprenyl has since shown promise as well against Alzheimer's disease, another common affliction of aging characterized by a gradual deterioration in mental and physical function.

Animal studies and research into the drug's effects on the body indicate that deprenyl may treat not only the diseases of aging but also aging itself. In the brain deprenyl acts as an antioxidant to protect brain cells from damage by free radicals. Laboratory animals that have been given deprenyl experienced significant extensions in both average and maximum life span (see Chapter 10).

Deprenyl researchers quickly noticed that enhanced sexual function among older male animals was a major indicator of the drug's ability to prolong youth. Deprenyl-treated male rats that normally would be too old to be sexually active suddenly began to fornicate like randy teenagers. While no studies on normal, healthy humans have yet focused on this apparent side effect, many men who have taken deprenyl, for Parkinson's as well as in order to increase longevity, say that it is an effective aphrodisiac. These men, chiefly over the age of 50, report that a mild boost in mood and a dramatic increase in sex drive lasts for several days after taking deprenyl.

Researchers have traced deprenyl's mood-boosting and sex-enhancing properties to its effect on certain neurotransmitters in the brain. Deprenyl is attracted to a "pleasure center" of the brain, where the neurotransmitters dopamine and noradrenaline are especially active. Drugs that increase brain levels of dopamine and noradrenaline, including certain antidepressants, the Parkinson medication L-dopa, and cocaine and amphetamine, are often noted for causing a temporary boost in libido. Continual use at high doses, however, may lead to sexual dysfunction. Incidentally, Prozac and other antidepressants (including the amino acid tryptophan) that work by boosting levels of serotonin rather than dopamine frequently have a deadening effect on sex drive.

Deprenyl is chemically related to amphetamine and to PEA, the substance found in chocolate that is associated with feelings of love. Unlike PEA, when deprenyl reaches the brain it does not directly trigger the release of neurotransmitters such as adrenaline, noradrenaline, and dopamine. Rather, deprenyl inhibits the action of the enzyme monoamine-oxidase (MAO). Since MAO breaks down neurotransmitters, substances such as deprenyl that inhibit MAO have the effect of allowing neurotransmitters to stay active longer. It so happens that MAO levels in the brain tend to rise as people grow older. By the same token, levels of certain neurotransmitters such as dopamine remain fairly stable up to age 40 or 45 but then tend to fall with increasing age. As dopamine levels fall so does the sex drive of men and possibly women. MAO inhibitors such as deprenyl allow neurotransmitter levels to remain constant, thus maintaining sex drive (as well as preventing diseases such as Parkinson's and possibly delaying aging).

Drug researchers say that deprenyl is unique among MAO inhibitors because it targets MAO-B, one of the two main types of MAO enzymes. Other MAO inhibitors, such as the antidepressant phenelzine (Nardil), work by inhibiting MAO-A. Unfortunately, inhibiting MAO-A can activate too many neurotransmitters, leading to symptoms such as nervousness. Taking MAO-A inhibitors can also cause some people to experience a dangerous side effect—a sudden rise in blood pressure—after eating certain foods (such as aged cheese) that are rich in the chemical tyramine. By inhibiting mainly MAO-B, deprenyl avoids this "cheese reaction." So far, deprenyl is the only widely prescribed MAO inhibitor that has this desirable ability to selectively inhibit MAO-B. Researchers note that deprenyl's effects on the body have not been fully explained yet, and the drug may well increase dopamine through mechanisms other than inhibition of MAO-B.

Deprenyl appears to be a nontoxic drug with a "remarkable safety record," according to Joe Graedon and Dr. Teresa Graedon, authors of *Graedons' Best Medicine*. It has not been responsible for even a single death. Research, however, is still in its infancy. Scientists have not had the opportunity to do long-term studies, and many people may wish to take a wait-and-see attitude before using it. Others feel that already enough is known about deprenyl to use it safely; indeed, since the 1950s hundreds of studies have been done on deprenyl in the United States, Canada, Europe, and elsewhere. At the low dosages recommended to boost longevity and sexual pleasure (1 to 10 mg, depending on age), deprenyl causes few side effects. At higher doses (above 10 mg daily), deprenyl has been known to cause a "speedy" feeling, anxiety, nausea, nightmares, and insomnia. Taking more than 10 mg per day may also cause deprenyl to act like other MAO inhibitors, dangerously increasing some people's blood pressure when they eat certain food. High doses thus should be accompanied by strict dietary warnings. Finally, high dosages don't improve the drug's effectiveness at promoting longevity or improving mood and sexuality. Clearly, this is another case where more is not better.

Deprenyl is most readily available in the United States as the prescription drug Eldepryl. Though doctors typically prescribe it for its FDA-approved use against Parkinson's disease (at dosages not to exceed 10 mg daily), some doctors will prescribe it for its cognitive-enhancing or antiaging effects (see "Resources" to learn how to locate doctors who will prescribe deprenyl and other "smart drugs"). Eldepryl comes in 5-mg tablets. A more useful and purer form of deprenyl is the liquid deprenyl that is being developed by a Florida company, Discovery Experimental and Development. Though Discovery has submitted liquid deprenyl to the FDA for approval, as of early 1995 it remains an unapproved drug in the United States. Liquid deprenyl is approved and available, however, without a prescription in Mexico and other foreign countries. It is legal for Americans to purchase it by mail order from these sources (see "Resources").

HOW TO USE DEPRENYL: Liquid deprenyl is more easily dispensed in small doses and thus is preferable to Eldepryl tablets (which need to be split into fifths to obtain 1-mg pieces). As a drug taken regularly to boost longevity as well as increase sex drive, scientists at Discovery recommend adjusting dosage according to age.

Age	Dosage
30–35	1 mg (one drop of the liquid) twice a week
35–40	1 mg every other day
40–45	1 mg every day
45–50	2 mg every day
50–55	3 mg every day
55–60	4 mg every day
60–65	5 mg every day
65–70	6 mg every day
70–75	8 mg every day
75–80	9 mg every day
80 and over	10 mg every day

Dosages of between 6 and 10 mg daily should be divided, with half taken in the morning and half in the early afternoon.

Scents and Sexuality

Scents and sexuality are intimately related in the animal world, from insects to mammals. Courtship and mating behaviors are often triggered by the sense of smell. Germaine Greer has noted, "The efficiency of absorption of therapeutic substances into the bloodstream by the nasal route has probably not received sufficient attention. Plant estrogens are known to exert a powerful influence upon animal behavior; the estrus [the period of female sexual excitement, or heat] of many species is triggered by the presence of plant estrogens in pasture in springtime, probably not by ingestion but by inhalation."

Many humans are also most definitely sexually aroused by smells. Indeed, it could be argued that the connection between scents and sex is the fuel that powers the multibillion-dollar worldwide perfume industry. Scientists have shown that smell receptors in the nose are linked by nerves to the limbic system, a ring-shaped area in the center of the brain. The limbic system is a primitive part of the central nervous system that, in addition to playing a role in smell, helps to regulate body functions and trigger memories and emotions. The overlapping of smell, emotions, and memories is a phenomenon that has drawn the attention of novelists as well as scientists, perhaps most notably in Marcel Proust's description in *Remembrance of Things Past* of the rich, savory, memory-evoking cupcakes known as madeleines.

More directly, scent-bearing molecules can also carry pheromones, literally "hormone-bearing" chemical substances. Many scientists believe that humans of both sexes secrete pheromones through apocrine glands at the base of underarm and genital hair. When another person's unique scent is inhaled through the nose and transmitted to the brain, it can act as an aphrodisiac or otherwise affect sexual behavior. For example, researchers at the Monell Chemical Senses Center in Philadelphia found that pheromones released from the armpits of men help regulate their partners' fertility.

The Mood-Setting Essential Oils

The subtle, sexual undertones of any particular fragrance are thus highly individual perceptions. The moods and emotions generated in one person by a fragrance may be related to the perfume of a cherished lover. What excites another person may be a smell reminiscent of the blooming gardenias outside the window of a once-secret trysting place. Try one of the essential oils mentioned below that has a reputation as sexually stimulating, but feel free to experiment with different scents and see what works for you. If used occasionally, the scent you choose can become associated with lovemaking and reinforce your sexy mood.

Some essential-oil producers now offer combination products for use in diffusers as well as massage oils that blend commonly used libido-enhancing essential oils such as Sandalwood, Ylang-ylang, and Patchouli. Look for products such as Sensuality. One of the other most popular single essential oils for creating a sexy mood is Jasmine.

Jasmine

Jasmine belongs to an olive-family genus containing hundreds of species of shrubs and vines with fragrant flowers of white, red, or yellow. The species most often cultivated for use in perfumes and aromatherapy are common jasmine (*Jasminum officinale*) and royal or Italian jasmine (*J. grandiflorum*). Though native to the Far East, jasmine is now cultivated in Europe and elsewhere, with the principal essential-oil producers being Egypt, Morocco, and India. Jasmine is widely used in perfumes, cosmetics, and some foods. The essential oil has traditionally been used to treat some skin conditions and for its mood-boosting and aphrodisiac properties.

Most people consider the exquisite fragrance of Jasmine to be an aphrodisiac that is also stimulating and uplifting to the spirit. Noted aromatherapist Robert Tisserand, author of *The Art of Aromatherapy*, says that Jasmine "produces a feeling of optimism, confidence, and euphoria. It is most useful in cases where there is apathy, indifference, or listlessness." Jasmine's voluptuous scent wafting through the bedroom has been known to spice up lovemaking.

The highest-quality Jasmine essential oil is steam-distilled from the flowers. Because the flowers yield relatively little essential oil, Jasmine is considered rare and precious, like Rose. It is also extremely expensive, costing as much or even slightly more than Rose. Typically it is sold in 1-ml or ¹/₁₆th-ounce containers. A number of producers also offer Jasmine as an "absolute," a more viscous solvent-extracted form well suited for use as a sensuous fragrance. Jasmine absolute also is considered rare and precious.

The two most popular ways to take advantage of essential oils' aphrodisiac properties are massage and vaporization. See "How to Use Essential Oils" in Chapter 2 for instructions.

Where to Start

Measuring the intervals between sexual activity in months rather than days? Try the following combination on a daily basis for a few weeks to see if it adds a spark to the dormant fire.

- One of the sexual-system balancers, such as ginseng for men and perhaps vitex for women
- Choline (100 to 200 mg; or 1,100 to 2,200 mg of phosphatidylcholine that is 90 percent pure; or 5 to 10 g, or 1 to 2 tablespoons of granules, of lecithin that is 20 percent phosphatidylcholine)
- An insurance-level multivitamin-multimineral supplement, providing not only vitamin E and zinc but also the other major nutrients, such as vitamins C and B complex, that have been shown to promote fertility

Beyond Herbs and Supplements

Some of the reasons for the common loss of sex drive that people experience as they age have to do with factors such as changing hormone levels, the debilitating effects of disease, or common drug interactions. But for many people the key to a better sex life is attitude and fitness. The best aphrodisiac, of course, is not a drug or an herb but an eager mind coupled with a rested, healthy body. Here are just a few brief suggestions for making the most of your love life at any age.

• Get plenty of exercise or regular physical activity. Compared to sedentary people, men and women who exercise regularly are more likely to say that they have active, satisfactory sex lives. Fitness may boost sexual response indirectly by elevating mood and improving self-esteem. Exercise can also have a positive impact on levels of hormones and neurotransmitters related to pleasure and sexual performance.

• Trade sensual massage with your partner. Giving and receiving a sensual massage can extend your concept of the erogenous zone from merely the genitals to the entire body. It can also transform your idea of the goal of sex from having an orgasm to stimulating the entire body.

• If busy schedules and the needs of small children seem to conspire to keep you and your partner celibate, consider setting aside a special time and place for sex, when you can be alone together and unlikely to be interrupted by phone calls or other distractions.

• Practice safe sex. Few things can turn off most sexual partners as quickly as anxiety about the long-term consequences of sex, whether these be pregnancy or sexually transmitted diseases.

• Consider psychological or partnership counseling with your lover to help recognize emotions, attitudes, or beliefs that are constraining the full expression of your sexuality.

Prevent Heart Disease

While the death rate from heart disease in the United States has gradually been falling over the past two decades, degenerative heart disease remains a major national health problem. It is still the leading cause of death in the United States and most other industrialized countries, accounting for more than one in three fatalities.

Clinical trials and population studies have identified many of the risk factors for heart disease, including critical considerations such as exercise and activity levels, smoking, and body weight. Clearly, a person who remains lean and physically fit and doesn't smoke is much less likely to suffer from heart disease than a sedentary, obese smoker. Other crucial factors include the types and amounts of dietary fat you eat, your cholesterol intake, the degree to which your blood tends to form clots, and your blood pressure. All of these are factors that can be affected by various healthful natural substances, including herbs, vitamins, and essential fatty acids.

Good and Bad Fat and Cholesterol

Fats and oils, or lipids, are compounds that the body needs for optimal function. In the body fats act as a concentrated source of energy, provide internal insulation from the cold, and serve as a cushion to protect bones and delicate internal organs from the rough-and-tumble of everyday life. Fats are also required for the delivery of such nutrients as the fat-soluble vitamins (A, D, E, and K) and the essential fatty acids. The National Academy of Sciences estimates that most people need at least 15 to 25 g of fat per day for these purposes.

A diet totally devoid of fats thus would be harmful to health. Not to worry—the average American obtains 40 percent or more of his or her calories in the form of fats, with many consuming in excess of 150 g of fat per day. The vast majority of the fats in food and stored in the body are in the form of triglycerides, so called because they are composed of three fatty acids and a glycerol molecule. Other categories of lipids include the phospholipids (necessary components of cell membranes) and the sterols, including cholesterol. Dietary fats can also be categorized according to degree of saturation, a molecular measure related to the proportion of sites on carbon atoms in the fat molecule that are occupied by hydrogen atoms. Animal fats tend to be highly saturated, while vegetable fats are more frequently polyunsaturated or monounsaturated. The American Heart Association and other public-health authorities now recommend that the percentage of calories from total fat intake should be 30 percent or lower, and that most fats should be unsaturated.

Cholesterol is a crystalline fatty alcohol that occurs naturally in the body. It is manufactured primarily by the liver from the food you eat, especially from saturated and polyunsaturated fat. How much cholesterol you have in your blood is also affected by how much preformed cholesterol you consume from animal foods. Contrary to popular perception, the amount of saturated fat you eat is usually a more important blood-cholesterol factor than your dietary cholesterol intake.

Cholesterol is a useful fat in the body, to a degree. It helps to form hormones and vitamins and serves as a necessary component in other bodily substances such as bile acid, which is necessary for the digestion of fatty foods. When serum cholesterol levels or blood triglyceride levels get too high, however, bad things start to happen to your heart and circulatory system. Excess cholesterol and triglycerides promote the accumulation of fatty deposits on the inner linings of the blood vessels, leading to a narrowing of the arteries (atherosclerosis) and an increased risk of heart attack or heart failure.

While total blood cholesterol (as measured in milligrams of cholesterol per deciliter of blood, or mg/dl) is important, an equally crucial factor is the relative levels of the different types of cholesterol. Cholesterol is carried around in the blood attached to proteins. The primary lipoproteins are the low-density lipoproteins (LDLs) and the high-density lipoproteins (HDLs). The HDLs are cholesterol removers. They collect cholesterol from artery linings and elsewhere and transport it to the liver. The liver metabolizes the cholesterol and sends it on its way, to be excreted eventually from the body. The LDLs, on the other hand, are cholesterol deliverers. They distribute the cholesterol to muscle and other bodily tissues, where an excess of cholesterol can have adverse effects.

Hundreds of scientific studies over the past few decades have confirmed that both a high total cholesterol level as well as a high level of LDL cholesterol relative to HDL cholesterol dramatically increase the risk of heart disease. If your total blood-cholesterol level is greater than 256 mg/dl (as is the case for some 40 to 50 million Americans), your risk of developing heart disease is five times greater than if it was below 220, approximately the American average. In general, if you lower your LDL level by 10 percent, you decrease your heart attack risk by 20 percent or more. Also, if you increase your HDL level by 10 percent, you decrease your heart attack risk by an even greater degree, often 30 to 40 percent.

The relative benefit of lowering cholesterol for those with levels that are already below average is more controversial, with some studies showing little net benefit. Other research, including some recent large-scale studies such as a study of over 9,000 Chinese men and women ages 35 to 64, indicates that even if your total cholesterol level is below 220, you can gain protection against future heart disease by relatively small reductions in overall cholesterol. It is fair to say that both conventional medical doctors and practitioners of natural medicine have in recent years begun to recognize that cholesterol has been somewhat overemphasized as an overall risk factor for heart disease.

New kits available from pharmacies and mail-order catalogs now make it easy to test your total cholesterol level at home. You need to draw a few drops of blood from a fingertip. The blood is placed in a little well on the testing device, and in 10 to 15 minutes a reading is available. (Critics point out that because the home kits tell you only total cholesterol, not HDL and LDL levels, they are of limited diagnostic use.) A single-use, disposable test runs about $20 to $25. Whether you test at home or at a clinic, be wary of relying on any single test result, since error rates in labs vary considerably, and results can be affected by factors such as recent stress.

Many medical doctors and their patients still rely on conventional drug therapy to lower cholesterol levels, even though dietary and lifestyle changes and natural supplements are safer and more effective. The most widely prescribed cholesterol-lowering drug in America is lovastatin, which works by inhibiting an enzyme required by the liver to produce cholesterol. The pharmaceutical producer Merck, which promotes its brand of lovastatin (Mevacor) in weekly news magazines as well as medical journals, states that the drug "is indicated as an addition to diet for many patients with high cholesterol when diet and exercise are inadequate." (The number of Mevacor users who do actually seriously attempt to lower their cholesterol levels with diet and exercise is open to debate.) Side effects include nausea, headache, weakness, muscle damage and pain, and blurred vision. Doctors recommend frequent liver-enzyme tests to monitor patients for liver damage.

Another popular cholesterol-lowering drug is cholestyramine (Questran), which works by reducing the amount of bile in circulation, thus promoting the liver's conversion of cholesterol into bile and in turn reducing the level of circulating cholesterol. Among the possible side effects of this drug are constipation, muscle pain, shortness of breath, and vitamin deficiencies.

Cholesterol-lowering drugs are expensive and of dubious long-term safety. Their track record in general has been less than inspiring, with some of them actually increasing the death rate from heart disease and other conditions. The authors of a study published in the *British Medical Journal* in 1992 said that the failure of cholesterol-lowering drugs to actually reduce mortality is cause for a moratorium on their use.

In Search of Teflon-Coated Platelets

Platelets are small, sticky blood particles that play a major role in how blood clots form. When you eat a high-fat, high-cholesterol diet, platelets can get more sticky. This increases their tendency to clump, or aggregate. This is a useful or even life-saving process when you have a cut and need blood clots to form to stop the bleeding. On the other hand, overly sticky platelets flowing through your blood vessels can lead to health problems.

When platelets form a blood clot within an intact blood vessel, the process is known as thrombosis. Thrombosis often occurs when sticky platelets encounter a rough area or lesion on the inside wall of an otherwise intact blood vessel. This encourages the buildup of a fatty, cholesterol-containing substance known as atheroma. Atheroma that sticks to the inside of blood-vessel walls and accumulates in raised patches is called plaque. Over time, this plaque buildup becomes harmful or even life-threatening. The inside passageway of the artery becomes increasingly narrow, preventing oxygen-carrying blood from adequately nourishing tissues. When the damaged arteries and tissues in question are those of the heart, you've got atherosclerosis. If a blood clot then comes along that is big enough to block the entire passageway, the result is a heart attack. Plaque buildup that interferes with the blood supply to the brain can lead to strokes, another leading cause of death in the United States.

Reducing the tendency of platelets to stick together thus can markedly reduce the risk of heart disease and heart attack. That is the thinking behind the recent recommendations from medical doctors that people should take low dosages of aspirin every day. Aspirin thins the blood by lowering platelet stickiness. A number of natural substances can also help reduce the risk of heart disease through their beneficial effects on platelet stickiness, often without the potential side effects of prolonged aspirin intake (such as an increased risk of peptic ulcer and stomach bleeding).

Platelet aggregation inhibitors should be avoided if you are taking anticlotting drugs, experience prolonged bleeding from cuts, or are planning surgery.

Toward Better Blood Pressure

An estimated 40 to 60 million Americans have some degree of elevated blood pressure, a condition that results when blood that is pumped from the heart exerts a higher-than-normal force on the inside walls of arteries. Also known as hypertension, high blood pressure is insidious in that its short-term symptoms are unremarkable (fatigue, headache), yet its long-term effects can be devastating: It significantly increases the risk of heart attack, stroke, and kidney failure. It is also insidious because medical authorities say that in nine out of ten cases of hypertension, the direct cause is unknown. (Some obvious causes include cancer, kidney and adrenal disorders, and certain drugs.)

The lack of specific knowledge about the cause of most high blood pressure does not mean that little is known about the conditions that are *associated* with it. On the contrary, recent research has established that a half-dozen or so factors are closely allied with high blood pressure. These include:

Obesity. Losing excess weight is among the most effective ways to lower blood pressure.

Excessive consumption of alcohol, caffeine, and refined sugar, accompanied by a low intake of fiber. Eating more fiber-rich whole foods, such as grains, beans, fresh vegetables, and fruit, is beneficial for hypertensives.

High intake of saturated fats. Regular use of monounsaturated oils such as olive oil may lower blood pressure, according to a joint U.S.-Italian study of almost five thousand men and women. Also, vegetarians and others who eat few animal fats typically have lower-than-average blood pressure.

Smoking. Overcoming an addiction to nicotine typically lowers blood pressure.

Unbalanced sodium and potassium consumption. Those who can reduce their intake of sodium compounds, including table salt, while increasing their consumption of potassium are likely to reduce their high blood pressure.

Prolonged exposure to high levels of stress. Using techniques such as meditation or biofeedback to reduce the worst effects of severe mental stress is an effective step in controlling blood pressure.

Inactivity. Being in good physical shape helps to keep blood pressure down.

The above factors are the main evidence that hypertension is primarily a disease of industrialized society. The good news is that the vast majority of people with high blood pressure who do address these diet and lifestyle factors will significantly reduce not only their blood pressure but also their risk of a whole host of killer diseases, from heart disease to cancer.

The blood-pressure norm for American adults is often considered to be 120 over 80 (120/80). The 120 refers to the pressure within arteries when the heart is contracting to pump the blood; the technical name is systolic blood pressure. The 80 refers to the pressure when the heart is resting between beats; doctors refer to it as the diastolic pressure. Because early blood-pressure gauges used mercury in a glass column to measure blood pressure, the figures are still expressed as millimeters of mercury (mm Hg). As a general rule, repeated readings in excess of 140/90 indicate a need to reduce blood pressure. Multiple readings are recommended because body position, recent exercise, time of day, and even nervousness from having your blood pressure taken can significantly affect the results. Doctors estimate that roughly 80 percent of those with the condition suffer from "mild" or so-called Stage 1 hypertension.

Readings of 160/115 or higher indicate severe high blood pressure and usually call for immediate medical attention and, frequently, prescription drugs. Check with your medical practitioner about using natural methods for lowering blood pressure in conjunction with conventional approaches. Also check with your doctor before attempting to reduce or discontinue any conventional drug therapy.

Because so many people find it difficult to make the necessary adjustments to their diet and lifestyle, drugs remain a major tool for treating high blood pressure. The hypotensive (blood-pressure-lowering) prescription drugs are now a significant category, representing substantial market shares for the pharmaceutical companies. Not only do doctors write a lot of prescriptions, but they also often need to use multiple drugs in conjunction with each other. Among the most commonly used drugs for high blood pressure are diuretics such as furosemide (Lasix). Diuretics make you urinate more frequently, draining your body of fluids and thus lowering pressure inside the arteries. Doctors also turn to different types of drugs to increase the diameter of blood vessels, such as diltiazem (Cardizem) and captopril (Capoten). The beta-blockers, such as propranolol (Inderal), lower blood pressure by reducing the force and rate of the heart's pumping action.

Each of these drugs comes with its own set of potential side effects, some of them serious. Side effects may also result when diuretics are combined with drugs that open blood vessels, which they often are. Some of the more frequently encountered side effects include drowsiness, dry mouth, fatigue, dizziness, headache, nausea, impotence, constipation, and depression. Some side effects, such as an increased cholesterol level, directly counteract the drugs' presumed benefit of lowering your risk of heart disease. Finally, as naturopath Michael Murray points out, "The two most definitive trials . . . have shown the drugs offer no benefit in protecting against heart disease in borderline-to-moderate hypertension."

In combination with dietary and lifestyle changes, the following natural substances offer a safe and effective way to attain optimal levels of blood triglycerides and cholesterol, platelet stickiness, and blood pressure. For starters, we'll look at a few of the herbs and nutritional substances that have the most wide-ranging effects on the cardiovascular system and the most dramatic benefits.

The All-Purpose Natural Substances for the Heart

Two sets of natural substances, the allium family of plants (principally garlic) and the essential fatty acids, deserve to be ranked ahead of all the other herbs and nutrients with beneficial effects on the heart.

Garlic

Garlic's reputation as one of the best herbs for the heart rests on a solid foundation. Not only have studies shown that garlic can lower blood levels of both total cholesterol and triglycerides, but garlic can also have a positive impact on blood pressure and platelet stickiness. Moreover, Japanese researchers recently identified components of garlic extract with considerable antioxidant properties, and American researchers have found that garlic does indeed significantly reduce the susceptibility of fats in the blood to oxidation. (This process, called lipid peroxidation, can have harmful effects on heart function.) What all this means is that regular consumption of garlic can dramatically reduce your risk of atherosclerosis and heart attack.

Numerous studies have demonstrated that members of the *Allium* genus, including garlic and onion, can reduce harmful LDL and raise beneficial HDL cholesterol. A noted population study on the alliums' effects on heart disease was done in India in the late 1970s. Researchers tested the blood cholesterol and triglyceride levels of members of the Jain community, who follow nearly identical vegetarian diets except for the amount of garlic and onion they consume. Researchers compared the cholesterol and triglyceride levels of three Jain populations: those who were heavy garlic and onion eaters (50 g per week of garlic and 600 g per week of onions); moderate garlic and onion eaters (10 and 200 g per week, respectively); and those who ate no garlic or onions. The scientists found that heavy garlic eaters averaged cholesterol and triglyceride levels of 159 and 52, respectively, while the corresponding scores for those with moderate allium consumption were 172 and 75, and for non–garlic-eaters 208 and 109.

Double-blind, placebo-controlled scientific studies have also found that garlic consumption more in line with Western norms for supplementation (the equivalent of one-half to one fresh clove per day) can also have significant effects on triglycerides and total cholesterol. For example, a Tulane University study in which subjects took 900 mg daily of standardized garlic tablets found a 6 percent reduction in total cholesterol over twelve weeks. A recent German study of over eight thousand subjects with cholesterol levels ranging from 221 to 230 attributed a 3 percent reduction to taking 600 mg of standardized garlic powder per day. Total cholesterol reductions in the 8-to-10-percent range would not be unexpected among those who consume between 2,500 and 5,000 mg of fresh garlic equivalent per day (approximately equal to eating one to two cloves of fresh garlic).

Studies done in Germany and elsewhere indicate that when garlic or onions are eaten with a fatty meal, blood platelets are less sticky afterward. Some researchers have found garlic to be equal to or more potent than aspirin as an inhibitor of platelet aggregation. Mirroring its effects on blood cholesterol and triglyceride levels, higher doses of garlic have a greater effect against platelet stickiness. Consuming 2,500 to 5,000 mg of fresh garlic equivalent per day, however, is enough to significantly reduce the likelihood that blood clots will form on damaged blood-vessel walls.

Garlic's ability to prevent excess platelet stickiness has been traced to its principal medicinal compound, allicin, and its breakdown products, such as ajoene. Researchers also recently isolated a potent member of the prostaglandin series from onions, marking the first time a plant has been identified as a prostaglandin source.

Garlic's benefits to the heart and circulation likely extend to include prevention and treatment of high blood pressure, according to human and animal studies. A number of European researchers found that people with high blood pressure who took moderately high doses of garlic (the equivalent of two or three cloves daily) experienced significant drops of 10 percent or more in overall blood pressure or diastolic blood pressure within three months. Because hypertensive patients have been shown to have low blood levels of certain amino acids that contain sulfur, some researchers speculate that garlic's beneficial effects may be due to its sulfur-containing compounds.

Even if you don't need to consume large amounts of garlic daily for therapeutic effects, you can benefit your heart by incorporating more garlic and onions into your diet. (Keep in mind that the heat from cooking inactivates garlic's enzymes and significantly reduces its medicinal effects.) For many people, taking daily doses of garlic supplements is the best way to help prevent heart disease.

HOW TO USE GARLIC: Garlic supplements come in a wide variety of powders, liquids, tablets, and capsules. Many are standardized for allicin content or fresh garlic equivalent. For better cardiovascular health, take 600 to 1,000 mg of pure or concentrated garlic or garlic extract powder, or 1,800 to 3,000 mg of fresh garlic equivalent. An average recommended dosage for allicin is 1,800 to 3,600 mcg per day.

Essential Fatty Acids

Nutritional scientists were faced with a mystery when they pondered the eating habits of the Inuit and other native peoples of the polar regions. The daily diet for an average Inuit was made up to a great extent of fatty cold-water fish and marine mammals. All of the reigning models of heart disease pointed to fatty diets increasing the risk of atherosclerosis. Yet the Inuit had extremely low rates of heart disease. Numerous studies over the past two decades have solved the mystery. A diet high in saturated animal fats definitely does increase the risk of heart disease. But diets rich in certain types of polyunsaturated fats containing what are now called the essential fatty acids, such as those found in large amounts in the Inuit diet, are actually strongly protective against heart disease.

Both the omega-3 and the omega-6 EFAs can affect cardiovascular function through their action on prostaglandins, various series of fatty acids naturally produced in the body. Prostaglandins have hormonelike actions that help to regulate diverse bodily processes, including cholesterol and triglyceride levels, platelet aggregation, blood pressure, and fluid balance.

Numerous studies have now established that diets lacking in EFAs are characterized by elevated total cholesterol and increased platelet stickiness. Researchers have repeatedly found that regular consumption of eicosapentaenoic acid (EPA) and docosahexaenoic acid (DHA), both omega-3 fatty acids, tends to raise HDL cholesterol and reduce triglyceride levels. Though the omega-6's have not been as widely tested as the omega-3's, there is also some evidence that gamma linolenic acid (GLA) lowers total cholesterol levels. Some studies have also shown that eating fish or taking EFA supplements can reduce platelet stickiness. A diet rich in EFAs, including plant-based GLA, helps to promote the formation of certain prostaglandins that have antiaggregative effects and to decrease levels of prostaglandins that encourage aggregation.

A recent placebo-controlled study of patients with angina pectoris (chest pains due to loss of blood supply to the heart) found that fish-oil supplements significantly reduced the number of attacks. The supplements also increased exercise tolerance and reduced blood fat levels.

High blood pressure is another symptom of a deficiency in essential fatty acids. A number of well-controlled studies have found that consuming cold-water fish or EFA supplements can reduce blood pressure in people suffering from hypertension. Though fewer in number, there are also some studies documenting a beneficial effect on blood pressure from the plant-derived omega-6 fatty acids, such as GLA. For example, a study of animals with stress-induced hypertension found that GLA was effective at lowering blood pressure. The omega-3 and omega-6 EFAs promote the widening of blood vessels and a reduction in blood pressure through their action on prostaglandins.

People who are taking anticoagulant drugs, or who have diabetes or a tendency to bleed, should check with a physician before taking essential fatty acid supplements.

See Chapter 2 for more information on types and sources of essential fatty acids.

HOW TO USE ESSENTIAL FATTY ACIDS: They are typically sold as liquids or oil-filled capsules (supplements may need to be refrigerated). An average daily dosage of fish-oil or plant-oil capsules to help prevent heart disease is 500 to 1,000 mg.

The Polyphenols and Flavonoids

This large class of plant constituents may play an important role in preventing heart disease. Flavonoids have been shown to help heal and strengthen capillaries and to lower overall cholesterol. Researchers have determined that many flavonoids can help prevent aggregation of platelets.

For example, a 1993 Dutch study reported in *The Lancet* examined the impact of overall flavonoid intake in over 800 elderly men. The researchers found that subjects who consumed the greatest amounts of flavonoids (primarily from tea, as it turned out, rather than fruits or other herbs) had a much lower risk of cardiovascular disease than those who consumed the least amounts. The benefits were still clear even after taking into account other known cardiovascular risk factors, such as weight, smoking, and blood pressure.

Bioflavonoid complex, and bioflavonoids in combination with vitamin C and other supplements, are typically found in tablet and capsule form. An average daily dose of the complex is 500 to 1,000 mg; of quercetin and rutin, 200 to 500 mg.

Some of the healthy-heart herbs rich in flavonoids include ginkgo, bilberry, European coastal pine, hawthorn, green tea, and red wine/grapes.

Ginkgo. In human and rabbit studies, ginkgo has been shown to counteract the platelet-aggregative effects of the bodily substance known as platelet-activating factor (PAF), notes herbal researcher Steven Foster. An average dosage of ginkgo is 40 mg three times daily of a standardized extract containing a minimum of 24 percent flavoglycosides.

Bilberry. An Italian study of anthocyanidins indicates that bilberry can lower blood cholesterol and triglyceride levels. An average dosage of an encapsulated extract product standardized for 20 to 25 percent anthocyanoside is 80 to 160 mg three times daily.

European coastal pine. The flavonoids in this tree extract are used to make Pycnogenol, a trademarked product that strengthens blood vessels and may reduce the risk of heart disease. An average daily dosage of Pycnogenol is 50 to 100 mg.

Hawthorn. Hawthorn deserves special attention because its traditional use for heart ailments has been confirmed by numerous studies in recent years. The plant is a rich source of polyphenols, including quercetin, vitexin, and catechin. Researchers have found that hawthorn can lower serum cholesterol, reduce blood pressure, and prevent palpitations (rapid heartbeat) and arrhythmias (irregular heartbeat). Some of these effects are due to its ability to dilate major blood vessels, including those in the heart, and increase the heart's pumping force. The herb is also a mild diuretic. Some studies indicate that hawthorn can actually help reverse atherosclerosis by reducing existing plaque deposits.

In Germany and other parts of Europe, hawthorn berry extract is used to make popular heart remedies, both OTC and prescription-strength. Most herbalists say that hawthorn needs to be taken for an extended period of time and that its actions are cumulative. Though hawthorn is relatively nontoxic and causes few side effects even at large doses, natural practitioners warn against using it after self-diagnosing some kind of existing heart problem. It shouldn't be taken along with the heart drug digitalis except with the approval of your physician. Some people take low dosages of hawthorn as a daily heart tonic, such as 250 to 500 mg of the dried powder, or 100 to 200 mg of encapsulated powder standardized to 1.8 percent vitexin.

Green Tea

Green tea's ability to inhibit aggregation of platelets and decrease arterial cholesterol helps protect the heart. The flavonoid catechin's effects in this regard have been compared to aspirin's, though catechin action may actually surpass aspirin action because catechin also inhibits the production of PAF. A noncatechin compound in green tea has also been shown to inhibit an agent in the body (thromboxane) that promotes platelet stickiness. A study of some six thousand Japanese women found a 50 percent reduction in the risk of stroke among those who drank five or more cups of green tea per day. An Israeli study of five thousand tea drinkers and a Japanese study using lab animals also indicate that green tea extracts can help lower cholesterol levels and possibly reduce high blood pressure.

Green tea that is brewed for only 2 or 3 minutes has moderate levels of caffeine (20 to 30 mg per cup) and a subtle, delicate flavor. Green-tea extract capsules are quickly coming onto the market; look for products such as Polyphenols 60, Green Tea-Power, and Preventin. Some green tea supplement manufacturers add extra caffeine and promote the product as "energizing."

If you brew green tea, don't drink it scalding hot, which may eliminate its benefits.

HOW TO USE GREEN TEA: It is predominantly available in teas and capsules. An average daily dose to obtain 50 to 100 mg of polyphenols is 3 to 5 cups of tea. Dosages of capsules depend upon polyphenol content, which may range from 15 to 50 percent. An average daily dose of the capsules standardized for 15 percent polyphenols is 300 to 600 mg; of the capsules standardized for 50 percent polyphenols, 100 to 200 mg.

Red Wine/Grapes

How is it that the French die from heart disease at a much lower rate than do Americans, yet eat a diet that often includes more cheese, butter, and other foods high in saturated fat? Since this so-called French paradox was pointed out by researchers in a study published in *The Lancet* in 1979, some nutritionists have tried to resolve the mystery by noting that the French drink considerably more wine than Americans. Those areas in France that drink the most wine, moreover, have lower heart disease rates than the teetotaling parts of France. Because alcohol is potentially relaxing and stress-relieving, and drinking it in low to moderate amounts tends to increase blood levels of the good HDL cholesterol, many health authorities assumed that alcohol itself could account for the observed reduction in heart disease—even though the authors of the 1979 *Lancet* study said that if wine does have a protective effect, "it is more likely to be due to constituents other than alcohol."

New findings may have begun to confirm these early suspicions that alcohol is not responsible for all of the presumed benefits. A team of researchers from the University of Wisconsin recently completed a study using blood tests on volunteers and found that red, but not white, wine substantially reduces the tendency of blood to clot. The findings have been corroborated in studies on dogs.

The researchers believe that the polyphenol and flavonoid compounds in red wine (particularly from the grape skins and seeds) may be the most beneficial agents, rather than the alcohol itself. The flavonoid quercetin in particular seems to mimic aspirin's ability to prevent clots from sticking to fatty buildups on artery walls. Flavonoids in grapes and wine also include the catechins, proanthocyanidins, and anthocyanidins. Young red wines have higher flavonoid contents than older wines; white wines have very low levels.

In the past few years the first red-wine supplements appeared on the American market. Others will surely follow if research continues to support the potential benefits of grape compounds. Look for products such as French Parad'ox and Wine & Tea Polyphenols. Grape-seed extract products are also starting to become available. Look for products standardized to deliver 50 to 100 mg of polyphenols.

HOW TO USE RED WINE/GRAPES: Red wine can be drunk as an alcoholic beverage, and the various extracts can be found as liquids or in capsules. An average daily dosage of the red wine extract capsules standardized to provide 40 to 60 mg of polyphenols (the approximate flavonoid content of two glasses of red wine) is 250 mg.

Herbal Heart Tonics

Garlic, essential fatty acids, and the aforementioned herbs rich in polyphenols all have wide-ranging beneficial effects on the cardiovascular system. Some herbs and nutritional substances seem to have more limited therapeutic actions but are still worth considering as part of an overall healthy-heart program. For example, deserving special mention in the battle against platelet stickiness and elevated cholesterol levels are guggul, ginger, fo-ti, and ginseng.

Guggul

Guggul products are derived from the resin of the small, thorny mukul tree (*Commiphora mukul*) of India's semiarid plains. Mukuls are related to the tree (*Commiphora molmol*) whose bark is the source for another gummy substance with healing properties, myrrh. Guggul gum is used to produce standardized or purified extracts called gugulipids. Heart drugs based on guggul extracts are sold in India, where almost all of the research on guggul has been done.

The studies indicate that guggul extracts can have dramatic effects on heart disease risk factors, with reductions in both triglycerides and total cholesterol of between 15 and 30 percent over three months. Guggul extracts reduce LDL cholesterol while raising HDL cholesterol. Some herbal authorities say that guggul extracts compare favorably with natural substances such as garlic and with conventional prescription drugs for lowering lipids in the blood. If it is also true, as preliminary studies indicate, that guggul extracts can reduce platelet stickiness, this herb would rank among the most important, since few substances have a positive impact on both blood fats and platelets.

Indian researchers report that guggul is safe to take even during pregnancy and in high doses. No side effects were noticed in one study that administered 4 to 5 g, an amount that is much higher than the average recommended daily dose.

Guggul is a new herb on the North American market. Most products available are capsules or tablets standardized for gugulipids, or for gugulipids' steroid compounds, the guggulsterones. The potency used in most of the studies is 25 mg guggulsterones per tablet. Look for products such as Gugulmax and Maximum Guggulsterones.

How to use guggul: An average daily dosage is 25 mg of guggulsterones two or three times daily.

Ginger

Ginger is most widely known as a digestive stimulant and nausea remedy, but it has also drawn attention recently for its ability to act as a heart tonic. A study published in the *New England Journal of Medicine* in 1980 found that ginger can help reduce cholesterol levels, possibly by limiting the amount of cholesterol the blood absorbs. Other researchers have found that, like green tea, ginger may inhibit thromboxane and thus help reduce platelet stickiness, possibly even rivaling the effects of such better-known clot-preventers as aspirin and garlic. Ginger's effect on blood pressure is unclear, though some researchers have found that the herb can lower it.

It is nontoxic and safe to take in large doses.

How to use ginger: It comes fresh or dried and in tablets, capsules, concentrated drops, tinctures, and extracts. An average daily dosage as a heart tonic is 500 mg of the dried herb, or 1 to 2 dropperfuls of tincture or concentrated drops.

Fo-ti

This popular Chinese tonic herb is often taken to promote longevity and overall health. Modern practitioners of traditional Chinese medicine also use it to treat dizziness, anemia, and elevated blood cholesterol. Laboratory studies done in China have confirmed fo-ti's ability to reduce cholesterol levels and prevent plaque formation. Fo-ti contains lecithin, a fatty compound that may partially account for the herb's effects. There is some evidence that the lecithin components choline and phosphatidylcholine can play a role in reducing blood-fat levels.

To lower cholesterol, researchers in China have administered relatively large doses of fo-ti (which they call *he shou wu*)—2 to 3 g three times daily of an extract-and-powder mix for up to six weeks. Whether there is a noticeable cardiovascular effect from taking much lower, tonic levels of fo-ti on an ongoing basis is unknown, but fo-ti is safe and nontoxic at such lower doses.

HOW TO USE FO-TI: It is sold dried and as powders, tablets, capsules, concentrated drops, tinctures, and extracts. An average recommended tonic dosage of the concentrated drops is ½ to 1 dropperful two or three times daily.

Ginseng

Ginseng is most widely used as a performance enhancer (see Chapter 4), stimulant (see Chapter 5), and sexual-system strengthener (see Chapter 7), but some studies on both animals and humans indicate saponins and other ginseng constituents also have a healthful effect on cholesterol levels and platelets. That is, ginseng helps in the transport and metabolism of cholesterol, thus lowering total cholesterol, decreasing LDL, and increasing HDL. Ginseng may also reduce platelet stickiness. Its effect on blood pressure is more unpredictable—in some cases it is normalizing, but in others it can cause an unwanted increase in blood pressure.

HOW TO USE GINSENG: It is sold as a whole root or powdered, and in capsules, tablets, tea bags, tinctures, and extracts. An average daily dosage for use as a heart tonic is 250 to 500 mg of capsules standardized for 5 to 9 percent ginsenoside. An average daily dosage of some concentrated extracts and ginseng products with higher standardized percentages may be as low as 100 to 200 mg.

Other Supplements for a Healthy Heart

There is also some preliminary evidence that a number of other nutrients can help reduce the risk factors of heart disease. For example, magnesium (an average optimal daily dose is 450 to 650 mg) and vitamin B_6 (consume as part of a daily dose of 50 to 100 mg of vitamin B complex) may help to inhibit platelet aggregation and reduce the likelihood of harmful blood clots. Vitamin B_6 is especially promising as an agent for preventing some forms of heart disease because of pyridoxine's ability to prevent an accumulation of homocysteine in the blood. Homocysteine is an amino acid that numerous studies have tied to an increase risk of atherosclerosis and stroke. According to a study published in early 1995 in the *New England Journal of Medicine,* when only 2 mg of B_6 was combined with 400 mcg of folic acid and 10 to 20 mcg of B_{12}, it reduced high blood levels of homocysteine and the risk of clogged neck arteries.

Two other natural substances that can improve cholesterol profiles are activated charcoal and niacin. Because they are typically used therapeutically to lower high cholesterol levels, we'll focus here on some other nutrients for everyday preventive use, including vitamin C, carnitine, chromium, and fiber.

Activated charcoal. This is pure carbon processed in a special way to make it highly absorbent of particles and gases in the body's digestive system. Activated charcoal slides through the intestines without itself being absorbed. It is taken internally to relieve gas pains, reduce flatulence, and absorb and excrete from the body poisons and other toxins (see Chapter 16). High dosages (25 to 50 g daily) of it for months at a time may lower blood cholesterol and blood fat levels, according to some preliminary research. The reductions can be significant, including up to a 40 percent drop in harmful LDL. Taking such high dosages, however, requires supervision, because activated charcoal can also bind with and eliminate medications and nutrients.

Niacin. This B-complex vitamin (B_3) helps the body produce energy, metabolize fats and carbohydrates, and manufacture fatty acids as well as sex and adrenal hormones. Deficiency causes pellagra, characterized by rough, cracked skin and diarrhea. Niacin is found in high amounts in brewer's yeast, peanuts and other legumes, sesame seeds, whole grains, fish, and meats. Therapeutically it is used in the treatment of schizophrenia, arthritis, and lack of blood circulation to the extremities. Perhaps its most promising therapeutic role is as an effective, inexpensive treatment for elevated blood cholesterol.

Numerous studies have established that large doses (2 to 3 grams daily) of niacin are effective at lowering total blood cholesterol, reducing LDL, and increasing HDL. The effect is quick (within a few weeks), dramatic (a 30 percent or higher increase in HDL), and long-lasting. Large, druglike doses of niacin, however, can cause side effects. These include the warm skin flush on the face and neck that most people notice from doses in excess of 50 to 100 mg at a time, as well as nausea, fatigue, and digestive problems. Niacin comes in various forms, including "flush-free" or "sustained-release" niacin, but megadoses of some of these won't lower cholesterol, while others can apparently increase the risk of toxicity to the liver. If you want to try niacin to lower your high cholesterol levels, arrange for monitoring by a physician or other health practitioner.

Vitamin C

A number of studies have found an association between blood levels of vitamin C and cholesterol. That is, people with high serum levels of vitamin C tend to have high blood levels of the good HDL cholesterol. The studies, however, that have attempted to confirm the next step— that supplementing with C actually lowers total cholesterol or raises HDL levels—have had mixed results. Some confirm this direct effect while others don't, suggesting that higher vitamin C consumption may accompany other factors (such as increased exercise) that cloud the cause-and-effect scenario. The research does suggest that even very moderate daily consumption of vitamin C (200 mg) is associated with higher levels of HDL compared to those who eat a low-C diet. Vitamin C's apparent beneficial effects may be due to its action as an antioxidant that protects HDL from harmful free radicals.

A study on hypertensive males in their thirties indicated that vitamin C may be an important factor in blood pressure. Those men with the lowest blood levels of vitamin C had the highest blood pressure readings. In another study researchers at Tufts University found that high intakes of vitamin C can reduce systolic blood pressure by up to 11 percent. More studies are necessary to confirm vitamin C's role in blood pressure, but consuming an optimal level of the vitamin cannot hurt.

HOW TO USE VITAMIN C: It comes in powders, tablets, capsules, and other forms. An average daily dosage for optimal heart health is 250 to 500 mg two or three times daily.

Coenzyme Q10

This vitaminlike compound with an affinity for the cardiovascular system has shown promise in the treatment and prevention of angina pectoris, cardiomyopathy (a type of heart failure often due to an enlarged heart or to reduced blood flow), arrhythmia, and other forms of heart disease. The conventional treatment for some of these heart conditions is difficult and expensive. For example, many patients with cardiomyopathy end up waiting years for a heart transplant. In many cases coenzyme Q10 offers a safe, inexpensive, and effective natural treatment for heart ailments. Among the common effects heart patients notice from taking coQ10 supplements are enhanced pumping action, more regular heartbeat, and increased exercise tolerance.

CoQ10 is an antioxidant and an essential nutrient for the heart. In humans coQ10 concentrates in the heart muscle, where it is needed in large quantities to help cells produce the energy needed to keep the heart beating. Studies of patients with heart disease have confirmed that many of them suffer from a deficiency of coQ10. Some conventional drugs taken to lower cholesterol have also been shown to have an adverse effect on coQ10 levels.

American cardiologists are just beginning to recognize coQ10 as a potentially useful therapeutic agent, although many still remain unaware of it. Critics of coQ10 contend that there is insufficient evidence for it in the form of large, controlled clinical trials, yet there have been dozens of studies that have shown benefit to heart patients from taking coQ10. For example, out of some 1,100 subjects with heart failure tested by Italian researchers in a recent study, 80 percent improved from supplementing their diet with coQ10. The nutrient has also been the focus of more than a half-dozen international medical symposia in recent years.

CoQ10 also reduces hypertension. One ten-week, placebo-controlled study done on hypertensive patients found that coQ10 could reduce systolic and diastolic pressure. Researchers say that coQ10 apparently has a beneficial effect on the function of blood vessels' walls. A typical therapeutic dose to lower high blood pressure is 30 mg three times daily.

Heart patients often take a coQ10 dose of 120 to 360 mg per day. Though a totally safe and nontoxic dose, it should be emphasized again that self-diagnosis and self-treatment of heart problems is not recommended.

How to use coenzyme q10: Coenzyme Q10 comes in capsules

ranging in size from 10 to 100 mg. An average daily dosage for optimal heart health and to prevent a coQ10 deficiency is 15 to 30 mg daily.

Vitamin E

One of the symptoms of vitamin E deficiency is thought to be increased platelet aggregation. A number of studies that have looked at people at high risk for developing blood clots (such as women taking birth control pills) have found that increased vitamin E consumption can decrease platelet stickiness and thus reduce the risk of heart disease. Vitamin E's antioxidant action is thought to protect prostaglandins that have antiaggregative effects. In addition, a recent double-blind study that tested a form of vitamin E called tocotrienol found that it caused a decrease of 15 to 22 percent in cholesterol levels after four weeks. Another recent pair of studies done by researchers at Harvard University found that people who take at least 100 mg of vitamin E daily (a level well below average supplementation) have up to 40 percent less heart disease than those who get less vitamin E.

HOW TO USE VITAMIN E: It comes in liquids and oil-filled capsules. An average daily dosage to help protect against platelet aggregation and high cholesterol is 400 to 600 IU.

Carnitine

Like coenzyme Q10, carnitine is a vitaminlike compound naturally present in the body (stored in muscle tissue) and essential to the functioning of the heart. Carnitine deficiency may result from excessive exercise, illness, and insufficient dietary intake. Bodily levels of carnitine tend to fall with advancing age. In the body carnitine plays an essential role in fat metabolism. It escorts fatty acids to their place of combustion, inside cells' mitochondria. Here, the burning of fats produces ATP, the energy-carrying compound needed by the heart for regular contraction. In essence, the heart depends upon carnitine for fuel. When insufficient carnitine is present, harmful fatty acids can build up in the heart rather than get burned, damaging cells and preventing the heart from functioning normally.

Recent studies have shown carnitine to be potentially useful in the treatment of heart conditions including angina pectoris, arrhythmia, and atherosclerosis. Carnitine doses in the range of 750 to 1,000 mg per day have been shown to reduce total blood cholesterol and triglycerides, increase HDL cholesterol, and improve the heart's exercise tolerance.

Carnitine is found primarily in animal foods, as its name would indicate. A number of studies suggest that the active, L-form of this amino acid derivative is safer and more effective than inactive D-carnitine or the mixed form, DL-carnitine. Almost all supplemental carnitine is L-carnitine.

HOW TO USE CARNITINE: It typically comes in capsules and tablets of 250 to 500 mg, and in liquid form. An average daily dosage to help prevent heart disease is 250 to 500 mg.

Chromium

Chromium is a trace element that is an essential part of glucose tolerance factor (GTF), a bodily substance necessary for proper insulin function. Chromium thus plays an important role in regulating the metabolism of fats and carbohydrates, including glucose (blood sugar). Studies indicate that chromium may also play an important role in preventing heart disease, since the mineral's effects on blood sugar can spill over to affect fat metabolism and blood-cholesterol levels. It is well established that people who suffer from diabetes have a significantly higher risk of heart disease. Population studies have found that high tissue levels of chromium are associated with lower rates of heart disease, and low tissue levels are associated with higher rates of disease. "Chromium may be only one of the factors accounting for the differences in rates of diabetes and atherosclerosis between cultures, but it is probably a major one," says Elson Haas, M.D., author of *Staying Healthy with Nutrition.*

Like niacin, one of chromium's partners in GTF, chromium has been used therapeutically to lower cholesterol. Some of the studies have used high doses (2,000 mcg daily), but researchers have also reported successful reductions in blood fats and cholesterol levels, and increases in the good HDL cholesterol, among subjects taking average daily doses (200 to 400 mcg) of chromium. Several promising recent studies have found that chromium may be the key to using niacin for cholesterol-lowering in a way that totally prevents the usual side effects associated with its therapeutic use. For example, a study done on elderly subjects found that 200 mcg of chromium and 100 mg of niacin significantly decreased LDL cholesterol.

Biologically active forms of chromium include GTF, chromium picolinate, and chromium polynicotinate. Chromium is often combined with other nutrients or included in multivitamin-multimineral supplements. Chromium supplements on the market include Chromoplex, Chromium Complex, and Performance Picolinate.

How to use chromium: Chromium supplements are widely available in tablets (usually 100 to 200 mcg), capsules, and liquids. An average daily dosage for adults to prevent heart disease is 200 to 400 mcg.

Fiber Supplements

Dietary fiber refers to certain parts of plants, especially components of the cell walls and substances in plant saps, that are mostly not digested when you eat them. Plants rich in various types of fiber include fruits, vegetables, nuts, legumes, cereals, and grains. Even though fiber does not directly provide nutrients or energy, how much or little you eat of it can nevertheless have wide-ranging health effects. Since the early 1970s dietary fiber has garnered increasing attention for its beneficial effects in preventing cancer, heart disease, and diabetes. Fiber can also play an important role in normalizing digestion and in the prevention or treatment of gastrointestinal problems ranging from constipation to Crohn's disease.

The two main types of dietary fiber are soluble and insoluble, which are defined by how they react when added to water. Insoluble fiber doesn't dissolve in water, whereas soluble fiber and water forms a gel-like substance capable of coating intestinal walls. Many plants contain both soluble and insoluble fiber, though one or the other may predominate.

Soluble dietary fiber includes gums and mucilages such as acacia gum (from the stems of an African tree, genus *Acacia*), guar gum (from the seeds of various legumes, genus *Cyamopsis,* especially one native to India and now grown in the United States), and glucomannan (from the root of a Japanese plant, *Amorphophallus konjac*). Other sources of gums and mucilages include beans, peas, and other legumes, certain trees, and some plant seeds or husks, particularly oats (*Avena sativa*) and psyllium (*Plantago ovata; P. psyllium*). Another class of soluble fiber is the pectins, predominantly from fruits such as apples and oranges. In general, soluble fiber is known for lowering cholesterol, aiding in weight loss (see Chapter 17), and possibly helping to control blood-sugar levels and thus diabetes. Insoluble dietary fiber includes the cell wall components cellulose and hemicellulose as well as the woody lignins. These are found mostly in wheat bran and rice bran, though oats and psyllium are also reliable sources. As a rule, insoluble fiber is more important than soluble fiber for maintaining gastrointestinal health (see Chapter 16).

A number of well-controlled, double-blind studies have shown that moderate amounts of added dietary fiber (15 to 30 g per day) can improve overall cholesterol levels by 5 to 10 percent. Other studies using high doses of soluble fiber (30 to 50 g or more) have shown quicker and more dramatic effects on overall cholesterol. Fiber decreases LDL and increases HDL. There is some evidence that even low doses of fiber (5 to 15 g daily) may benefit people whose cholesterol levels are in the normal range. Increasing dietary fiber also tends to decrease blood pressure and to improve glucose tolerance. (As noted in the discussion of chromium, positive effects on blood sugar can boost cardiovascular health.) Fiber helps to reduce cholesterol by inhibiting its synthesis or binding to cholesterol-containing bile in the intestines and then eliminating it from the body. A recent study suggests that psyllium's cholesterol-lowering effect is greatest when it is taken with meals rather than between meals, because of the increased bile levels in the intestines during meals.

Fiber is best obtained through foods, but if you can't get enough in your diet, taking supplements may increase your heart health. Soluble-fiber supplements include pectin, oat bran, psyllium, and guar. Many supplement companies offer products combining soluble and insoluble fiber from various sources. Look for products such as Fiber-Plex, Fiber Plus, Maxi-Fiber, Fibersol, and Super Fiber.

Don't overdo supplemental fiber. Start with up to 4 or 5 grams per day and gradually increase your intake if necessary as your body adjusts. Some people who take high levels of supplementary fiber (usually over 30 g per day) may experience mineral deficiencies due to impaired absorption of nutrients. You should also drink healthy amounts of water (6 to 8 glasses per day) to prevent fiber supplements from leading to constipation.

How to use fiber supplements: Fiber comes in powders, tablets, capsules, and liquids. An average dosage of the supplements for better heart health is one teaspoon (or 4 to 6 g in capsules or tablets) two or three times daily, taken at meals with water or other liquid.

Special Considerations for Maintaining Healthy Blood Pressure

Mention blood pressure and diet, and most people think immediately of sodium. Typical Western diets that feature large amounts of processed foods are usually high in salt (sodium chloride). Excessive consumption of sodium has long been recognized as a risk factor for hypertension, though recent studies indicate that salt's role has been exaggerated and that it is misleading to regard sodium as the single most important factor in high blood pressure. Some 30 to 40 percent of the population is especially susceptible to sodium's fluid-retaining effects. In addition, when it comes to high blood pressure, scientists are now finding that other minerals, particularly potassium, calcium, and magnesium, may be equally as important to the equation. Optimal levels of zinc, niacin, and vitamin C may also help maintain proper blood pressure. Nutritionally oriented practitioners often recommend a number of substances to help prevent or treat high blood pressure, including essential fatty acids, bioflavonoids, shiitake mushrooms, and the amino acid taurine. There is also some evidence for the efficacy of coenzyme Q10.

If you have high blood pressure, you should consult with a knowledgeable practitioner of natural medicine before attempting to treat it. An herbalist may recommend a program that makes use of some herbs that in general are used only under the supervision of an herbal practitioner. Herbs such as mistletoe (*Viscum album*), black cohosh (*Cimicifuga racemosa*), and hawthorn are strong remedies with potentially widespread effects on the cardiovascular system beyond a reduction in blood pressure. An herb that is safe to try on your own and has shown promise as a blood pressure normalizer is celery.

Potassium

Sodium and potassium play related roles in controlling fluid balance in the body. Without sufficient potassium to help the body secrete sodium, sodium builds up and exerts its harmful effects. Thus, to reduce high blood pressure most people need not only to lower sodium intake but also to increase potassium consumption. Indeed, some studies indicate that potassium intake is a stronger factor in determining blood pressure than is sodium intake. Various population studies confirm a beneficial effect on blood pressure from increases in potassium consumption. Researchers speculate that the reason why high blood pressure is more prevalent among African-Americans compared to white Americans is tied to the generally poorer, more potassium-deficient diet of African-Americans.

Some studies have found that people taking conventional drugs to lower blood pressure can reduce or even completely eliminate the need for them by adjusting their diet to include optimal levels of potassium. (Never abruptly discontinue drug therapy for high blood pressure; consult with your doctor about how to reduce dosages.)

There is no RDA for potassium, though it is possible for deficiency symptoms, such as muscle weakness and confusion, to occur. An optimal level of intake is probably not less than 3 to 4 g per day, much higher than the average daily consumption in the standard American diet. Fruits and vegetables are the foods with the best ratio of potassium to sodium. Especially high in potassium and low in sodium are potatoes, oranges, peaches, cantaloupes, lima beans, avocados, and bananas. For example, one medium banana contains anywhere from 450 to 650 mg of potassium and only a milligram or two of sodium. Studies of people who eat bananas on a regular basis find that, on average, they have lower blood pressure and a reduced risk of stroke.

How to use potassium: It is available over-the-counter in 99-mg tablets. Because you need a prescription to get potassium supplements in dosages higher than 99 mg, most people can best benefit from potassium by increasing their consumption of fruits and vegetables rather than by taking potassium supplements. (One bite of banana provides about the same potassium as you get in a 99-mg tablet.)

Calcium and Magnesium

Like sodium and potassium, calcium and magnesium are bodily partners in the battle against high blood pressure. Some researchers even contend that calcium and magnesium are more important than sodium and potassium in controlling blood pressure. Calcium plays an important role in regulating heartbeat; magnesium helps to control how blood vessels dilate.

Studies have shown that low levels of both of these nutrients are associated with high blood pressure, while populations that eat diets rich in calcium and magnesium generally have lower average blood pressures. Furthermore, when subjects with high blood pressure are given extra calcium and magnesium, blood pressure tends to fall. In a four-year study of 58,000 women, researchers found that subjects who consumed an average of 800 mg of calcium per day had a lower risk of high blood pressure than those who consumed an average of 400 mg. Consuming at least 300 mg of magnesium also significantly reduced women's risk of hypertension. In another clinical trial, 95 percent of subjects who took magnesium supplements reduced their systolic blood pressure by an average of 12 points, and diastolic pressure by an average of 8 points.

How to use calcium and magnesium: These minerals are widely available separately as powders, tablets, and capsules, and can sometimes be found combined. Many nutritionists recommend that they be taken in approximately a 2:1 ratio of calcium to magnesium. Therapeutic dosages to lower high blood pressure are on the order of 1,000 to 1,500 mg calcium and 500 to 750 mg magnesium per day. As a preventive measure, take approximately 750 mg calcium and 375 mg magnesium daily.

Celery

Both the whole plant and, more commonly, the seeds of this crunchy stalk vegetable (*Apium graveolens*) have been a noted Chinese and Ayurvedic medicinal herb. The ancients used celery for its nourishing and restorative properties and to treat rheumatism, gout, and digestive complaints. Celery has also been recommended in order to stimulate milk flow in new mothers and to promote weight loss. More recently it has been recognized as a potential aid in the battle against hypertension. Studies have confirmed that celery seed is a diuretic, potentially useful in treating high blood pressure. A potent essential oil distilled from the seeds can also help to lower high blood pressure, apparently by relaxing smooth muscles in blood vessels. A University of Chicago study found that lab animals given tiny amounts of butyl phthalide, a compound found in the oil, experienced a 12 percent drop in systolic blood pressure over a four-week period. The compound also lowered cholesterol levels. A Chinese study on 16 people with hypertension also reported positive results using celery seed.

Celery seed can be toxic in extremely large amounts. It is also best not to use it during pregnancy. Most herbalists recommend that you work with an herbalist or naturopath if you want to use therapeutic doses of celery seed for treating high blood pressure. Just eating a few stalks of the vegetable every day, though, may help to keep blood pressure normal.

How to use celery: It is available in tablets, tinctures, and concentrated drops. A safe dosage for occasional use as a preventive measure is ¹/₂ to 1 dropperful of the concentrated drops.

Where to Start

The following formula offers many benefits beyond promoting better heart health:

- Garlic (600 to 1,000 mg of pure or concentrated garlic or garlic extract powder; or 1,800 to 3,000 mg of fresh garlic equivalent; or 1,800 to 3,600 mcg allicin per day)
- An insurance-level multivitamin-multimineral supplement, with optimal levels of vitamins C, E, and B complex, the mineral chromium, and the nutrient coenzyme Q10
- One of the polyphenol-flavonoid supplements, such as green tea or red wine extract (equivalent to approximately 50 to 100 mg of flavonoids per day)

Beyond Herbs and Supplements

Combine your intake of natural substances with attention to various lifestyle factors to achieve the best results for overall cardiovascular fitness.

- Achieve and maintain your optimal weight. Numerous risk factors for heart disease, from high blood pressure to inactivity, are closely related to being overweight.
- Stay fit. Your heart is a muscle. Use it or lose it, as the saying goes.
- Avoid excessive consumption of alcohol and caffeine.
- Reduce your intake of saturated fats and high-cholesterol foods while increasing your consumption of fiber-rich whole foods, such as grains, beans, fresh vegetables, and fruits. The best way to increase your intake of dietary fiber is to eat plenty of these foods. Though supplements can also help, they shouldn't be used as a substitute for healthful foods.
- Don't smoke. Smoking increases threefold your risk of suffering a heart attack. As harmful as cigarette smoke is to your lungs, it is worse for your heart.
- Reduce your levels of stress, or learn how to use techniques such as meditation or biofeedback to control your usual reaction to stress.

Lower Your Cancer Risk

Cancer is a type of cellular riot that may be touched off by a variety of instigators, from food to tobacco smoke to industrial pollutants. When one of these cancer-causing substances, or carcinogens, influences bodily tissue in a particular way, cells start to go out of control. They grow and multiply without doing the job that cells in their bodily neighborhood have always done. Over time these cancerous cells may form a hard lump or tumor that has a malignant effect on surrounding tissues, diverting nutrients to its own growth. Through obstruction and chemical mayhem, the tumor eventually begins to prevent nearby blood vessels, nerves, bones, and other tissues and organs from performing their necessary functions. Cancer cells may spread through the blood to other parts of the body, where they act as outside agitators to start whole new cellular riots. When uncontrolled growth starts in another place as well, the cancer is said to have metastasized, signifying an advanced stage of the disease. The riot has become a revolution, and your body is soon to be its first—and only—victim.

The process lives on, of course, as does the proliferation of carcinogenic substances. Cancer is an adaptable disease, capable of acting through diverse mechanisms and striking various parts of the body. Oncologists, medical doctors who study and treat cancer, have identified more than a hundred types of cancer, from common ones such as those that cause tumors in the lungs, breasts, colon, prostate, stomach, and pancreas, to rarer conditions that affect the testes or certain blood cells.

Cancer is neither a uniquely human disease nor a strictly modern one. Pets, farm animals, and even animals in the wild sometimes get cancer, and paleontologists have determined that cancer also occasionally struck prehistoric humans. The incidence of cancer, however, has no doubt risen in modern times. Aging and average longevity are factors—some gerontologists consider cancer a natural byproduct of advancing years. Certainly diet, lifestyle, smoking, alcohol, and environmental pollutants are also major considerations in increasing cancer rates. Doctors diagnose more than a million new cases each year in the United States, where it is responsible for one in five deaths, second only to heart disease as a cause of death.

In his seminal 1986 *New England Journal of Medicine* article "Progress Against Cancer?" John C. Bailar III challenged the notion that the multibillion-dollar war on cancer was being won. Actually, he pointed out, cancer cure rates were barely better for many forms of the disease than they had been decades earlier. "We should not build a long-range research program on the assumption we'll find fully effective cures," he said. "We gave that a good shot, and now it's time to get serious about another approach—prevention. If we can convince the American people that their hope lies in preventing the disease we will save more lives than any of these drugs ever will."

While the cancer establishment treated Bailar's findings as heresy, his central message remains salient almost a decade later. Cancer is a complex illness, one that may take years to develop to the point at which symptoms are evident. By then, even the best conventional treatments are fighting a desperate, pitched battle. After studying the potential for vitamin A derivatives to both prevent and possibly treat cancer, cancer researcher Frank L. Meyskens, Jr., said, "We propose a general strategy which defines precancer and cancer as a continuum from normality to abnormality in which the modalities of prevention and treatment are blurred." Anything that can help the body to engage its remarkable healing forces against cancer during the disease's earliest stages, or its preventive forces even before that, will show worthwhile returns.

Though the line between prevention and treatment may not be as stark as is sometimes proposed, it is necessary to emphasize that cancer is a serious medical condition that can benefit from natural remedies but should not be self-diagnosed or self-treated. The focus of this chapter is natural remedies for the prevention end of the cancer continuum, not the treatment end. An excellent, balanced presentation of alternative cancer treatments is contained in *Choices in Healing: Integrat-*

ing the Best of Conventional and Complementary Approaches to Cancer by Commonweal founder Michael Lerner (see "Resources").

The Cancer-Prevention Diet

It is now widely accepted that diet is an important factor—perhaps the single most important factor—in protecting against cancer. In a few cases greatly increased cancer risks have been linked with specific types of foods. For example, the notoriously high levels of stomach cancer in parts of China and Japan have been reliably traced to habitual local consumption of salt-cured, smoked, and pickled foods. More commonly, diets lacking in healthful nutrients such as fiber, vitamins and minerals, and garlic have been tied to increased cancer risks.

In recent years dozens of studies have also linked diets rich in fruits and vegetables with a reduced risk of cancer. Many commonly eaten vegetables in particular seem to help protect against cancer, especially the cruciferous vegetables. These mustard-family, *Brassica* genus plants, including broccoli, Brussels sprouts, cauliflower, cabbage, kale, collard greens, and radishes, all contain what are now being called phytochemicals or phytonutrients (*phyto* is Greek for "plant"). Phytochemicals are plant-derived compounds with important health effects. The cruciferous vegetables are the source of various phytochemicals that have been shown to prevent cancer or even inhibit tumor growth. For example, researchers at Johns Hopkins University in Baltimore have found that sulforaphane, isolated from broccoli, stimulates certain cellular enzymes. These enzymes help to remove carcinogenic molecules from cells; they also slow the growth of tumors in laboratory animals. Sulforaphane consumption has been tied to a reduced incidence of breast cancer.

Brussels sprouts, cabbage, and other cruciferous vegetables also contain various compounds—glucobrassicin, benzyl isothiocyanate—that are thought to reduce the risk of cancer. According to Devra Lee Davis, a senior science advisor at the U.S. Public Health Service, "There is growing evidence that these natural products can take tumors and defuse them. . . . They can turn off the proliferative process of cancer."

The National Cancer Institute has recently begun a multimillion-dollar project to study phytochemicals. Researchers will be studying not only compounds from cruciferous vegetables but also polyphenols and flavonoids, such as those found in citrus fruits, strawberries, grapes, raspberries, and other plants. Some of these phytochemicals have been found to neutralize carcinogens before they can affect cells' DNA and cause biomolecular havoc. Plants such as tomatoes, pineapples, and green peppers are also rich in compounds that help to disrupt cellular processes that can result in cancer.

All of this research activity, of course, has not been lost on the supplement manufacturers. Although in general the newly identified phytocompounds have not yet been synthesized, extracted, or concentrated for inclusion in supplements, they probably soon will be. The large category of supplements known as green-food concentrates (see below) probably do already have some of these compounds. And new forms of whole-foods supplements, such as one called The Vegetable Bin, have already started to hit the market. For example, the manufacturer of Vegi-Power Broccoli tablets says these are the "first to be certified to contain four of broccoli's key compounds," with one tablet equaling 11,000 mg of fresh broccoli.

These and many other natural substances, including vitamins and minerals, herbs, nutritional substances, and medicinal mushrooms, can be taken on a regular basis to substantially reduce the risk of cancer.

The Cancer-Prevention Vitamins and Minerals

Cancer specialists sometimes recommend a number of nutritional compounds in druglike doses as part of a conventional approach to treating cancer. For example, megadoses of the B-complex vitamin folic acid have been successfully used in the treatment of cervical cancer. Derivatives of vitamins D and A may also help reverse some cancers—the vitamin-A-based drug tretinoin recently was shown to cause remission in nine out of ten patients suffering from the rare cancer known as acute promyelocytic leukemia. In addition, nutritionally aware oncologists have found various vitamins and nutrients to be valuable in supporting and promoting the health of patients undergoing conventional cancer treatments. Vitamins and minerals are sometimes recommended as adjuncts to conventional treatment, and deficiency states are recognized as impeding recovery.

Some of the vitamins and minerals frequently mentioned for their role in helping to prevent cancer include the following:

Vitamin D. Studies have linked higher vitamin D levels with a reduced risk of various cancers, including skin, breast, prostate, and (when combined with calcium) colon and rectal cancer. Vitamin D is one of the fat-soluble vitamins capable of building up to toxic levels in the body. Your skin makes it naturally if you expose yourself to about 15 or 20 minutes of sunlight every day or so. People who live in cold climates or who get little regular sun exposure may benefit from 400 to 800 IU daily in supplements.

Calcium. As just noted, this mineral may help protect the colon and rectum from cancer. An optimal supplement level to help prevent cancer is 800 to 1,500 mg daily. (Many nutritionists recommend combining calcium and magnesium supplements in approximately a 2:1 ratio, as in 750 mg calcium and 375 mg magnesium; higher levels of magnesium in the diet have also been associated with lower cancer risk.)

Zinc. Optimal blood levels of zinc have been linked with improved protection from cancers of the esophagus and prostate. An average daily dosage of zinc to help prevent cancer is 17 to 25 mg.

Medical researchers have also identified anticancer properties in numerous B vitamins. In addition, the antioxidant vitamins and minerals have demonstrated significant potential in the prevention of cancer.

Vitamin B Complex

Studies indicate that riboflavin possibly protects against cancer of the esophagus and that vitamin B_{12} may reduce the risk of lung cancer even among smokers. Perhaps the most promising anticancer B vitamin is B_6, found in supplements as pyridoxine. Pyridoxine is crucial to proper immune function, and deficiency has been tied to increased risk of cancer. A B_6-based compound has even shown preliminary success in helping to inhibit melanoma, a deadly form of skin cancer. According to alternative cancer therapy expert Michael Lerner, in humans "metabolic disorders resembling vitamin B_6 deficiency states are found in Hodgkin's disease, and bladder and breast cancer. One study suggested that vitamin B_6 supplementation to correct the metabolic abnormality might prevent recurrence of bladder cancer."

Taking individual B vitamins can cause an imbalance in other B vitamins. Many nutritionists recommend taking B vitamins as part of an insurance-level multivitamin or as B complex.

How to use b complex: It is available in liquids, tablets, and capsules. An average dosage for preventing cancer is 25 to 50 mg once or twice daily.

The Antioxidant Cancer-Fighters

Until recently, the cancer-preventive effects of the antioxidant vitamins and minerals, including vitamin A/beta carotene, vitamin C, vitamin E, and selenium, were almost unquestioned. Antioxidants are well known to protect against cellular damage caused by free radicals such as those derived from fatty foods and tobacco smoke, including the kind of damage that can lead to the development of cancerous tumors. Numerous studies supported antioxidant theory, including a large-scale study that the National Cancer Institute reported in 1993. Researchers determined that a battery of antioxidant supplements, including vitamin E, beta carotene, and selenium, lowered the incidence of cancer mortality by 13 percent among 29,000 adults in China. The antioxidants also lowered the rate of stomach cancer by 21 percent and overall mortality by 9 percent.

Antioxidants and cancer, however, briefly became the center of controversy in early 1994, when the *New England Journal of Medicine* published the results of a long-term study involving 29,000 male Finnish smokers. The researchers had tested for the presumed anticancer effects of beta carotene and vitamin E when taken by these subjects over the course of five to eight years. What the researchers found— that both beta carotene and vitamin E supplements "may actually have harmful as well as beneficial effects"—was all the more surprising since other studies had not hinted at any such potential risks. (Some studies had, of course, not confirmed actual benefits.) The Finnish study found that the incidence of lung cancer was 18 percent higher in those who took beta carotene supplements (20 mg, or 33,000 IU daily) than those who didn't. And while vitamin E lowered the risk of prostate cancer, it apparently increased the risk of death from heart disease.

The immediate results received wide publicity. Somewhat less attention was paid, however, to a number of questionable aspects of the Finnish study subsequently pointed out by reviewing scientists. Critics of the study pointed out that many of the subjects had extremely high risks for cancer, since they were middle-aged men who had been pack-a-day smokers for an average of 36 years and who also reported high daily alcohol intakes. (Those subjects who stopped smoking during the study were kicked out and not counted.) The researchers used beta carotene supplements colored with a carcinogenic substance. Also, it is possible that the study didn't proceed long enough to really measure the long-term effects of beta carotene.

The level of vitamin E administered (50 IU daily) was so low that any therapeutic effect at all would be truly surprising. Some critics said that the beta carotene level was also insufficient, though others admitted that if there were adverse effects from taking beta carotene, they may be due to beta carotene crowding out other healthful carotenoids. It should be noted that the subjects who had the highest *dietary* intakes of beta carotene (and, presumably, other carotenoids) at the start of the study did actually have lower cancer rates compared to those who consumed less of the nutrient.

Even the study authors admitted that their findings "may well be due to chance." Antioxidant authorities pointed out that these nutrients may protect against the early stages of cancer and thus would not be expected to show results in a study such as this one of longtime smokers.

Given these criticisms, and the fact that this is the only study out of approximately two hundred that has suggested such supplementation could cause some harm, many researchers have concluded that the results of the Finnish study are some kind of fluke. Nutritionists and most other practitioners of natural medicine feel that there is good reason to ignore the findings of the Finnish study and to continue to recommend antioxidants, including beta carotene and E, to help prevent cancer.

Vitamin C

The role of vitamin C in cancer has been controversial since the famous study conducted by Linus Pauling and E. Cameron and reported in 1976 in the *Proceedings of the National Academy of Sciences*. They found that administering 10 g of vitamin C daily in divided doses to "hopelessly ill" cancer patients allowed them to live significantly longer than those who did not take extra C. In the years since, similar studies have reported inconsistent results for vitamin C as an adjunct to cancer treatment.

Researchers have documented a stronger association, however, between a high intake of vitamin C and a reduced risk of future cancers, particularly of the mouth, esophagus, stomach, cervix, and breasts. Vitamin C was shown to offer significant protection in some 33 of 46 population studies surveyed by Gladys Block, Ph.D., of the National Cancer Institute. Block says, "While it is likely that ascorbic acid, carotenoids, folate and other factors in fruit and vegetables act jointly, an increasingly important role for ascorbic acid in cancer prevention would appear to be emerging."

Chemists have traced some of vitamin C's ability to reduce the risk of cancers of the esophagus and stomach to the nutrient's effect on nitrosamines. Nitrosamines are carcinogenic organic compounds found in tobacco smoke, contaminated drinking water, and certain foods. Nitrosamines are also formed in the stomach after you eat nitrates and nitrites, preservatives sometimes used to cure meats. Vitamin C inhibits the formation of nitrosamines. Animal studies have also suggested that vitamin C may reduce certain cancer-causing compounds associated with the breakdown of estrogen. Vitamin C's supportive role in forming collagen, a fibrous protein found in various tissues, may also have a preventive effect on the spread of cancerous cells.

How to use vitamin c: Vitamin C comes in a wide variety of powders, tablets, and capsules. An average cancer-preventive dosage is 250 to 500 mg two or three times daily.

Selenium

This trace mineral, needed by the body in minute amounts, is a potent antioxidant and immune booster. It is also the most important cancer-prevention mineral. Population studies have provided dramatic proof that selenium helps to prevent cancer. Selenium is found in fish and in plants that have been grown in selenium-rich soil. High soil levels of the mineral have been linked to low cancer rates of local people, and low soil levels to high cancer rates. Animal studies using selenium have also confirmed that it helps prevent cancer, with the best results occurring when test subjects are started on supplements early in life.

Take selenium in combination with vitamin E for increased cancer-prevention effect.

How to use selenium: Selenium is widely available in tablets and capsules ranging in size from 50 to 200 mcg. An average daily dosage for cancer prevention is 100 to 200 mcg.

Vitamin A/Beta Carotene

At least three dozen population studies have linked reduced cancer rates with a high intake of either vitamin A or, more frequently, its vegetable-based precursor beta carotene. A low vitamin A/beta carotene intake is associated with an increased risk of various cancers, particularly lung cancer but also cancers of the esophagus, stomach, bladder, colon and rectum, and cervix. According to cancer researcher

Peter Greenwald, in nine retrospective studies looking at cancer incidence and vitamin A or beta carotene intake, "a significant increase in cancer risk at various sites was associated with diminished vitamin A intake. Risks reported for groups with low vitamin A intake were about twice those for the high intake groups." Results have not been uniform, but many animal studies have also found that an increased intake of vitamin A/beta carotene helps to protect against some cancers.

Beta carotene's effectiveness as an antioxidant that neutralizes free radicals generated by singlet oxygen (see Chapter 10) and the ability of both vitamin A and beta carotene to boost the immune system may account for much of the nutrient's anticancer power. According to Ralph W. Moss, Ph.D., author of *Cancer Therapy*, "Beta-carotene slowly reaches more parts of the body for a longer time and gives more protection than plain vitamin A. It is considered one of the most promising natural anti-cancer agents."

The cancer-preventive effects of vitamin A/beta carotene have prompted researchers to test high dosages of beta and alpha carotene as well as retinoids and other vitamin A derivatives as cancer treatments, with some success. A number of clinical trials have shown that beta carotene can promote regression of precancerous lesions in the mouth.

Taking high doses of preformed A (such as 100,000 IU daily for months, or 500,000 to 1,000,000 IU daily for two to three weeks) can allow it to accumulate in the body and cause potentially serious adverse health effects. On the other hand, the body converts to vitamin A only as much beta carotene as it needs. Extra beta carotene is stored, but the only adverse effect of such storage is a slight orange tinge to the skin.

How to use vitamin a/beta carotene: It comes in a wide variety of tablets and capsules. An average daily cancer-preventive dosage is 5,000 to 10,000 IU of vitamin A plus 25,000 to 50,000 IU (15 to 30 mg) of beta carotene or, even better, beta carotene plus mixed carotenoids.

Vitamin E

Vitamin E's use in conventional cancer treatment has been mainly to enhance the effectiveness of chemotherapy and radiation therapy, though there is some evidence that E may also impede the growth of some existing cancers. With regard to prevention, animal and human studies indicate that vitamin E may lower the risk of breast, lung, and liver cancer. Population studies have found that people who have high blood levels of vitamin E also have lower rates of cancer, and vice versa. And like vitamin C, vitamin E has been shown to inhibit the formation of cancer-causing nitrosamines.

Often overlooked in the controversy surrounding the aforementioned Finnish study is that a relatively low daily dose of vitamin E (50 IU) reduced prostate cancer rates for these heavy smokers.

According to prominent vitamin E researcher K. N. Prasad, "Studies suggest that vitamin E may be one of the important anti-cancer agents which could play a very significant role in the prevention and treatment of cancer."

Taking vitamin E in combination with vitamin C and selenium may enhance all of these nutrients' cancer-preventive effects.

How TO USE VITAMIN E: It comes in liquids and oil-filled capsules. An average daily dosage to help prevent cancer is 400 to 600 IU.

Herbs That Lower Your Cancer Risk

A number of plant- and nutrient-based compounds are either currently being used in cancer treatment or are on the verge of mainstream acceptance for that purpose. For example, the rosy or Madagascar periwinkle or catharanthus plant (*Catharanthus roseus;* formerly *Vinca rosea*) is the source of two alkaloids used in prescription drugs to treat pediatric leukemia and Hodgkin's disease. Just recently researchers have identified the bark of the Pacific yew tree (*Taxus brevifolia*), and possibly the needles of other *Taxus* species, as the source for the compound taxol. Preliminary studies strongly indicate that taxol may cause partial or even complete remission of advanced cases of ovarian and breast cancer, and the FDA has recently approved taxol for the treatment of these conditions. Both of these anticancer remedies require large quantities of the plant material in order to obtain even tiny amounts of the sought-after compound. Thus, these plants are not used as herbs per se, nor are these substances appropriate for cancer prevention. Fortunately, there are some readily available herbs that can be taken on a regular basis to help reduce your risk of cancer. Chief among these are garlic and astragalus.

Garlic

Ancient Greece's medical pioneer Hippocrates recommended garlic for its anticancer effects, and so have many others since then. Various animal, human, and population studies done over the past thirty years have confirmed that garlic, onions, and other allium plants do have the ability to ward off cancer. For example, researchers in China recently completed one of the most dramatic epidemiological studies on garlic consumption. They analyzed the diet of 1,800 Chinese, including almost 700 with stomach cancer, and found that the more garlic and other alliums study subjects ate, the lower their risk of stomach cancer. Conversely, those Chinese suffering from stomach cancer had low average rates of garlic consumption. Summarizing their study in the *Journal of the National Cancer Institute,* the researchers concluded that a diet high in garlic "can significantly reduce the risk of stomach cancer."

Another population study demonstrating anticancer effects for an allium used as a base the stomach cancer rates among whites who live in the area of Georgia that produces Vidalia onions. They suffer from markedly (50 to 67 percent) lower levels of stomach cancer compared both to other Georgia residents and to Americans as a group.

Various animal studies have also found that garlic can reduce the risk of cancer. In one, researchers injected mice with tumor cells. Those mice who had been injected with garlic-treated tumor cells outlived the ones injected with untreated cells.

Garlic and onions contain an abundance of compounds potentially responsible for these cancer-preventive effects, especially allylic sulfides and dozens of other sulfur-containing chemicals. Sulfide compounds enhance the action of cellular enzymes capable of neutralizing carcinogens. Garlic and onions are also rich in flavonoids and the cancer-fighting mineral selenium.

HOW TO USE GARLIC: Garlic supplements come in a wide variety of powders, liquids, tablets, and capsules. Many are standardized for allicin content or fresh garlic equivalent. To help protect against cancer, take 600 to 1,000 mg of pure or concentrated garlic or garlic extract powder, or 1,800 to 3,000 mg of fresh garlic equivalent. An average recommended dosage for allicin is 1,800 to 3,600 mcg per day.

Astragalus

Recent studies done in both the United States and China suggest that this immune-boosting Chinese herb (see Chapter 3) may have some cancer-preventive effects. The studies, performed at the University of Texas System Cancer Center in Houston and the Chinese Academy of Medical Sciences in Beijing, tested astragalus not as a cancer preventive but as a remedy to reduce the adverse effects of chemotherapy for cancer. The researchers found that astragalus extract dramatically increased the anticancer activity of certain immune-system cells. They also determined that oncologists should be able to obtain better results while using lower amounts of the potentially toxic chemotherapy drug in conjunction with the extract.

Practitioners of traditional Chinese medicine have a term, *fu–zheng* therapy, for this ancient approach to cancer and other diseases. Basically, *fu–zheng* means "fortifying the constitution," enhancing the body's overall immune-boosting capabilities and thus promoting its ability to fight off disease. Since testing began almost two decades ago, astragalus has been the most promising *fu–zheng* herb for use with cancer patients undergoing chemotherapy. It has boosted patients' immune response and increased survival rates. Astragalus is one of the premier tonic/adaptogens (see Chapter 13), useful in strengthening and balancing various bodily functions.

How to use astragalus: Astragalus is sold fresh or dried and in capsules, concentrated drops, tinctures, and extracts. An average dosage is 1 dropperful of tincture or concentrate two or three times daily, or 500 to 1,000 mg of the powdered herb in capsules.

The Polyphenols and Flavonoids

These potent plant constituents are found in almost all fruits and vegetables, especially citrus fruits, dark-colored berries, and various herbs (see Chapter 2). The polyphenols and flavonoids are effective antioxidants and have been shown to slow the proliferation of cancer cells. In the body flavonoids protect healthy cells from cancer-causing hormones such as estrogen and thus reduce the likelihood of tumor formation.

Bioflavonoid complex, and bioflavonoids in combination with vitamin C and other supplements, are typically found in tablet and capsule form. An average daily dosage of the complex is 500 to 1,000 mg; of the flavonoids quercetin and rutin, 200 to 500 mg.

Another rich source of flavonoids is Pycnogenol, a patented blend of compounds derived from the bark of the European coastal pine tree. Pycnogenol is a powerful antioxidant. Studies done mostly in Europe indicate that it helps to prevent varicose veins, capillary fragility, and poor circulation, and probably reduces the risk of skin cancer. Pycnogenol comes in tablets and capsules. An average daily dosage is 50 to 100 mg. Grape seed extract products provide the same type of beneficial flavonoid compounds.

One of the herbs rich in polyphenols and flavonoids that has recently been shown to have dramatic anticancer effects is green tea.

Green Tea

In 1994 the *Journal of the National Cancer Institute* published findings from a carefully controlled study involving almost 2,500 Chinese. Researchers found that women who were regular drinkers of green tea had a 60 percent lower risk of esophageal cancer than women who didn't drink green tea, once smoking, alcohol, and dietary factors were taken into consideration. The protective effect was only slightly lower for men. Each year, cancer of the esophagus claims the lives of more than 10,000 Americans. (Note that studies have also found that in areas where green tea is traditionally drunk scalding hot, the population suffers from *increased* rates of esophageal cancer. Allow green tea to cool slightly before drinking.)

Though other population studies have also produced mixed results, most do suggest that green tea may also help protect against cancers of the lungs, skin, liver, pancreas, and stomach. Studies done on animals have found that green tea can protect against skin cancer. Surveys indicate that green tea consumption may be an important factor in why Japanese smokers have a much lower death rate from lung cancer compared to American smokers. An animal study in which green tea apparently led to significantly fewer lung tumors in mice bolsters the case for its protective effect.

Green-tea-extract capsules are among the hottest new supplement products in natural-food stores. They may be sold as simply green-tea extract or given names such as Polyphenols 60 and Preventin. Some green-tea supplement manufacturers add extra caffeine and promote the product as "energizing." The caffeine content of extract capsules without added caffeine is usually 5 to 15 mg.

Steep the leaves or tea bags only two or three minutes to obtain a subtle, delicate flavor and to keep caffeine levels low (20 to 30 mg per cup).

How to use green tea: It is predominantly available in teas and capsules. An average daily dosage to obtain 50 to 100 mg of polyphenols is 3 to 5 cups of tea. Dosages of capsules depend upon polyphenol content, which may range from 15 to 50 percent. An average daily dosage of the capsules standardized for 15 percent polyphenols is 300 to 600 mg; of the capsules standardized for 50 percent polyphenols, 100 to 200 mg.

Medicinal Mushrooms Against Cancer

Medicinal mushrooms are a rich source of various polysaccharides that have been shown to boost immunity (see Chapter 3) and may help prevent cancer. Shiitake is the most widely taken medicinal mushroom to help fight cancer, but the following may also help. They're available in natural-food stores in various forms, including the dried mushroom and various powders and capsules; follow dosage directions on the label.

Reishi. Several species of ganoderma have traditionally been used by the Chinese to prevent or treat cancer of the esophagus and other organs. Studies show that certain steroidlike compounds in reishi can help kill liver cancer cells. Reishi extracts have also been shown to boost the immunity of cancer patients.

Zhu ling. Practitioners of traditional Chinese medicine use this medicinal mushroom in some cancer-fighting remedies.

Enokitake. According to Andrew Weil, M.D., author of *Natural Health, Natural Medicine,* the polysaccharide flammulin from enokitake may be a potent immune booster and cancer fighter. "Japanese scientists have demonstrated [flammulin's] anti-tumor activity in animals and believe that high consumption of enokidake by growers and their families in the vicinity of Nagano City, the center of cultivation in central Japan, is responsible for lower cancer rates in that region. I often recommend that people with cancer or high risk of cancer eat this mushroom regularly," Weil says.

Shiitake

In Japan, shiitake is widely perceived to be an effective remedy, with applications in both the treatment and prevention of cancer. Studies have shown that the polysaccharide lentinan, derived from shiitake, may improve the outcome of surgery for breast cancer or of chemotherapy for cancers of the gastrointestinal tract. Lentinan is now an approved drug in Japan to reduce the adverse effects of conventional cancer treatments, and some researchers have found that lentinan or shiitake extracts can actually shrink tumors.

According to Lerner, studies indicate that even consuming average supplemental levels of shiitake mushrooms can provide potent anti-cancer properties. He says, "Some of these compounds act in a manner similar to interferon or boost the activity of interferon-like protein polysaccharides, which attack and destroy cells. They also interfere with the initiation and promotion stages of carcinogenesis."

HOW TO USE SHIITAKE: Shiitake is available fresh and dried (add it to soups and other dishes that call for edible mushrooms) and in capsules, tinctures, and extracts. An average dosage in capsule form is 500 mg two or three times daily.

How to Choose

If your diet, lifestyle, or family history suggests you have an increased likelihood of developing certain cancers, some combinations of supplements may be more effective than others at reducing your risk. Here are some common types of cancers and suggestions for appropriate natural substances to take on a regular basis.

- Colon: fiber supplements and the beneficial live bacteria
- Breast: the antioxidant nutrients and herbs, vitamin B complex, and vitamin D/calcium
- Stomach: garlic and the antioxidant nutrients and herbs
- Esophagus: vitamin C and zinc
- Lung: the antioxidant nutrients (especially beta carotene) and herbs, and green tea

Nutritional Supplements Against Cancer

One of the most controversial nutritional substances frequently taken for its potential role in the treatment or prevention of cancer is animal cartilage, particularly that from sharks. These fish are atypical in that their skeletons are composed primarily of cartilage rather than bone. And, as a popular book title promoting the anticancer effects of shark cartilage states, sharks don't get cancer. Since most other bony fish do get cancer, does this mean that shark cartilage can actually help prevent or treat cancer?

The answer is quite possibly yes, though research is still sketchy at this point. One study done by scientists at the Massachusetts Institute of Technology and published in *Science* in 1983 found that "shark cartilage contains a substance that strongly inhibits the growth of new blood vessels toward solid tumors." Scientists have identified the substance in shark cartilage (and, in much lower concentrations, in cartilage derived from cows) that slows the process of angiogenesis, the growth of new blood vessels. The substance, dubbed angiogenesis inhibition factor (AIF), has the effect of denying a tumor the blood-derived nutrients and oxygen it needs to grow.

A number of studies have now confirmed that preventing blood-vessel growth is a potentially useful therapeutic approach for existing cancers of the brain, lungs, and other organs. Cartilage supplements, however, should not be used by anyone for whom new blood-vessel development is healthful, including pregnant women and anyone with heart disease or vascular disease. For this reason, their regular use as a cancer preventive is considered controversial. They are widely available in natural-food stores.

(Eating a diet rich in miso, tofu, and other soy-based foods may have an effect similar to that of taking shark cartilage. German researchers recently announced that they had isolated a chemical called genistein in soybeans that prevents capillaries from growing and bringing oxygen and other nutrients to a tumor. They speculate that genistein's antitumor effects may be the reason why Japanese men who move to the West and significantly reduce their consumption of soy-based foods experience a marked increase in prostate cancer risk.)

Though nutritional substances play a relatively limited role as exclusive treatment agents, they offer a much wider range of benefits as treatment adjuncts and as cancer preventives. The following five nutritional substances have been shown to play a significant role in optimal health. Though definitive cancer studies are lacking, and it is still too early to say for sure, it is likely that these can reduce the risk of cancer at least a little. With the possible exception of arginine for some people, all of these substances are safe and nontoxic at the dosages recommended below.

Coenzyme Q10. This versatile vitaminlike compound has been shown to reduce the adverse effects of chemotherapy. It comes in capsules ranging in size from 10 to 100 mg, and an average daily dosage for optimal health is 30 mg.

Organic germanium compounds. The Japanese-developed Ge-132 and other organic germanium compounds improve oxygenation of tissues and restore the normal function of immune-boosting cells. Preliminary studies done on mice indicate that taking organic germanium compounds may help prevent cancer. It comes in powders, granules, and tablets, as well as capsules ranging in size from 25 to 250 mg. An average dosage for optimal health is 50 to 100 mg daily.

Arginine. A number of studies (exclusively on animals rather than humans, unfortunately) have indicated that this amino acid with immune-boosting properties (see Chapter 3) may prevent cancer or even slow the development of existing tumors. Among those who should avoid supplemental doses of arginine, however, are pregnant or lactating women, anyone with kidney or liver diseases, and people under the age of 20. Arginine may reactivate latent herpes viruses in some individuals. It is widely available as a single ingredient in capsule and powder form. An average dosage for optimal health is 250 to 500 mg two or three times daily, with meals.

Essential fatty acids. Large doses of the omega-3 and omega-6 fatty acids from fish oils and some plants have also been shown in animal studies to reduce the risk of breast and some other cancers. EFAs are typically sold as liquids or oil-filled capsules (supplements may need to be refrigerated). An average daily dosage of fish-oil or plant-oil capsules for optimal health is 500 to 1,000 mg.

Beneficial live bacteria. A number of nutritional authorities are now recommending acidophilus, bifidus, and other beneficial live bacteria products (see Chapter 2) to reduce the risk of colon cancer. While only a few studies have been done that support this recommendation (including a study on intestinal microflora and its connection to colon cancer published in the medical journal *Infection* in 1982, and a more recent study at Tufts University), it makes biochemical sense. The premise is that by preventing an imbalance in intestinal flora, beneficial live bacteria reduce the level of harmful intestinal bacteria that might otherwise promote the formation of carcinogens. Also, taking beneficial live bacteria supplements can ensure that your intestines harbor the enzymes necessary to neutralize nitrosamines and other cancer-causing compounds. Acidophilus and bifidus come in tablets, powders, capsules, and liquids. An average dosage to maintain a healthy intestinal tract is ½ to 1 teaspoon of powder or liquid daily, or 2 to 3 billion viable organisms.

Two other broad categories of very safe nutritional substances increasingly taken for their ability to help prevent cancer are fiber and green-food concentrates.

Fiber Supplements

Evidence has been accumulating for 25 years that the type of low-fiber, high-fat diet widely eaten in the industrial world increases the risk of cancers of the colon and rectum and possibly the breast and prostate as well. The pioneering population studies of D. Burkitt and H. Trowell, authors of the medical classic *Western Diseases: Their Emergence and Prevention,* suggested that increasing the consumption of dietary fiber, the mostly indigestible parts of vegetables, fruits, and whole grains, could protect against cancer. Subsequent population studies as well as some clinical trials have added weight to the fiber-cancer connection. For example, one recent four-year trial found that increased intake of dietary fiber led to fewer precancerous growths in the rectum.

While some researchers maintain that fiber's cancer-preventive effects are still unproven, the scientific consensus is that insoluble fiber in particular is an effective anticancer agent. "The evidence documenting the protective effect of dietary fibre on colon cancer is overwhelming," conclude Joseph Pizzorno, N.D., and Michael Murray, N.D., authors of the *Encyclopedia of Natural Medicine*. The National Cancer Institute and the American Cancer Society also recommend a high-fiber, low-fat diet to help prevent some forms of cancer.

Researchers have proposed a number of bodily mechanisms that might be responsible for fiber's cancer-preventive effects. In general, fiber helps to maintain a healthful condition within the gastrointestinal system, thus reducing the volume of toxins formed in the intestines that may be cancer precursors. Fiber may also promote the quick transit of potentially carcinogenic substances through the intestines and out of the body. Increased fiber intake may reduce certain types of free radicals. Fiber's apparently beneficial effect on breast cancer may be due to its tendency to increase elimination of estrogen. As a rule, insoluble fiber is more important than soluble fiber for maintaining gastrointestinal health and preventing cancer.

Many supplement companies offer products combining soluble and insoluble fibers from various sources. Look for products such as Fiber-Plex, Fiber Plus, and Super Fiber.

How to use fiber supplements: Fiber comes in powders, tablets, capsules, and liquids. An average daily dosage of the supplements is 4 to 6 g; take with plenty of water or other liquid.

Green-Food Concentrates

Green-food concentrates are chlorophyll-rich supplements. Most are derived from microalgae (such as spirulina, blue-green algae, or chlorella) or from the young grasses of cereal plants (such as barley, wheat, and alfalfa). They are particularly rich in such nutrients as vitamins, minerals, enzymes, and trace elements. Chlorophyll acts as an antioxidant and may have medicinal benefits against cancer and immune problems. Chlorophyll has not garnered a lot of scientific attention, but a few studies support an anticancer effect. According to Sheldon Saul Hendler, M.D., Ph.D., author of *The Doctors' Vitamin and Mineral Encyclopedia,* chlorophyll "has been identified as one of the factors that inhibit the mutation-promoting effect of carcinogens requiring metabolic activation."

Other phytochemicals found in green-food supplements may also have cancer-preventive effects. Green-food concentrates, for example, are rich in not only beta carotene but also many of the other carotenoids. One study done by a Japanese biologist found that a compound in barley-grass extract (apparently not chlorophyll) helped to protect cells from damage due to a carcinogen and to X rays.

HOW TO USE GREEN-FOOD CONCENTRATES: Green foods come in powders, tablets, capsules, juices, liquid concentrates, and extracts. Follow label directions for dosage.

Where to Start

Natural substances offer a multitude of choices in the fight against cancer. The following four supplements provide a firm base for reducing your risk.

- A potent multivitamin-multimineral supplement, or an ACES antioxidant supplement (one that combines vitamins A/beta carotene, C, and E, and the mineral selenium), to cover the micronutrients most often cited for their anticancer effects
- Garlic, a multipurpose herb that is more widely available and that has been more thoroughly studied for its anticancer effects than astragalus
- Green tea, the extract of which is a rich source of cancer-fighting compounds
- Shiitake, a potent (though expensive) anticancer substance

Beyond Herbs and Supplements

The allure of a magic bullet for cancer—a single substance, whether natural or not, to cure (or even prevent) all forms of the disease—is powerful. But in all likelihood cancer is too diverse and complex a disease ever to succumb to a single therapeutic agent. Cancer deserves a multidimensional approach to both treatment and prevention. Take steps throughout your life to lower your risk of cancer, using natural substances such as those just mentioned as well as commonsensical dietary and lifestyle practices.

• Eat a variation of the low-fat, high-fiber diet that population studies indicate is most likely to reduce your risk of breast, prostate, and colon cancer.

• Consume at least a half-dozen servings per day of fresh vegetables and fruits, for their numerous proven cancer-fighting compounds as well as for compounds that are probably important but haven't yet been identified. This alone could reduce your risk of certain cancers by 50 percent or more.

• Avoid regularly eating large amounts of smoked, salt-pickled, and salt-cured foods, which can increase your risk of cancer of the stomach and esophagus.

• Don't smoke. Lung cancer is the leading cause of death by cancer among American men, and the vast majority of these deaths are directly attributable to smoking. Tobacco use also increases the risk of bladder cancer.

• Drink alcohol in moderation only. Excessive drinking increases the risk of cancers forming on the tongue and the esophagus.

• Avoid obesity. According to the American Cancer Society, if you are overweight, you have an almost 50 percent higher cancer risk than similar people of normal weight.

• Participate in moderate exercise or physical activity. Sedentary women are more likely than those who are fit to suffer from breast, ovarian, and other cancers. Men also gain cancer protection from exercise and fitness.

Extend Your Life

Humanity's pursuit of longevity—and ultimately immortality—has attracted geniuses, crackpots, mystics, and quacks. They have sought to add years to their own and others' lives by transmuting lead into gold, trudging around Caribbean swamps in search of a fountain of youth, and living on a diet limited to air and one's own saliva.

Recent members of this rogue's gallery of longevity-searchers include the infamous Edouard Brown-Sequard. In 1889 this 72-year-old professor electrified his elderly compatriots at the College de France by claiming he had regained youthful vigor (enough to "pay a visit" to his young wife) after injecting himself with the watery extract of crushed dog testicles. Soon thousands of physicians were injecting similar extracts into patients, and probably themselves as well. Alas, the extract didn't work, and Brown-Sequard's experiments were dismissed by medical journals as "senile aberrations."

Schemers and charlatans since then have nevertheless tried similar tactics. There was Serge Veronoff, a Russian physician who transplanted ape testicles into old men; John Romulus Brinkley of the United States, who in the 1920s transplanted goat testicles; and Elie Metchnikoff, a Russian émigré to France who sought to emulate the long-lived people of the mountainous regions of southern Russia. He downed prodigious quantities of sour milk and yogurt faithfully for his last eighteen years before dying at 71 in 1916.

Despite the considerable efforts of these quixotic individuals, the upper limit for human life remains about 115 to 120 years. One thing these longevity researchers did accomplish was to make intellectually and medically disreputable the idea of extending life or postponing old age. Only since the 1940s, with the establishment of the fields of geriatrics and gerontology, have researchers undertaken a more systematic study of aging and life span. The knowledge gained about how and why we age has offered firmer groundwork for speculation on extending maximum life span. A growing number of longevity scientists and nutritional researchers now say that the disappointments of the past may fade quickly as new studies on aging bear fruit.

"Our studies show no reason why the symptoms of old age cannot be postponed until we're 90 or 100 years old," says Dr. Kathleen Hall, a gerontology research scientist. "It's more than just a theoretical possibility," she adds, "because science has identified several substances that can extend our years of peak functioning. The benefits discovered in the laboratory are finally coming home."

Do We Have to Age?

In the effort to determine how aging might be retarded, researchers have developed the concept of *biomarkers,* physical indicators of age. Dozens have been identified, but the most important include: the amount of air one can take in and breathe out in one breath; cardiac output—the amount of blood the resting heart pumps; degree of kidney function; rate of bone loss; aging of skin, as determined by wrinkles, age spots, how far skin will stretch, and how fast it will snap back to normal; rate of wound healing; flow of chemicals that transmit nerve impulses in the brain; rate of resting pulse; and degree of decline in the sensory-nerve system.

Exactly why these and other physical functions collapse with age is still a medical and scientific mystery, though not for lack of credible theories. There are at least two hundred theories of aging, and as yet none can totally explain the complexities involved. Three of the more widely held theories are:

Cross-linking. Over time the process of metabolism results in cellular byproducts known as cross-linking agents. These chemical agents seize separate molecules in body tissues and bind them together rigidly. For instance, as the fibrous protein collagen in the skin undergoes continuous chemical change, cross-linking occurs and leads to wrinkling, age spots, and so forth.

Immune function. Normally the body provides antibodies that recognize and destroy abnormal or foreign cells. As the function of the immune system diminishes with age, it can lead to trouble in two ways: by allowing abnormal cells to proliferate in the body, and by mistakenly attacking normal cells as well.

Free radicals. These are molecules that may be either formed within cells or taken into the body (from foods or cigarette smoke, for example). Free radicals act, as longevity researcher Dr. Roy Walford has put it, as "the great white sharks in the biochemical sea." Free radicals possess an extra electrical charge, a free electron, and are thus highly reactive, allowing them to oxidize and damage blood vessels, cell membranes, and skin and other tissues. The body produces scavengers —antioxidants—which help to control these molecular marauders, but the rate of antioxidant production decreases with age.

The good news is that all of these aging theories admit the possibility of human intervention in the process, if not its total negation. Individuals can take numerous steps, including making simple adjustments in diet and additions to one's supplement use, to reduce the effects of these factors in aging. It is possible to prevent cross-linking (see Chapter 15 for ways to reduce cross-linking in the skin), to support the immune system (see Chapter 3), and to increase antioxidant function. And, to some extent, studies confirm that improvements in these areas can extend average life span.

The bad news is that immortality is not around the corner. That's because some other theories of aging impose limits not likely to be affected by individual actions. In the early 1960s, gerontology researcher Dr. Leonard Hayflick discovered that skin cells grown in a lab will divide only about fifty times. If they are frozen, for instance, after twenty dividings, when unfrozen they will "remember" and divide only thirty more times. (Cancer cells are an exception; given the right environment, they will divide indefinitely.) Hayflick's discovery overturned a widely held tenet of gerontology: that cells are inherently immortal if given an ideal environment. Instead, it seems that an inborn clock ticks away within each cell and ultimately determines when old age occurs.

Another recent theory of aging looks at limits to DNA repair. DNA molecules, which are largely responsible for cellular health, suffer damage over time both from within (when cells divide there can be random mistakes in the way their DNA is copied) and from without (from ultraviolet light, X rays, and other factors). If a DNA molecule is damaged, its instructions to the cell get garbled, possibly resulting in such aberrations as cancer. Some evidence suggests that a species' life span is related to its ability to repair its genetic material. Humans live twice as long as chimps, for example, and our genetic repair rate is almost twice as great.

While immortality may have to wait, many people are nevertheless taking steps to increase the likelihood of surviving into their tenth decade and beyond. The following longevity nutrients and herbs can play an important role in any such program. If you accompany these natural substances with a basically healthy lifestyle, including proper diet and regular activity, you increase the odds that your later years will also be healthy years. The goal is not reaching the magic century mark by living the last decades of life in suffering and immobility, but to stay healthy, engaged, and vital well beyond today's norms.

Nutritional Substances for Increasing Life Span

Because aging is such a complex and multifaceted process, any supplement program to slow it really should start by making sure that all of the twenty or so indisputably essential vitamins and minerals are being provided at optimal levels. But if you want to prioritize, the evidence today suggests that the antioxidants are the principal longevity-enhancing nutrients.

Many studies in recent years have established that antioxidants can protect the body from the harmful effects of free radicals, including most of the conditions that cause the vast majority of deaths in the United States today—heart disease, cancer, and stroke. Though the next step in scientific proof—showing that increasing individuals' intake of antioxidant nutrients and herbs can extend average or maximum life span—will be more difficult to achieve, preliminary findings are encouraging. For example, recent research done by Japanese teams revealed that two antioxidant products have increased life span in mice and rats. If more such findings are made, they will ensure that the antioxidant nutrients remain one of the best-selling categories in the supplement field.

Beta Carotene

The vitamin A precursor beta carotene, as well as other carotenoid plant pigments, plays important roles in health unrelated to its vitamin A action. Beta carotene, gamma carotene, and other carotenoids, such as lycopene, have recently gained increased respect among scientists as antioxidants. (Vitamin A itself is a relatively weak antioxidant.) Studies have established that these carotenoids are among the most powerful neutralizers of singlet oxygen, a type of cell-damaging, free-radical-generating molecule found in air pollution and elsewhere. When it is absorbed by the body and concentrated in the skin and brain, singlet oxygen may cause cancer, premature aging, and other adverse effects. In contrast to vitamin E, beta carotene is not destroyed in the reaction with singlet oxygen and thus can neutralize it many times over. Beta carotene can also scavenge free radicals generated by singlet oxygen.

A 1984 primate study reported in the *Proceedings of the National Academy of Sciences* found that "tissue levels of carotenes [have] a better correlation with maximum life span potential than any other factor that has been studied." Numerous population and clinical studies have found that beta carotene boosts immunity and protects against diseases associated with aging, including cancer of the lungs and other organs, cataracts, gastric ulcers, and possibly heart disease.

Beta carotene is nontoxic, since the body converts to vitamin A only as much beta carotene as it needs. Extra beta carotene is stored, but the only adverse effect of such storage is a slight orange tinge to the skin. Although most beta carotene supplements offer only beta carotene, some newer products offer beta carotene in combination with alpha carotene and other carotenoids. The green-food concentrates (such as the algae products spirulina and chlorella, and the young green shoots of barley and wheat) naturally have a range of carotenoids, albeit in relatively low levels.

How to use beta carotene: It comes in a wide variety of tablets and capsules. An average daily antioxidant dosage of beta carotene or, preferably, beta carotene plus mixed carotenoids, is 25,000 to 50,000 IU or 15 to 30 mg.

Vitamin C

Some studies have found vitamin C to be the most effective antioxidant found in human blood. Because it is water-soluble, vitamin C is a powerful free-radical scavenger in the areas between cells. It protects the brain, certain blood cells, and other parts of the body in ways the fat-related antioxidants (such as vitamin E) can't. Vitamin C neutralizes hydroxyl free radicals that might otherwise damage DNA. It interrupts free-radical chain reactions, protects vitamin E from free radicals, and improves the body's ability to use selenium, another important antioxidant.

Numerous studies have tied high levels of vitamin C in the body to reduced risk of cancer, heart disease, cataracts, and other degenerative diseases. Some studies have also tied optimal vitamin C levels to increased life expectancy.

How to use vitamin c: Vitamin C comes in a wide variety of powders, tablets, and capsules. An average optimal dosage is 250 to 500 mg two or three times daily.

Vitamin E

Vitamin E plays an important antioxidant role, offering long-term protection of certain parts of the body from the harmful effects of free radicals. For example, a recent study, involving more than eight hundred subjects, conducted by ophthalmology researchers at Johns Hopkins University found that the risk of a certain type of eye cataract was dramatically smaller among those who had the highest blood levels of vitamin E. Vitamin E's antioxidant effects are thought to shield the sensitive eye cells from free-radical damage triggered by cigarette smoke and other agents.

Vitamin E has also been shown to help protect the skin, lungs, brain, and liver from free-radical damage. Vitamin E is found in the fatty membranes of cells, where it serves to protect them from the effects of oxidation. Vitamin E's positive effects on free-radical scavenging are compounded by the fact that it protects some hormones, vitamin A, and other substances from oxidation. "Vitamin E also protects DNA against free-radical attack, which if unrepaired could lead to cancerous mutations, cell death, or faulty cell reproduction, which could hinder cell function," notes Nancy Bruning, author of *The Natural Health Guide to Antioxidants*.

Animal studies have found that vitamin E can increase average life span. Even a low level of supplementation (50 to 100 IU daily) in some studies has been shown to have a significant protective effect against such diseases as cancer and heart disease.

(The vitaminlike nutrient coenzyme Q10 is sometimes included in antioxidant formulas, since coQ10 enhances the antioxidant activity of vitamin E. An average dose of coQ10 is 15 to 30 mg.)

How to use vitamin e: It is sold as a liquid and in dry and oil-filled capsules. An average daily dosage is 400 to 600 IU.

Selenium

Selenium plays a prominent role as a cofactor in an important enzyme that scavenges free radicals in the body. Without sufficient selenium your body can't produce glutathione, and without glutathione it can't produce the antioxidant enzyme glutathione peroxidase. Glutathione peroxidase neutralizes various common free radicals, such as hydrogen peroxide, that result from oxidation of fats.

Numerous studies have found that people who live in areas where the food is grown in selenium-deficient soil have increased rates of cancer, and that people who live in areas where food is grown in selenium-rich soil have decreased rates of cancer. Other studies have found that selenium could increase the life span of test animals. According to Sheldon Saul Hendler, M.D., Ph.D., author of *The Complete Guide to Anti-Aging Nutrients,* "Selenium is remarkable in that the best evidence suggests that it can have inhibitory effects on *all* of the major hypothesized aging mechanisms. That it can play a very important role in helping to reduce the incidence of many diseases associated with aging appears certain. Adequate selenium intake is unquestionably necessary if one is to attain optimal health and full life span potential. Man's ability to extend 'maximum life span' beyond presently defined limits remains unproved; if there *are* micronutrients that can help break the present 'life span barrier,' selenium has to be accounted one of the prime contenders."

HOW TO USE SELENIUM: Selenium is widely available in tablets and capsules ranging in size from 50 to 200 mcg. An average daily dosage for optimal antioxidant action is 100 to 200 mcg. Take selenium in combination with vitamin E for increased effect.

Promising Potential Life Extenders

Two additional substances deserve mention before we take a look at herbs. N-acetyl cysteine (NAC) is another nutrient that protects the body from the aging effects of oxidation. The life-extending effects of deprenyl, on the other hand, have been traced to its effects on neurotransmitters. Deprenyl is one of the new generation of "smart drugs." Unlike all of the other substances in this chapter, it is not an herb or a nutrient, but rather a synthetic drug. Because it is relatively safe and nontoxic, it is included here.

N-Acetyl Cysteine

N-acetyl cysteine is closely related to the sulfur-containing amino acid L-cysteine, found in beans, eggs, fish, and nuts. Along with selenium, L-cysteine is an important cofactor in the formation of glutathione peroxidase, one of the body's most powerful antioxidant enzymes. Without adequate blood levels of cysteine, the body cannot produce certain glutathione-containing substances that protect the heart and other internal organs from free radicals. A recent study published in the *Journal of Applied Physiology* found that taking even moderate daily levels of NAC (800 mg) increased the body's ability to scavenge free radicals. The researchers concluded that athletes who work out intensively or to the point of exhaustion, thus increasing the risk of harm from exercise-generated oxygen radicals, would benefit by taking NAC.

Both NAC and L-cysteine are available as nutritional supplements. L-cysteine, however, is potentially toxic and unstable in the body. It needs to be taken with megadoses of vitamin C to prevent it from increasing the risk of forming kidney stones. N-acetyl cysteine is a more stable, more powerful antioxidant nutrient. It strengthens cell membranes and helps to protect them against damage from heavy metals and pollutants.

Cysteine levels in the body often fall with advancing age, and a number of studies have indicated that increased cysteine consumption can dramatically extend the life span of animals.

HOW TO USE N-ACETYL CYSTEINE: It comes primarily in powders and 600-mg capsules. An average antioxidant dosage is 400 to 1,200 mg daily.

Deprenyl

Deprenyl is the generic name for a popular "smart drug" that also seems to boost libido. (It is available by prescription in the United States as the drug Eldepryl.) Animal studies, including one conducted by deprenyl's developer, Hungarian scientist Jószef Knoll, indicate that deprenyl may increase longevity as well. In a 1983 study that also established a "true aphrodisiac effect" for deprenyl, Knoll and colleagues found that deprenyl extended rats' maximum life span by almost 40 percent. Other animal studies also have found that deprenyl extends average life span. One deprenyl user reported in *Smart Drugs II,* "I take deprenyl, although I have never noticed any effects from it whatsoever. I take it on faith, because the research I've seen about its life-extending effects look so convincing."

Deprenyl works by enhancing the brain's production of the neurotransmitter dopamine. Bodily levels of dopamine generally fall with advancing age, often leading to depressed mental function (see Chapter 11).

Deprenyl can be purchased in liquid form in foreign countries; Eldepryl comes in 5-mg tablets. In the United States, the only FDA-approved use of the drug is to treat Parkinson's disease, for which doctors usually recommend a dosage not to exceed 10 mg daily. See Chapter 7 for more information on deprenyl's actions and safety, and for how to use it. See "Resources" for how to obtain liquid deprenyl by mail order.

Melatonin

This pineal-gland hormone, widely recognized as a safe insomnia remedy, is gradually gaining acclaim for its even more dramatic effects on health, particularly in the realm of boosting immunity and helping to prevent killer diseases such as cancer and osteoporosis. Melatonin thus may significantly increase longevity.

For reasons that are unclear, melatonin secretion in humans and animals greatly decreases with advancing age. Recent studies have tied falling melatonin levels to suppressed immunity. Scientists have also shown that administering supplements of the hormone to aging lab animals suffering from depressed immune function helps to restore natural immunity. Similarly, researchers have found that melatonin levels are depressed among cancer patients, and that supplements may help to prevent cancers of the breast and other organs. In addition, medical researchers are exploring a potential role for the hormone as an adjunct therapy in the treatment of some existing tumors.

How melatonin promotes immunity and helps fight cancer has not been fully determined. It has some direct antioxidant effects on free radicals, in particular neutralizing the harmful hydroxyl radical. One researcher has even stated that aging "can be regarded as a process caused by hydroxyl radical pathology and melatonin deficiency." Melatonin is also thought to play a role in the regulation of calcium levels and to affect the pineal gland itself by promoting the release of certain chemicals associated with immune function.

Some of the most promising scientific investigation into melatonin's ability to promote longevity has been done on laboratory animals fed a nutrient-dense but calorie-restricted diet. Numerous studies involving such "undernourishment without malnourishment" have proven it to be among the most reliable ways to increase both maximum and average life span. It is a difficult regimen for humans to follow—gerontology researcher Roy Walford, M.D., author of *Maximum Life Span*, is among the few trying it. Recent studies, and the administration of melatonin to animals fed a normal diet, suggest that increased melatonin secretion—one of the effects of caloric restriction—may be a primary reason why caloric restriction leads to prolonged life. Researchers have also determined that, unlike caloric restriction begun late in life, melatonin supplementation begun late in life is nevertheless effective at substantially increasing life expectancy. Some researchers suggest that the effectiveness of other nutrients that promote longevity, including deprenyl, may be due in part to their ability to promote the secretion of melatonin.

Studies indicate that melatonin is safe and causes relatively few side effects even when taken in doses much higher than recommended. Melatonin should not be taken by women who are pregnant or lactating, or by anyone suffering from kidney disease. Because it may affect growth-hormone levels, melatonin should also be avoided by anyone under the age of 20.

Unless you're a shift worker who sleeps during the day, melatonin should always be taken at night, to support the body's natural melatonin secretion pattern and enhance your body's natural biorhythms. To promote longevity, most people find that melatonin works best when taken at the same time each night, within an hour of bedtime.

HOW TO USE MELATONIN: Melatonin comes in 750 mcg (0.75 mg) and 3 mg pills. An average daily dosage to promote longevity is 0.75 to 1.5 mg; for elderly people, 1.5 to 2.25 mg.

The Longevity Herbs

Two prominent herbs of the Orient often cited as longevity enhancers include fo-ti (which the Chinese call he-shou-wu) and gotu kola. According to Foster and Chongxi in *Herbal Emissaries*, "Over the centuries he-shou-wu's reputation has bordered on the mythical for its power to produce longevity, increase vigor, and promote fertility."

The Chinese and Indian herb gotu kola likewise enjoys a reputation as a revitalizing and tonic herb that can slow the aging process. According to legend, gotu kola was the fountain of youth used by a famous Chinese herbalist said to have lived to the age of 256. Scientists have not yet studied the life-span-enhancing potential of fo-ti or gotu kola. Fo-ti and gotu kola are widely accepted in Asia for their strengthening and balancing effects on overall health.

Astragalus, reishi, and a number of other such "tonifying" and "adaptogenic" herbs (see Chapter 13) also have a reputation for enhancing longevity. Chief among these traditional life-extending herbs is ginseng, which, according to one of the earliest Chinese herbal books (*The Classic of Herbs*), can lead to longevity through continuous use. Today ginseng remains widely used for its positive effects on numerous bodily systems.

Another set of herbs, those rich in polyphenols and flavonoids, share with antioxidant nutrients the ability to reduce the harmful effects of free radicals. "The antioxidant and free radical scavenging activities of flavonoids are quite remarkable," note Joseph Pizzorno, N.D., and Michael Murray, N.D., authors of *Encyclopedia of Natural Medicine,* "but the fact that different flavonoids have a preference for specific tissues means that different flavonoid-rich plants should be used for different conditions." They also point out that flavonoids from plants exhibit "an extremely broad range of antioxidant activity" against a wide variety of free radicals, especially when compared to the nutritional antioxidants. We'll look here at some antioxidant herbs with important protective effects relating to the digestive system (garlic), brain and central nervous system (ginkgo), and liver (milk thistle).

Ginseng

Ginseng's energizing and strengthening effects have attracted people to it for thousands of years. In the East it is sometimes called "the root of immortality," and it enjoys widespread use as a tonic herb. Ginseng is even found in rejuvenation preparations now popular in Europe. Studies have shown that certain ginseng compounds, such as various flavonoids, maltol, and vanillic acid, have antioxidant properties. Ginseng has a stimulating effect on the immune system and reduces both physical and mental fatigue. It also protects cells from damage by X rays, radioactivity, and toxic substances.

HOW TO USE GINSENG: Ginseng comes in myriad forms, including as a whole root and in capsules, tablets, tea bags, tinctures, and extracts. An average dosage of capsules standardized for 5 to 9 percent ginsenoside is 250 to 500 mg. An average dosage of some concentrated extracts and ginseng products with higher standardized percentages may be as low as 100 to 200 mg.

Garlic

The many life-extending benefits garlic offers, including reducing the risk of heart disease and some types of cancer, are usually attributed to garlic's unique sulfur compounds. Garlic, and to an even greater degree its plant cousin the onion, contains flavonoids with potential antioxidant effects. The vitamin C and the high level of selenium in garlic also contribute to its antioxidant action.

HOW TO USE GARLIC: Garlic supplements come in a wide variety of powders, liquids, tablets, and capsules. Many are standardized for allicin content or fresh garlic equivalent. An average daily dosage is 600 to 1,000 mg of pure or concentrated garlic or garlic extract powder, or 1,800 to 3,000 mg of fresh garlic equivalent. An average recommended dosage for allicin is 1,800 to 3,600 mcg per day.

Ginkgo

Ginkgo's reputation among the Chinese for extending longevity may derive in part from its own success as a plant. *Ginkgo biloba* is the oldest living tree species, having survived an estimated 150 million years. This "living fossil" must be doing something right to have adapted to eons of changes in climate and predation. Scientists have determined that ginkgo extract contains various flavonoids (such as rutin) that are potent antioxidants, as well as other biologically unique compounds. Ginkgo's well-known ability to protect capillary health and scavenge free radicals is especially useful in promoting optimal function of the thyroid, circulatory system, and brain. Many of its most dramatic clinical effects are related to alleviating symptoms associated with aging, from poor memory to poor hearing.

HOW TO USE GINKGO: Ginkgo comes in tablets, capsules, concentrated drops, tinctures, and extracts. An average dose is 40 mg three times daily of a standardized extract containing 24 percent ginkgo flavoglycosides.

Milk Thistle

The flavonoids in this herb are potent free-radical scavengers with an affinity for the liver, the organ we depend upon for assistance in digestion, waste elimination, prevention of infection, and numerous other roles. Milk thistle extracts have been shown to increase the regeneration of liver cells and to boost the liver's ability to filter blood and break down toxins. According to Christopher Hobbs, author of *Milk Thistle: The Liver Herb,* the standardized milk thistle flavonoid extract silymarin "stabilizes liver cell membranes and prevents toxins from disrupting the liver's function. The liver then transforms the poison into a water-soluble substance that can be excreted from the body."

Milk thistle extract products have long been popular liver remedies in Germany and other parts of Europe. People take them both for preventive purposes and in the aftermath of exposure to toxins, whether from food poisoning, industrial chemicals, or radiation. Damage from more everyday toxins, such as alcohol and drugs, can also be reduced by milk thistle. The extracts have been shown to boost the immune system as well.

Milk thistle comes in powders, tablets, capsules, concentrated drops, and tinctures. Almost all of the research has been done using milk thistle extracts standardized for at least 70 percent silymarin. Look for products such as Thisilyn and Siliverin.

How to use milk thistle: An average daily dosage is 175 to 200 mg of extract standardized for 70 to 80 percent silymarin.

European Coastal Pine and Grape Seed

Extracts from these substances are rich in the flavonoids known as proanthocyanidins, which have been shown to be potent antioxidants capable of retarding aging and reducing the risk of various diseases. Studies done by Japanese researchers indicate that proanthocyanidins are many times more powerful than vitamins C and E as scavengers of certain free radicals.

European coastal pine extract is sold as the trademarked product Pycnogenol. Grape-seed extracts are available in products such as Proanthanol, Proflavanol, and OPC Plus.

How to use european coastal pine and grape seed: These extracts typically come in 20-to-50-mg tablets and capsules, some with added vitamin C and other flavonoid-rich herbs. An average daily dosage of proanthocyanidins is 50 to 100 mg.

Where to Start

Taking the following three supplements offers multiple health benefits and an increased potential for longevity.

An ACES antioxidant nutrient supplement. ACES supplements include the antioxidant vitamins A/beta carotene, C, and E, and the mineral selenium. Many supplement producers make tablets and capsules in this combination, and they are widely available in natural-food stores.

Melatonin. The minute doses necessary and the fact that it works with the body to support its natural functions make this an easy-to-take, safe, and effective longevity aid, especially for those middle-aged and older. Melatonin is also less expensive and more readily available than deprenyl and NAC.

Garlic. Its proven ability to reduce the risk of heart disease makes it especially important in the United States, where heart disease is widespread.

Beyond Herbs and Supplements

Extending life is a multifaceted project involving not only the individual—on the levels of body, mind, and spirit—but the family, the community, and society at large. Taking the right nutrients provides a solid foundation for longevity, but you still have to build a sturdy edifice by paying attention to diverse factors that range from your interpersonal relationships to the cleanliness of the air you breathe. According to Kenneth Pelletier, Ph.D., author of *Longevity: Fulfilling Our Biological Potential,* "The same factors which determine the quality of life also have a profound influence upon the quantity of life." Fortunately, many of the factors that determine both longevity and overall health are within your control.

• Keep your weight down and your nutrition up. Undernourishment without malnourishment is one of the most promising lines of longevity research. The idea is to stay thin but nevertheless to get optimal levels of all the necessary nutrients. Population studies confirm that being thin seems to reduce the risk of dying prematurely—a recent report on an ongoing study of 21,000 men found that those who weighed around 20 percent less than the national average for their height and age had the lowest rate of premature death. An insurance-level nutritional program is a must for anyone considering a low-calorie diet.

• Avoid the health-destructive habits most likely to shorten your life. Among the most obvious habits to avoid are smoking, excessive alcohol intake, a sedentary lifestyle, unsafe sex, and not wearing a seatbelt.

• Emulate the centenarian lifestyle. A number of studies have been done on individual centenarians and on communities where the elderly remain vigorous and active. They suggest that the average centenarian has led a stable and orderly life, remained physically active, approached things in a level-headed and pragmatic way, and refused to dwell on guilt or remorse. Such people also take care of their own health, rarely need to see health professionals or doctors, and expect to live a long and healthy life.

11

Boost Your Brain Power

There are no drugs, prescription or over-the-counter, that conventional American medical doctors use to enhance memory or learning in normal, healthy persons. The FDA has no category for such substances and has never approved any drug for such a use. Medical practitioners do, however, often recommend a number of therapeutic substances, from nutrients to prescription drugs, to help improve the mental function of victims of Alzheimer's disease and other conditions associated with age-related loss of mental capacity.

These substances work in various ways in the body, some of which haven't been well explained yet. Brain-related mechanisms that have been identified for their ability to boost mental function include the following:

Circulation and oxygen supply to the brain. Anything that reduces the flow of blood to the brain has a negative impact on mental function. The effect may be as benign as temporary dizziness or as serious as unconsciousness and death. Limited blood flow to the brain (cerebral insufficiency, the doctors call it) may be a factor in certain diseases of aging, including Alzheimer's, that are characterized by poor concentration and memory. By the same token, agents that tend to increase the flow of blood (by dilating blood vessels in the brain, for example, or otherwise improving their carrying capacity) and the delivery of essential nutrients and oxygen to brain cells can potentially have a positive effect on cognition, learning, and memory.

Nutrient and antioxidant levels. Just as there are vitamins and minerals crucial for the heart or the eyes, the brain requires optimal levels of fuel (from glucose) and various nutrients to perform its diverse functions. When a bodily deficiency of certain nutrients deprives the brain of necessary nourishment, mental function can suffer. The person may become confused, forgetful, and unable to concentrate. Also, antioxidants—such as the vitamins A/beta carotene, C, and E, the mineral selenium, and various nutritional substances and herbs—are capable of neutralizing harmful free radicals generated in the brain before they damage nearby cells.

Neurotransmitter levels in the brain. Studies have shown that the neurotransmitters dopamine, adrenaline, and noradrenaline all have potential effects on alertness, mood, and concentration. Perhaps even more crucial to certain aspects of mental function is the neurotransmitter acetylcholine, low levels of which have been tied to problems relating to memory, learning, and attention span. Neurotransmitter levels in the brain often fall with age. Nutrients, drugs, and other substances that increase neurotransmitter production, or protect these neurotransmitters from breakdown, can promote better mental clarity.

Until very recently, much of the impetus for learning how to improve brain function came from medical researchers dedicated to alleviating the problems of aging. But today a much broader segment of society has recognized the value of operating at peak mental ability. Some of these are people who are dissatisfied with caffeine's actions and are seeking more reliable ways to improve learning ability, promote short-term memory, and increase attention span. Whether the goal is to achieve better grades, become more successful at business, or just talk more articulately about one's interests, an increasing number of people wish to take advantage of brain-boosting substances.

The widespread desire for increased mental clarity, and the research into substances that can affect cognition, memory, learning, and even creativity among normal, healthy people, have reinforced each other in recent years. As a result, there are now a variety of substances in the field to choose from, including brain-boosting vitamins, minerals, nutrients, and herbs. For the more adventuresome, there is also a new class of drugs called "smart drugs" or nootropics (a word coined in the early 1970s from the Greek for "mind-turning") that seem to improve mental function in promising new ways.

Nutritional Substances for the Thinking Person

Many people new to the idea of using supplements to enhance learning, memory, and cognition prefer to try nutritional supplements or herbs before taking "smart drugs" such as deprenyl, piracetam, and Hydergine. On the one hand, the nutritional supplements are more readily available and less expensive. On the other, some of the "smart drugs" have been more extensively tested for cognitive effects. Both types of product are relatively safe and nontoxic, though in general the nutritional supplements are preferable on this score because they play broader roles in supporting the health of other organs and bodily systems. Vitamins and minerals in particular also have much wider margins of safety between optimal dosages and potentially toxic ones.

Severe nutritional deficiencies have been known to cause mental problems, and it is possible that even marginal deficiencies can prevent the optimal functioning of the brain. The following are the nutrients that are most often recommended for their positive effects on memory, learning, and cognition.

Vitamin B complex. Various B vitamins play a role in the synthesis of acetylcholine, including thiamine, pantothenic acid, and B_6. The B-complex vitamins also promote the smooth operation of the nervous system and assist in the metabolism of carbohydrates and proteins in the brain. Researchers have linked deficiencies of folic acid, B_{12}, and other B vitamins to cognitive impairment, memory loss, mental confusion, and depression. An optimal dosage of vitamin B complex is 25 to 50 mg once or twice daily.

Vitamin C. This is another nutrient that the body needs to produce neurotransmitters, including acetylcholine and noradrenaline. High levels of vitamin C also help to protect brain cells from oxidation. Vitamin C has been associated with intelligence in studies, though a cause-and-effect relationship has not been established. For instance, one study found that subjects with lower average blood levels of C scored more poorly on IQ tests than did subjects with higher average blood levels of the vitamin. Deficiency has been known to cause problems with memory and cognition. An optimal dosage is 250 to 500 mg two or three times daily.

Zinc. The brain maintains high levels of this mineral, which works with enzymes there to help prevent damage from free radicals. Optimal zinc levels improve neurotransmission. A recent study found substantial effects on mental function among head-injury patients who were given supplemental zinc over three years. Assessment using a specialized cognitive scale revealed that zinc significantly improved test scores and promoted speedier recovery from the head injuries. Otherwise healthy subjects on zinc-deficient diets have also been shown to have lower average scores on memory and attention tests. Finally, one of the signs of a zinc deficiency is mental lethargy. An optimal dosage is 17 to 25 mg daily.

Magnesium. Magnesium assists in the functioning of the nervous system and the transmission of nerve signals. Deficiency can lead to confusion and learning problems, and high doses have been used to improve depression and poor memory in the elderly, dementia victims, and people with Alzheimer's disease. Magnesium also plays an important role in keeping the brain supplied with adenosine triphosphate (ATP), the body's principal energy-carrying chemical. An optimal daily dosage of magnesium is 450 to 650 mg, usually taken in conjunction with approximately twice those quantities of calcium.

It is likely that the cumulative effects on thinking processes of these four nutrients, along with others usually consumed in insurance-level multivitamin-multimineral products, are greater than any individual effect. Two similar studies confirmed this premise in 1988, one in California and one in England. Both found that vitamin and mineral supplements given to schoolchildren increased average nonverbal IQ scores (verbal IQ scores were not affected) when compared to the scores of a control group. One of the studies found that over the course of the school year the supplement-takers gained an average of seven points more than the control group. When the California study was replicated in 1991 with 615 schoolchildren over a three-month period, it again found statistically significant increases in nonverbal IQ scores.

Beyond Vitamins and Minerals

A number of vitaminlike compounds, amino acids, and other natural substances have also been shown to have positive effects on neurotransmitters or other agents affecting brain function. Among the most widely used of these substances are choline, acetyl-L-carnitine, DL-phenylalanine, and DMAE. These and the just-mentioned brain-boosting vitamins and minerals are often combined in supplement products such as MegaMind, Extension I.Q., The Mental Energy Formula, and Herba Choline Brain Formula. Some of these products also include the "smart herbs" ginkgo and ginseng.

Choline/Phosphatidylcholine/Lecithin

Choline and its parent substances phosphatidylcholine and lecithin can directly affect brain levels of the neurotransmitter acetylcholine.

Choline's connection to acetylcholine is so important that it is some-times referred to as the "memory nutrient." Increased blood levels of choline, from eating choline-rich foods (such as soy-based foods or egg yolk) or taking choline supplements, helps more choline reach the brain, where it assists in the production of acetylcholine. Choline also plays a role in forming healthy nerves.

Studies have found that choline supplements promote better recall and clearer thinking in some but not all Alzheimer's patients. Alzheimer's researchers were disappointed when choline did not pan out as a dramatic cure for the condition, since it was thought at the time that low acetylcholine levels were a primary cause of Alzheimer's. The mechanism that results in this malady is now realized to be more complex. Many nutritional practitioners believe, however, that it is likely that timely choline supplementation can help *prevent* the condition.

Some human and animal studies have confirmed that choline can improve memory in normal, healthy subjects. For example, choline seems to improve students' ability to recall long lists or sequences of words. Choline also had a positive impact on rats' ability to remember mazes, even if the choline doses were administered only during in-fancy. One recent study done by researchers at Florida International University on 41 healthy people who took 500 mg of choline daily found that after five weeks those subjects taking the nutrient experi-enced only around half as many memory lapses as subjects taking a placebo. People who use choline for its brain-boosting effects fre-quently report better overall thinking capacity, improved short-term memory, and increased ability to concentrate.

See Chapter 2 for more information on the distinctions between choline, phosphatidylcholine, and lecithin.

How to use choline/phosphatidylcholine/lecithin: Choline is available in powders, tablets, capsules, and liquids. An average daily dosage is 100 to 200 mg. Phosphatidylcholine typically comes in cap-sules; an average daily dosage of phosphatidylcholine that is 90 percent pure is 1,100 to 2,200 mg. Lecithin comes in granules, oil-filled cap-sules, and liquids; an average daily dosage of lecithin that is 20 percent phosphatidylcholine is 5 to 10 g, or 1 to 2 tablespoons of granules. Taking choline with 25 to 50 mg of vitamin B complex may improve its brain-boosting effects.

Acetyl-L-Carnitine

This naturally occurring compound is a relative of carnitine, the vitaminlike substance used to maximize fat-burning, to boost strength and endurance, and to support the functioning of the heart. Acetyl-L-carnitine (ALC) is found in milk and other foods. As a supplement, it has been used to increase alertness, elevate mood, and expand attention span in people suffering from Alzheimer's disease, age-associated memory impairment, and cerebral insufficiency. There is also some recent evidence that normal, healthy people who take it experience better memory and increased verbal and cognitive abilities. It may enhance longevity. How it works is not well known, but it is thought to increase the actions of acetylcholine or dopamine.

ALC is relatively safe and nontoxic at average dosages. Some users take 1,000 to 2,000 mg daily without apparent adverse effects. Nevertheless, it is not recommended for use by pregnant or breast-feeding women.

ALC is not a widely available supplement at this time. Carnitine is more readily found in natural-food stores and may have similar effects —it is necessary for the production of acetylcholine, and studies on Alzheimer's patients have shown it has a positive effect on memory. The supplement maker Source Naturals of Santa Cruz, California, sells ALC in 250-mg tablets; Smart Products in San Francisco (see "Resources") sells it in 500-mg capsules. It is also produced in a liquid by some companies.

How to use acetyl-l-carnitine: An average brain-boosting dosage to begin with is 250 to 500 mg.

DL-Phenylalanine

The L- form of this essential amino acid is well known for its stimulant effects, increasing alertness and concentration by stimulating the production of the neurotransmitters dopamine, adrenaline, and noradrenaline. While the D- form is usually taken for chronic pain, there is also some evidence that D-phenylalanine has a memory-boosting effect. Therefore, the mixed form (DL-phenylalanine, or DLPA) may be the best way to try phenylalanine as a brain booster.

Phenylalanine is a common ingredient in "smart drinks" sold at special bars set up for all-night "raves" and the like.

Phenylalanine should be avoided by pregnant and lactating women, people with high blood pressure, and those taking MAO-inhibitor

antidepressants. It should also be avoided by people with phenylketonuria, a genetic disorder of phenylalanine metabolism. As with most
other stimulants, its potential side effects include excessive stimulation,
insomnia, and anxiety. In general, avoid using single amino acids for
longer than two or three weeks at a time.

HOW TO USE DL-PHENYLALANINE: It comes in powders and capsules.
An average brain-boosting dosage is 500 to 1,000 mg.

DMAE

DMAE is short for dimethylaminoethanol, a compound that occurs
naturally in the brain and is found in sardines and some other fish. As a
brain boosting supplement and nervous system stimulant DMAE is
taken to increase alertness and energy levels and elevate mood. Studies
indicate it can also have positive effects on attention span, memory,
and learning ability. Those who have used DMAE report that it enhances concentration, planning, and decision-making. Its medical uses
are limited, though studies suggest it may be useful in the treatment of
learning disorders and neuromuscular conditions such as tardive dyskinesia.

In the body DMAE is a precursor of choline. Increased choline
levels in turn help the brain to produce more acetylcholine, accounting for DMAE's effects on memory, learning, and alertness. DMAE
also has antioxidant properties.

In 1983 the FDA questioned Riker, the maker of the DMAE-
related prescription drug Deaner, about Deaner's effectiveness as a
remedy for children with attention-deficit disorder. Though many
parents of hyperactive children preferred Deaner to Ritalin, Riker
decided to pull Deaner off the U.S. market rather than invest the ten
years and $220 million necessary to research the drug for FDA ap-
proval. Deaner (also known as Deanol) is still sold in other countries
and can be mail-ordered from the United States (see "How to Obtain
'Smart Drugs,'" below). It is considered to be somewhat more potent
than the over-the-counter DMAE products sold in this country.

To a greater extent than with the aforementioned brain-boosting
nutrients, some nutritional authorities question the safety and effectiveness of DMAE. Sheldon Saul Hendler, M.D., Ph.D., the author of
The Doctors' Vitamin and Mineral Encyclopedia, says that while DMAE is
a choline precursor and potential regulator of acetylcholine in the
brain, evidence for its effects on life span are conflicting. Hendler says
that Deaner "certainly should not be used as a dietary supplement, as

some 'life extension' enthusiasts have suggested." The authors of *Smart Drugs II*, Ward Dean, M.D., John Morgenthaler, and Steven Fowkes, counter that the "overwhelming lack of side effects" from DMAE argue for its acceptability as an everyday nutrient. Some people have been known to take high doses (500 to 1,000 mg daily) for extended periods with no adverse effects, while others experience anxiety, excessive nervousness, headaches, or other side effects from even average doses.

To be on the safe side, pregnant or lactating women, and anyone who suffers from convulsions, epilepsy, or manic-depression, should avoid using DMAE. It is recommended that you start with a low dosage (25 to 50 mg) and increase it only if necessary and if you experience no effects, adverse or otherwise. Elderly people, whose acetylcholine levels are naturally lower, may need to take slightly higher than average doses for best results. The full brain-boosting effects of DMAE may not be apparent until after several weeks of daily use.

The most common form of DMAE is DMAE bitartrate, which contains 37 percent DMAE and 63 percent tartaric acid.

How to use dmae: It comes in powders, liquids, tablets, and capsules. An average daily dosage for those new to DMAE is 100 mg of DMAE bitartrate (providing 37 mg of DMAE).

"Smart Drugs"

"Smart drugs," or nootropics, are compounds whose principal effects are on the brain, where they act to enhance memory or learning without either stimulating the central nervous system or causing notably adverse side effects. Unlike the herbs and nutritional substances discussed throughout this book, the substances being considered here are truly drugs, available at U.S. pharmacies only by prescription. Some people may choose not to use them for this reason alone. If so, there are plenty of other options in the form of brain-boosting nutrients and herbs. We include the discussion of three "smart drugs" because, in general, they are safe and nontoxic, possibly as safe as the brain-boosting nutrients. Even an FDA paper admitted that they have not caused any reported injuries among the estimated 100,000 Americans using them. Whether these deserve to be prescription drugs is also controversial. In many other countries, including some in Europe, these substances are widely available over the counter. It is certainly worthwhile consulting with your physician before using any of these "smart drugs" regularly, though you may have to educate him or her about them.

The following substances may be taken on their own or in conjunction with one another. Their actions are sometimes enhanced when used together. It is often necessary, however, to take lower-than-average doses when combining these drugs, even with brain-boosting nutrients.

Deprenyl

Deprenyl and selegiline are generic names for a prescription drug (Eldepryl) that is approved for use in the United States for the treatment of Parkinson's disease, a brain disorder that is sometimes helped by drugs that increase dopamine action. Studies of patients with Parkinson's show that deprenyl can improve their memory, attention span, learning, and cognitive and motor functions.

Researchers have determined that deprenyl has an apparently unique effect on an enzyme, monoamine oxidase B (MAO-B), that breaks down dopamine and other neurotransmitters. By selectively inhibiting this action of MAO-B, as well as directly stimulating the brain to produce more dopamine, deprenyl increases alertness and energy levels. Deprenyl is also an antioxidant that protects brain cells from damage by free radicals. Some people who use deprenyl as a "smart drug" report becoming more assertive, ambitious, confident, and capable of coping. Deprenyl's effects on cognition, however, are thought by some to be secondary to its ability to elevate mood, stimulate sexuality (see Chapter 7), and enhance longevity (see Chapter 10).

Deprenyl is most readily available in the United States as Eldepryl, which comes in 5-mg tablets. Though Eldepryl's only FDA-approved use is for Parkinson's (at a dosage not to exceed 10 mg daily), a select few doctors are willing to prescribe it for its "smart drug" effects. A more useful form of deprenyl (because it is more easily divided into small dosages) is the liquid deprenyl that is being developed by a Florida company, Discovery Experimental and Development.

According to Discovery, "Deprenyl is not normally a fast-acting product. Results from the administration of deprenyl normally take between one and six months of continual usage."

See Chapter 7 for more information on deprenyl's actions and safety, and for how to use it. See "Resources" for how to obtain liquid deprenyl by mail order.

Piracetam and Pyroglutamic Acid

Piracetam is the generic name for one of the pioneering "smart drugs," Nootropil. Developed in Europe in the early 1970s, Nootropil remains internationally popular as a "smart drug" for everyday use, with annual worldwide sales in excess of one billion dollars in 1990. Because the Nootropil patent has expired, piracetam drugs are now available from a number of pharmaceutical companies. Despite its apparent safety and effectiveness, piracetam is not available by prescription or over the counter in the United States. It can be purchased from overseas sources (see "How to Obtain 'Smart Drugs,'" below). Piracetam and other drugs with similar molecular structures, such as oxiracetam and pramiracetam, are all derived from the same acetylcholine-affecting substance, pyrrolidone.

Studies on animals and humans have found that piracetam increases learning speed and ability, reaction time, and alertness. Researchers have noticed that children with learning disorders gain some benefit from piracetam. For example, a study of dyslexic children found that those who received the drug experienced improvements in reading and writing speed and ability. Unlike some of the other "smart drugs," which were developed to alleviate severe mental dysfunctions such as dementia and Alzheimer's, piracetam is first and foremost a drug for normal people (though it has attracted the attention of Alzheimer's researchers). Piracetam seems to enhance memory and overall mental performance without causing any adverse reactions.

Piracetam accomplishes this through its effects on the brain's metabolism of glucose and production of energy-carrying ATP. Piracetam stimulates an enzyme in the brain to produce more ATP. Piracetam also affects levels of acetylcholine and other neurotransmitters and boosts the brain's use of oxygen. Finally, piracetam has been found to affect the right and left hemispheres of the brain in a way that, as one researcher terms it, "superconnects" the two, possibly resulting in greater feelings of creativity.

Piracetam rarely causes "speediness" or any other side effects, even in doses much larger (5 to 6 g daily for long periods) than average. According to the authors of *Smart Drugs II*, "Piracetam's absence of any known toxicity makes it an ideal candidate for over-the-counter sales." Some users report minor side effects such as nausea, insomnia, and gastrointestinal problems.

Some substances that are chemically related to piracetam are available as nutrients in the United States. The pyrrolidone compound pyroglutamic acid (PCA), or pyroglutamate, is an amino acid found in meat, vegetables, and other foods. In the body PCA is concentrated in the brain. As a nootropic, it seems to function much as piracetam does. Studies of pyroglutamate performed on both animals and humans have shown it has a positive effect on mental function, increasing memory and learning.

Because it is a naturally occurring amino acid, the sale of PCA is not restricted by the FDA. PCA is available (as L-arginine pyroglutamate) from amino acid producers, such as JM Pharmacal of Campbell, California. Pyroglutamic acid is also included in some brain-boosting nutritional formulations, such as Deep Thought, made by KAL of Woodland Hills, California; Mental Edge, made by Source Naturals; and Memory Boost, which comes in a powdered drink formula and in capsules and is made by Vitamin Research Products of Carson City, Nevada. (VRP also sells pyroglutamic acid in powder and capsules.)

For increased effect, many people combine piracetam with choline, DMAE, or other nutrients that enhance acetylcholine production. Piracetam's effects are usually noticeable within an hour.

HOW TO USE PIRACETAM AND PYROGLUTAMIC ACID: Piracetam typically comes in 400- or 800-mg tablets or capsules. An average recommended dosage for enhanced mental function is 800 to 1,600 mg per day, in divided doses. Pyroglutamic acid comes in powders and capsules, usually 500 mg. An average dosage is 250 to 500 mg two or three times daily.

Hydergine

Hydergine is the name the Sandoz Pharmaceuticals company gave in the early 1950s to the semisynthetic drug it developed from the plant-based compound known as ergoloid mesylates. In recent years, with the expiration of the Hydergine patent, a number of European pharmaceutical companies have come out with competing prescription drugs, such as Hydroloid-G, based on ergoloid mesylates. Some authorities maintain that Hydergine is a more effective "smart drug" than these latecoming generics, which haven't duplicated exactly the original formula. Hydergine remains the most popular formulation of this compound. It is the only one mentioned in the *Physicians' Desk Reference* (*PDR*), which describes Hydergine's approved use in the United States as a treatment for "symptomatic decline in mental capacity of unknown etiology."

Hydergine has an interesting pedigree. It was created in 1950 by Dr.

Albert Hofmann, the Swiss biochemist who twelve years earlier had first synthesized another innovative drug, LSD. (Hofmann didn't discover LSD's remarkable hallucinatory powers until he inadvertently ingested some five years afterward, in 1943.) Hofmann's work on what became the most famous psychedelic of the sixties foreshadowed his development of what today is one of the most famous and widely consumed "smart drugs" of the nineties. The formulas for both LSD and Hydergine were based on the structure of some alkaloid compounds found in ergot, a fungus (*Claviceps purpurea*) that naturally grows in grainlike masses on the kernels of rye and other cereals.

Ergot is a toxin that caused outbreaks of gangrenelike poisonings or convulsions in Europe and precolonial America, and may have even been partially responsible for episodes of mass hysteria such as those that resulted in witch burnings. Ergot alkaloids, however, have significant medicinal potential. The ergot alkaloids that Hofmann spent much of his life researching have since been developed into other drugs, including ones widely used to prevent and treat migraine and to stimulate uterine contractions.

Though in much of the rest of the world it is best known as an all-purpose brain booster, Hydergine is approved in the United States for symptomatic relief of declines in cognitive skills, mood, self-care ability, and motivation associated with a relatively narrow set of conditions related to dementia, cerebral insufficiency, and Alzheimer's disease. Medical uses in Europe also extend to using it to treat the effects of a lack of oxygen to the brain, such as occurs with near drownings, heart attacks, and drug overdoses.

The normal, healthy people who are using Hydergine as a "smart drug" report that it improves alertness, concentration, and memory. Hydergine users say they feel more intelligent and well-spoken. Overall mood is also improved. Studies that have been done on Hydergine confirm that it can increase mental clarity, stimulate short-term memory, and alleviate mild depression.

The specific mechanisms by which Hydergine works are still being researched. An increase in cerebral blood flow and oxygen supply to the brain accounts for some of its effects. Hydergine is an antioxidant and metabolic booster in the brain. Like ALC, Hydergine may help reduce accumulation in the brain of lipofuscin, a fatty pigment that builds up with aging and can interfere with proper brain function. There is also some evidence that Hydergine has a positive effect on nervous-system function and neurotransmission.

Hydergine would appear to be one of the safest prescription drugs available. No serious side effects have been noticed in people regularly taking high daily doses (12 to 15 mg). Hydergine has one of the shortest listings in the entire *PDR* under contraindications, precautions, and adverse reactions, categories that for many drugs require whole columns of print. The only contraindications are hypersensitivity to the drug and psychosis; the only precaution is to attempt a careful diagnosis; the only adverse reactions are sublingual irritation from sublingual use, transient nausea, and gastric disturbances. Users report that these effects occur only rarely.

Hydergine is often used in reduced dosages with piracetam.

HOW TO USE HYDERGINE: Hydergine comes in a liquid and in tablets and capsules of 0.5 and 1 mg. Most doctors recommend starting with a daily dosage of 1 to 2 mg. (Note that while the highest dosage approved by the FDA is 3 mg per day, in Europe it is often used in daily dosages of up to 9 mg.)

How to Obtain "Smart Drugs"

The overwhelming majority of American doctors will not write you a prescription for deprenyl (as Eldepryl tablets) or Hydergine for purposes other than those approved by the FDA, and the FDA has not approved these drugs (or any others) for enhancing cognitive function. Only a few dozen physicians in the United States are knowledgeable about unapproved uses for these drugs.

Deprenyl, Hydergine, piracetam, and various other nootropics are more easily purchased through foreign sources. If you visit Mexico, Spain, Belgium, Japan, or some other countries, you can buy "smart drugs" in drugstores without a prescription. It is also possible to order these drugs from overseas through mail-order sources.

You need to consider certain legal and regulatory restrictions when you mail-order drugs from overseas. Since 1988 the FDA and the U.S. Customs Service have allowed Americans to mail-order from foreign sources up to a three-month supply of drugs that are legal in the country of origin yet unapproved or "experimental" in this country. (This leeway was granted in response to protests from AIDS activists who felt they were being denied access to potentially life-saving drugs.) In 1992 the FDA issued an "import alert" on a half-dozen foreign importers who were found to be either shipping more than a three-month supply or advertising their products in the United States. An import alert allows the Customs Service to confiscate shipments from these suppliers. According to Beverly A. Potter, Ph.D., and Sebastian Orfali, authors of *Brain Boosters,* "The import alert confirmed that the FDA would maintain its policy of allowing shipments of small quantities of unapproved drugs for personal use. However, the FDA emphasized that this is a policy and not a law, which means that permitting shipments to pass through U.S. customs is left to the discretion of the FDA's field offices. In short, any shipment of unapproved drugs can be detained arbitrarily." Even with these hurdles to consider, tens of thousands of Americans are successfully obtaining "smart drugs" from overseas sources.

The Cognitive Enhancement Research Institute in Menlo Park, California (see "Resources"), maintains up-to-date lists of U.S. physicians knowledgeable about these drugs, foreign mail-order suppliers, and suppliers who have been hit with import alerts by the FDA.

Herbs for Better Brain Function

Anyone who has used coffee, tea, guarana, cola, or maté can attest to the ability of these caffeine-containing herbs to increase alertness and concentration. Indeed, caffeine or caffeine-containing herbs are often included in brain-boosting products. While caffeine is certainly stimulating to the central nervous system, it offers some drawbacks when it comes to being a brain booster. For one, caffeine is a potent alkaloid with a relatively high potential for abuse. Many regular coffee drinkers are dependent on it and experience withdrawal symptoms when it is not available. Also, high doses often have unwanted side effects, including anxiety, insomnia, and irritability. Perhaps more important, caffeine's effects on overall mental function are not all positive. Some controlled studies have shown it actually reduces recall.

Safer herbs with more positive overall effects on thinking, memory, and attention include ginkgo, ginseng, and possibly gotu kola.

Ginkgo

Ginkgo has a well-established ability to increase circulation to parts of the body, including the legs, ears (see Chapter 14), and genitals (see Chapter 7). This revered Chinese herb, however, is most widely taken for its ability to increase circulation to the brain, an action that has been exploited for both its therapeutic and cognitive-enhancing effects. Many medical conditions of the elderly that are associated with poor blood flow to the brain have been shown to be improved by ginkgo, including Alzheimer's disease, hearing loss, and dizziness. For example, a recent double-blind, placebo-controlled study of elderly subjects suffering from mild to moderate memory impairment found that administration of a ginkgo extract for six months had "a beneficial effect on mental efficiency," according to the researchers. Other studies of elderly patients have found that ginkgo can slow the rate of mental deterioration and reduce forgetfulness.

Studies have also found that younger, healthier people can benefit mentally from taking ginkgo on a regular basis. Ginkgo has been shown to increase concentration, quicken information recall, and improve alertness. The authors of one study, in which subjects experienced an improvement in short-term memory, concluded, "These results differentiate *Ginkgo biloba* extract from sedative and stimulant drugs and suggest a specific effect on memory processes."

Ginkgo's positive effects on mental processes are not due solely to its ability to stimulate blood flow in the brain. It is an antioxidant that can protect brain cells from harmful free radicals. Ginkgo may also boost metabolism, neurotransmission, and electrical activity in the brain.

Most herbalists recommend taking ginkgo on a daily basis for an extended period of time to best enhance mental function.

HOW TO USE GINKGO: Ginkgo comes in tablets, capsules, concentrated drops, tinctures, and extracts. An average dosage is 40 mg of a standardized extract containing 24 percent flavoglycosides three times daily.

Ginseng

Much of ginseng's popularity is due to its ability to increase physical performance under stress and boost overall energy levels. Ginseng also has positive effects on alertness, mood, and mental performance. Animal studies and human studies done on nurses, students, soldiers, senior citizens, radio operators, and others have found that ginseng can improve attention and concentration, raise scores on arithmetic and other types of mental tests, and increase understanding of abstract concepts. Ginseng seems to allow animals and people to work longer and harder at mental tasks while making fewer mistakes. In addition to affecting the central nervous system, ginseng boosts circulation and metabolic activity in the brain and helps to balance blood-sugar levels.

Commercial ginseng products vary tremendously in potency; high-quality extracts are reliable providers of the herb's active ingredients.

HOW TO USE GINSENG: Ginseng comes in myriad forms, including as a whole root and in capsules, tablets, tea bags, tinctures, and extracts.

An average brain-boosting dosage of capsules standardized for 5 to 9 percent ginsenoside is 500 to 1,000 mg. An average dosage of some concentrated extracts and ginseng products with higher standardized percentages may be as low as 200 to 400 mg.

Gotu Kola

This is an herb traditionally used in India for strengthening the nervous system and boosting energy levels. In recent years it has also gained a following for its ability to improve memory and enhance mental function. The scientific evidence for this effect is slim but promising. There was one study done in India on mentally retarded children that found improvements in attentiveness and concentration after three months, and a recent study on rats that showed an improvement in learning and memory, but otherwise gotu kola's reputation as a psychic energizer and brain booster rests on word of mouth among users.

Gotu kola does not contain caffeine, as the similarly named herb kola does.

How to use gotu kola: It is sold dried and in capsules, concentrated drops, tinctures, and extracts. An average dosage of the concentrated drops or tincture is 1/2 to 1 dropperful two or three times daily.

Mindful Essential Oils

Essential oils that are dispersed in the air can quickly reach the brain through the olfactory system and affect mood and mental function. Some businesses have even begun to experiment with adding scents to office air-handling systems to increase workers' productivity and mental sharpness. Though such efforts have a somewhat disturbing Big Brother aspect to them, there is no reason not to choose your own essential oils for brain-enhancing effects.

Producers of aromatherapy products have developed various combination oils and other products for boosting brain power. Look for products such as Concentrate, Focus, Creativity, Mental Power, Clear Mind, Inspiration, and the humorously named Brain-Dead. Many of these are available as oils and aromatic mists for diffusing, and as lotions for massage or other topical application. Some are also available as a smelling salt for direct inhalation.

Probably the three most popular essential oils for use in the combination products are Rosemary, Peppermint, and Basil. All of these, especially Basil, are also excellent as individual oils for maximizing mental performance.

Basil

The aromatically scented leaves of this white-flowered annual herb (*Ocimum basilicum* and other species) have long been a popular cooking herb. It also has a respected place in the traditional healing practices of China, India, and parts of Africa. Originating in India, basil spread throughout the world and is now widely cultivated. The light yellow essential oil, steam-distilled from the leaves and flowering tops, is used in the food industry and in aromatherapy.

The essential oil has a reputation as a digestive regulator, aphrodisiac, menstrual-cycle balancer, and migraine remedy. When it is inhaled or applied topically, Basil also seems to increase mental function and brighten mood. "It clears the head, relieves intellectual fatigue, and gives the mind strength and clarity," said Austrian aromatherapy pioneer Marguerite Maury.

Basil is not recommended for use during pregnancy.

Vaporization, inhalation, and massage are the most common ways to take advantage of essential oils' mentally stimulating properties. See "How to Use Essential Oils" in Chapter 2.

Where to Start

The following are two of the safest and most popular ingredients in commercial brain-boosting formulas. Each is also readily available as a single supplement.

- Choline/phosphatidylcholine/lecithin (daily, 100 to 200 mg of choline; 1,100 to 2,200 mg of phosphatidylcholine that is 90 percent pure; or 5 to 10 g, or 1 to 2 tablespoons of granules, of lecithin that is 20 percent phosphatidylcholine)
- Ginkgo (40 mg of a standardized extract containing 24 percent flavoglycosides, three times daily)

Beyond Herbs and Supplements

The brain is a remarkable organ of control, capable of regulating the body's complex web of organs, systems, and senses. Whether the brain is considered to *encompass* the mind or to *be encompassed* by it, it is also the principal organ for controlling bodily health, capable of making decisions that may either undermine or optimize the health and longevity of other organs as well as itself. Here are some of the ways you can empower it toward self-preservation.

• Get regular exercise or participate in regular physical activity. Exercise helps to maintain a healthy circulatory system, including blood-vessel tone and blood flow in the brain. By delivering more oxygen to the brain, you can boost your mood (an important factor in mental function) and improve your short-term memory. One study of 30 people found that those who did regular endurance and strength workouts over a nine-week period performed better on memory tests than those who didn't work out.

• Just as a high-fat, low-fiber diet can lead to clogged arteries of the heart and thus to heart disease, it can also lead to clogged arteries of the brain and an increased risk of stroke. A plant-based, low-fat, high-fiber, nutrient-dense diet helps to keep maximum blood and oxygen circulation in the brain.

• Sufficient sleep is crucial for keeping the brain functioning at its best. "All you have to do is rest," said Jean Molière. "Nature herself, when we let her, will take care of everything else."

• Conscious relaxation or meditation for 10 to 15 minutes or so during the day can reinvorgorate mental processes.

• Chronic substance abuse, especially addictive use of tobacco or alcohol, is harmful to the brain and overall intellectual function. Smoking decreases blood flow to the brain. It is well established that alcoholism frequently leads to memory loss (both short-term, as in "the lost weekend," and long-term), learning disabilities, and other mental problems. (Keep in mind as well that many medical drugs, singly or in combination, can have adverse effects that include confusion, memory loss, and difficulty concentrating.)

12

Calm Your Nerves

Given the widespread use of caffeine and other stimulants, the prevalence of high-stress jobs, and the quickening pace of modern society, it should not come as a surprise that many people have a difficult time staying calm during the day, relaxing after work, or falling asleep at night. Living with a constantly overexcited nervous system can detract from life's simple pleasures, put a strain on personal relationships, and lead to anxiety attacks. It can also eventually lead to medical problems more serious than occasional insomnia, including peptic ulcers and heart disease.

If you want to be more relaxed, try one of the numerous safe and effective strategies that don't involve taking a drug or natural remedy, such as meditation, regular exercise, or changing work habits. For various reasons, many people who are feeling nervous, anxious, restless, or just plain wired also choose to ingest relaxing substances. Indeed, some of the most popular psychoactive drugs in the world are relaxants, including alcohol. While alcohol obviously plays other roles as well, particularly that of a social lubricator, it shares a number of significant drawbacks with conventional drugs taken for relaxation. These drawbacks include toxicity, addiction potential, an increase in accidents, next-day hangovers, and a wide range of side effects, from headaches to memory loss. Not infrequently, the drugs end up causing more problems than the nervousness or insomnia they are taken to cure. Fortunately, there are numerous natural alternatives, from herbs to amino acids to nutritional supplements, that are safe and effective substitutes for conventional relaxants.

Agents that calm you down or reduce your energy level, whether prescription drugs, herbs, or nutritional supplements, can be classified in a number of ways. An *antispasmodic* affects the muscles more than the nerves, reducing muscle tension and spasms and thereby indirectly causing the mind and body to slow down. A *sedative* soothes the nervous system and exerts a calming effect on the mind, relieving nervousness and irritability. To a lesser extent it also reduces the action of organs and muscles. A *hypnotic* is an agent that induces sleep. In practice, the distinction between sedatives and hypnotics is minor. Many calming agents cause restfulness and relaxation at a low dose and induce sleep at slightly higher doses. Medical authorities frequently combine the terms and refer to certain drugs, including alcohol and most sleeping pills, as *sedative-hypnotics*. The term *tranquilizer* may refer to any agent that induces tranquility, but in medical practice it is usually reserved for more potent drugs, the so-called minor and major tranquilizers (a somewhat misleading distinction, since these categories of tranquilizers are not chemically related). The minor tranquilizers are the popular antianxiety and anti-insomnia drugs such as diazepam (Valium) and chlordiazepoxide (Librium). The major tranquilizers, such as chlorpromazine (Thorazine), are potent drugs that are generally reserved for treating psychoses and for managing out-of-control patients.

From Booze to Downers

Alcohol is the king of drugs, in all likelihood having reigned the longest as the most popular mind-altering substance in the world. Biochemically, it is a sedative-hypnotic that quiets the nervous system, slows reflexes and muscle response, and promotes sleep. Recent studies indicate that if alcohol is used in moderation, its relaxing, stress-relieving effects may help lower the risk of heart disease. Both as a sedative and as a hypnotic, however, alcohol has its limitations. In low doses—a drink or two—alcohol often has a somewhat stimulating effect. Especially if you're drinking with other people, you are likely to feel more happy, uninhibited, and socially at ease. A few more drinks brings increased sedation as well as loss of motor control, a greater likelihood of accidents, and decreased brain function. As a hypnotic, alcohol can promote sleep if used occasionally, but if used regularly, it can interfere with normal sleeping and dreaming patterns. Alcohol also has contradictory effects on sexual desire, is potentially fatal in overdoses, and can increase the risk of heart disease, cirrhosis, and other degenerative conditions when regularly consumed to excess.

Among the most potent pharmaceutical depressants are the sedative-hypnotics of the barbiturate class. The first one, barbituric acid, was discovered in 1864, though it wasn't until the early years of the twentieth century that the barbiturates became popular as sleeping pills. Barbiturate drugs now number in the hundreds. The most widely used barbiturates today are the short-acting ones, such as secobarbital (Seconal), whose effects last 6 to 7 hours rather than the 12 to 24 hours of phenobarbital (Donnatal), for instance. Barbiturate abuse is not uncommon, and they're popular street drugs. They act like alcohol for many people, initially causing drunkenness rather than relaxation or sleepiness. Some users experience a hangover the next day. The list of side effects that may be caused by barbiturates, from breathing difficulties to depression, is lengthy. Taking barbiturates in high doses, or drinking alcohol before or after taking them, can be fatal.

The so-called minor tranquilizers are a relatively new class of prescription drugs, dating back only to the development in the mid-1950s of meprobamate (Miltown). With the advent in the 1960s of the benzodiazepines, which include Librium and Valium, tranquilizer use spread into all corners of society. Doctors wrote prescriptions almost indiscriminately for housewives (these are the pills that the Rolling Stones referred to derisively as "mother's little helpers"), students, the elderly, businesspeople, and anyone else complaining of everyday nervousness or anxiety. By 1990 American doctors were writing an estimated 60 to 80 million prescriptions annually for various minor tranquilizers.

"The pharmaceutical industry," notes Andrew Weil, coauthor of *From Chocolate to Morphine,* "has tried hard to convince doctors and patients that these chemicals are revolutionary drugs that specifically reduce anxiety, making people calm and relaxed. In fact, the minor tranquilizers are just another variation on the theme of alcohol and other sedative-hypnotics, with the same tendency to produce adverse effects and dependence." Minor tranquilizers can eventually interfere with normal sleeping and dreaming patterns. Tolerance to them can at times develop relatively quickly. Common side effects include headache, nausea, memory loss, and depression.

Another popular type of conventional depressant is the over-the-counter (OTC) insomnia remedy. These drugs are basically antihistamines packaged and marketed to take advantage of what is normally an unwanted side effect: drowsiness. OTC insomnia remedies usually contain either diphenhydramine (Sominex, Compōz) or doxylamine (Ultra Sleep). In addition to drowsiness, some people also experience the additional side effects that accompany these medicines, including dry mouth, headache, sluggish thinking, and morning hangover. Also, some people are stimulated rather than relaxed by antihistamines. People who suffer from asthma and glaucoma should not take these drugs. High doses of them have also been known to lead to delirium.

The Herbal Relaxants

Humanity has been using herbs for their calming effects for millennia. There are dozens of herbs that can safely and effectively calm frazzled nerves, reduce anxiety, relax major muscles, and help induce sleep. Some herbs can directly depress the central nervous system, while others affect mainly the muscular or digestive system. According to Paul Bergner, editor of *Medical Herbalism,* "Although no clinical proof is available, practitioners often observe that the overall health of a patient taking these herbs will improve over several weeks of taking them. One possible mechanism for the improvement in health is that most herbs used for nervous disorders also have bitter properties. Bitter herbs improve liver and digestive function, resulting in improved uptake of nutrients."

In general, herbal relaxants are milder in their effects on mood and behavior when compared to prescription sedatives and other conventional depressants. You won't experience the giddy alcohol-like high of some drugs. Nor will you, however, experience these stronger drugs' negative effects: hangover; interference with normal sleeping, dreaming, and waking patterns; potential for addiction; risk of death if mixed with alcohol; and so forth. Even though the calming herbs and nutrients are generally safe and nontoxic, they should be treated with respect, kept away from children, and not relied upon on a daily basis.

Herbs for relaxation can be taken in various forms. Capsules and tablets are popular, as are liquids such as concentrated drops and tinctures. Brewing an herbal tea for sipping a half hour or so before bedtime can be soothing, though in general teas deliver only a low dose of an herb's constituent chemicals. Some people like to pour powdered herbs or a few cups of herbal tea into a warm bath, or a footbath, to help promote sleepiness.

Herbal companies often combine the herbs described below in formula remedies for nervous tension and insomnia. In general, federal regulations prohibit health claims for herbs and prevent herbal manufacturers from using the product label to educate consumers about the herbs' effects. Product names can be descriptive, however, so look for herbal combinations that go by names such as Stress-Release, Good-Nite, Peaceful Night, Stress Master, Deep Sleep, Stay Calm, Arko-Sleep 2000, Stress-Ezzz, Naturest, Silent Night Formula, and Relax & Sleep. Some formulations may also include other herbs such as corn poppy (*Papaver rhoeas*), wood betony (*Stachys officinalis*), black cohosh (*Cimicifuga racemosa*), and wild lettuce (*Lactuca virosa*), as well as nutrients such as vitamin B complex, calcium, and magnesium.

The following is a top-ten list of the herbs most commonly used as relaxants and sleep-inducers in the West. The average doses offered here are for helping to promote sleep. Experiment with slightly lower amounts if you want to induce relaxation.

Among the following ten herbs, chamomile, passionflower, lemon balm, and catnip are those most often used to help calm children. Reduce the adult dosage—children's dosages are usually one-half (for 10- to 14-year-olds), one-third (for 6- to 10-year-olds), or even less, depending on the child's size. Check with a knowledgeable practitioner if you have any doubts about the safety of an herb for your child.

Note that because calming herbs can cause drowsiness, depending on dose and on factors unique to every individual, it is best to avoid using them before driving an auto or operating heavy equipment. At the very least, get to know their effects on you before undertaking such activities.

Valerian

Valerian is sometimes referred to as the herbal Valium because of the similarity in name (*valerian* comes from the Latin *valere,* "to be strong or well") and use (as an antianxiety drug, muscle relaxant, and sleeping pill). There the similarities end: valerian is a natural plant remedy, while Valium is a trade name for a synthetic prescription drug (diazepam). Valerian is also safe, non-habit-forming, and nontoxic while diazepam may cause a wide variety of adverse reactions and has significant potential for leading to psychological or physical dependence. A number of studies have also suggested that use of minor tranquilizers such as diazepam, meprobamate, and chlordiazepoxide during the first trimester of pregnancy increases the risk of congenital malformations.

Valerian products are prepared from the strong-smelling root of a European perennial (*Valeriana officinalis*) that now grows throughout the northeastern United States. Herbalists have been using it medicinally for at least a thousand years, and it has gained widespread popularity as the most useful calming remedy in Europe. German companies, for example, market more than a hundred OTC herbal remedies containing valerian. Valerian relaxes both the nervous and digestive systems. It is a mild but effective tranquilizer, sedative, and hypnotic. It is sometimes used as an antispasmodic to relax muscles and relieve back spasms. People take it to prevent insomnia, reduce nervous excitability and anxiety, lower high blood pressure, and relieve tension headaches. It can also help relieve stomach and menstrual cramps, and constipation or indigestion from nervous tension.

Numerous double-blind, placebo-controlled scientific studies have confirmed valerian's relaxant effects. Several studies have found that the herb is as effective as some barbiturates for reducing the time needed to fall asleep. Tests show that valerian neither interferes with the quality of sleep nor causes morning grogginess, as do the synthetic tranquilizers.

Although valerian's sedative action has been confirmed in studies of the whole herb, exactly which of the plant's active constituents are responsible for its effects has yet to be positively determined. Valerian contains a volatile oil and a number of other compounds (valepotriates) that at one time were thought to be responsible for the plant's calming effects. A notable 1988 German study found that while the whole herb depressed the central nervous system, the isolated oil and the valepotriates did not. "Possibly a combination of volatile oil components, valepotriates or their derivatives, and as-yet-unidentified water-soluble constituents is responsible," notes Varro E. Tyler, Ph.D., in *The Honest Herbal.* Further research is necessary to pinpoint valerian's mechanism of action. In the meantime, supplement producers generally use the whole herb, with extracts often being standardized for tiny percentages of essential oil or the related valeric acid.

While valerian is not addictive and does not cause significant side effects at recommended dosages, it shouldn't be used in large amounts or on a daily basis for an extended period of time. For unknown reasons, a small minority of people react to it by being stimulated rather than calmed. If that is the case with you, use any of the other relaxing herbs mentioned below.

Valerian is probably the most common herbal component of combination formulas that go by names such as Eurocalm, Herbal Calm, and Forty Winks.

HOW TO USE VALERIAN: Valerian is sold dried and as a coarse powder for making tea. It can also be found in tablets, capsules, concentrated drops, tinctures, and extracts. An average dose is 1 to 2 dropperfuls of the tincture or concentrated drops or 200 to 300 mg of the liquid or solid extract.

Passionflower

Passionflower preparations are made from the leaves, flowers, and fruits of a creeping vine (*Passiflora incarnata*) native to the southeastern United States and Central America. It has traditionally been used as an analgesic and as a sedative, an effect confirmed by animal studies. Many users report that passionflower can help induce a contemplative state or mild euphoria, and it can relieve headaches or muscle spasms that are due to nervous tension. It is a popular natural sedative in Europe, and is recognized by German drug regulators as an effective remedy for "nervous anxiety." It is also sometimes recommended as a digestive aid and menstrual-pain reliever. It is not an aphrodisiac, despite its name (which derives from the plant's resemblance to symbols of the biblical Passion—Jesus's crown of thorns and his wounds).

Passionflower is gentle enough for children who are nervous and for the elderly suffering from insomnia.

HOW TO USE PASSIONFLOWER: It is sold dried and in concentrated drops, tinctures, and extracts. An average dosage of the solid extract is 150 to 300 mg; an average dosage of the concentrated drops is 1 to 2 dropperfuls.

Hop

Hop is a climbing plant (*Humulus lupulus*) whose conelike fruits are best known for preserving beer and giving it its bitter flavor. Hop is powerfully scented, and English growers noticed that hop gardens located next to infants' bedrooms could exude an odor capable of lulling babies to sleep. Today hop is known to affect both the nervous and digestive systems. It is often combined with chamomile for use as a digestive stimulant, especially for indigestion, tense bowel states, and other complaints caused by anxiety. It is also recognized as a gentle sedative and hypnotic for easing anxiety and tension, reducing restlessness, and (often in combination with valerian and other herbs) preventing insomnia. Herbalists consider it to be milder than valerian.

Scientists have identified a number of active constituents with potential sedative effects, including lupulin, found particularly in a pollenlike substance produced by the plant.

How to use hop: Tens of millions of Americans use hop on a daily basis, in the form of that familiar fermented, alcoholic beverage beer. Almost all of the relaxant effect in beer, however, is from the alcohol. Herbal hop products, both dried and liquid, are available in natural-food stores. An average dosage of the concentrated drops is 1 to 2 dropperfuls.

An unusual, traditional way to use hop is as an ingredient in a "sleep pillow" or "dream pillow." These are small pillows or muslin bags that are loosely filled with hop, lavender, chamomile, or other dried herbs known to contain volatile oils with potential sedative effects. Historians report that England's King George III used this ancient form of sleep therapy. As your head presses on the pillow tiny amounts of these volatile oils are released as fragrances and inhaled through the nose. The olfactory system reacts to chemical inputs and transports signals to special sections of the brain that act to relax the central nervous system. You'll need to renew the herbs every two months or so. (See "Resources" for a mail-order source of sleep pillows.)

California Poppy

California poppy (also known as golden poppy) is a yellow-flowering plant (*Eschscholtzia californica*) that is the state flower of California, but Californians are behind Europeans in recognizing the medicinal properties of this plant. The whole plant is used to make herbal remedies that produce a calming and quieting effect on the central nervous system. According to Michael Moore, author of *Medicinal Plants of the Pacific West,* California poppy "is a surprisingly effective herb for use with anxieties, jittery nervousness—a sort of controlled heebie jeebies, with skin hypersensitivity and peripatetic movements." He adds that it is not as "overtly sedative" as valerian.

California poppy is in the same family (Papaveraceae) as the opium poppy, the source of narcotic alkaloids such as morphine and codeine. The active alkaloids in California poppy, however, are much less potent and not addictive. Although California poppy is distinct from opium poppy, it is "chemically similar enough to cause a possible false positive in urine testing for opiates," Moore says.

California poppy is safe enough for children. Many parents have found it works well, singly or in combination with chamomile, to calm a restless or overexcited child.

HOW TO USE CALIFORNIA POPPY: This herb is not as widely available in tablet and capsule form as valerian, passionflower, and most other sedative herbs. It is more commonly found in concentrated drops and liquid tinctures. An average dosage is 1 to 2 dropperfuls.

Lemon Balm

Lemon balm preparations are derived from the lemony-smelling leaves of a perennial mint plant (*Melissa officinalis*) native to Europe. Also known as melissa, balm, bee balm, and sweet balm, it has traditionally been used to relieve nervousness and anxiety. Herbalists also recommend it to alleviate nervous headaches, settle mild upset stomachs, and treat cold sores and genital lesions caused by the herpes simplex viruses. Studies confirm that lemon balm relaxes the nervous system and. is an effective though mild herbal sedative. Its sedative action is largely attributed to volatile terpenes such as citronellal. Along with catnip, California poppy, and chamomile, lemon balm is among the gentlest of the calming herbs.

People with thyroid conditions should avoid using lemon balm, since two studies have shown that it may interfere with a hormone that stimulates the gland.

HOW TO USE LEMON BALM: This is another herb that is more popular in Europe than in the United States. An average dosage of the concentrated drops is 1 to 2 dropperfuls.

Kava Kava

Kava kava, or simply kava (*Piper methysticum*), is derived from the roots and rhizome of a large shrub related to black pepper that is widely cultivated in Samoa, Fiji, and elsewhere in the South Pacific. The British explorer Captain James Cook gave kava kava a botanic name that translates as "intoxicating pepper," indicating a usage that native peoples of the area have long exploited. They ferment fresh kava kava root into an alcoholic beverage that is drunk during various religious and cultural rituals. For example, it is shared by parties to a dispute to relax them and help them to come to an equitable resolution. Kava kava is also a social and recreational drink, said to induce a mild euphoric or even hallucinogenic state, to enhance dreams, and to heighten sexuality.

The principal active ingredients in kava kava are pyrones and kavalactones. Studies have shown that these chemicals can relax skeletal muscles, depress the nervous system, and cause changes in motor function. In Europe, herbal producers are using chemicals derived from kava kava to develop semisynthetic sedatives.

Fresh kava kava root is not generally available outside the South Pacific. The dried root taken in tablet or tea form is not so much intoxicating as relaxing. For most people kava kava simply reduces anxiety and nervousness, while for a few it seems to promote a pleasant, dreamy state.

HOW TO USE KAVA KAVA: In the United States kava kava is sold as the cut and sifted root or as a coarse, dry powder for brewing into tea. You can also find it in capsules, as a liquid extract, and in concentrated drops. An average dosage of the concentrated drops is 1 to 2 dropperfuls.

Chamomile

Chamomile, an ancient and widely used herb, is the flower of either of two annual plants: German chamomile and Roman chamomile. Taken as a tea, it has long been used to treat anxiety and insomnia. In Europe more so than the United States, chamomile has also enjoyed widespread use taken internally for digestive problems and applied topically to irritated skin, cuts and scrapes, sore muscles, and burns. As a mild soporific, chamomile seems to calm the nervous, digestive, and muscular systems. Many people find it a handy remedy for stress and nervous indigestion.

Chamomile is safe and gentle enough for use on restless or irritable children. Although chamomile is in the same large Compositae family as plants (such as ragweed) that cause allergic reactions, and some medical authorities claim chamomile also poses a significant allergic threat, this is simply not true. A 1984 review of worldwide medical records found allergic reactions to be extremely rare—a mere five instances over the past century (none fatal) are attributed to German chamomile, the type most commonly sold in the United States. Michael Castleman, author of *The Healing Herbs,* says that "the only people who should think twice about using this herb (and its close relative, yarrow) are those who have suffered previous anaphylactic reaction from ragweed."

HOW TO USE CHAMOMILE: Chamomile is available in a variety of herbal forms but in this country is most commonly consumed as a soothing, late-night tea.

Ashwagandha

Ashwagandha is one of the most widely used herbs of Ayurvedic medicine, the traditional healing practice of India. It is derived from the roots and leaves of a small branching undershrub of the nightshade family that grows abundantly in the arid highlands of Himalayan India. Ayurvedic practitioners have used ashwagandha for over 2,500 years as a general tonic and system balancer (see Chapter 13). It is now growing in popularity in the United States, where it is used to protect the body from the adverse effects of stress and to reduce anxiety. Taken after work, it acts as a mild sedative to help reduce nervousness and promote relaxation without causing sluggishness.

Although studies done over the past few decades have isolated dozens of compounds in ashwagandha, including alkaloids and withanolides, the plant's action as a sedative is still unexplained.

How to use ASHWAGANDHA: Within the past few years a number of American herbal companies have begun to market ashwagandha in capsules. Many are standardized for 2 to 5 mg withanolides, as are the preparations preferred in clinical studies. An average recommended dosage is 150 to 300 mg ashwagandha.

Catnip

Catnip preparations are derived from the fresh leaves or flowering tops of a mint-family perennial (*Nepeta cataria*) that excites cats but has the opposite effect on people. It is used as a mild sedative, but is not a marijuanalike intoxicant, despite rumors dating back to the late 1960s. Catnip also relieves menstrual cramps and is taken as an aid for indigestion and upset stomach. "Weak, cool catnip infusions may be given cautiously to colicky infants," notes Castleman in *The Healing Herbs*.

How to use CATNIP: It is available dried and as capsules, concentrated drops, and extracts. An average dosage of the concentrated drops is 1 to 2 dropperfuls.

Skullcap

Skullcap preparations are made from the whole flowering tops or the leaves of a North American perennial (*Scutellaria lateriflora*) in the mint family. The name derives from the shape of the plant's calyx. Skullcap has a reputation as a safe and mild relaxant that affects the nervous and musculoskeletal systems. While some studies have identified sedative effects, others have not, causing some herbal conservatives to regard skullcap as relatively inactive. People take it to relieve insomnia and the related problems of anxiety, restlessness, nervous tension, and excess stress; some herbalists recommend it as an antispasmodic to relieve menstrual cramps and reduce muscle spasms. It is more frequently combined with other herbs such as valerian, chamomile, or hop than used by itself to treat anxiety or insomnia.

How to use skullcap: An average dosage of skullcap is 1 to 2 dropperfuls of the tincture or concentrated drops.

Choosing and Combining the Calming Herbs

Many of the abovementioned herbs have overlapping effects. Some people may find one or another slightly better for certain purposes, such as inducing sleep, relaxing muscles, and reducing anxiety. The following chart offers a summary of the effects most often cited by herbalists for these herbs.

	Inducing sleep	Relaxing muscles	Calming anxiety
Valerian	•	•	•
Passionflower	•	•	•
Hop	•		•
California poppy	•		•
Lemon balm		•	•
Kava kava			•
Chamomile			•
Ashwagandha			•
Catnip	•	•	•
Skullcap			•

You can combine any of the above herbs to take advantage of their unique effects. "A nerve tonic formulated from several herbs may be much more effective than any of the herbs taken alone," notes Paul Bergner. While it is often simpler to buy ready-made combination products at natural-food stores, an easy way to combine calming herbs is to use tinctures or concentrated drops. For example, to promote sleep combine 1 dropperful each (yielding approximately one teaspoon total) of valerian, passionflower, and hop.

Valerian remains the king of the herbal relaxants. If you want to try only one herb, start with it.

The Calming Essential Oils

Many herbalists and aromatherapists recommend essential oils—concentrated aromatic liquids—to help relax the body and calm the mind. Essential oils are volatile and can readily be evaporated or dispersed into the air, where they are inhaled and quickly sent to parts of the brain that affect mood and behavior. A number of essential-oil producers now offer combination products, including massage and bath oils, that blend calming essential oils such as Lavender, Ylang-ylang, and Chamomile. Look for products with names such as Tranquility.

Lavender

The leaves and blue flowers of lavender, an evergreen Mediterranean shrub (*Lavandula officinalis*), contain a high concentration of volatile oils. Although the plant has long been traditionally used as a dried herb to treat coughs and the common cold, it is now more widely used as an essential oil for its relaxing, skin-soothing, and immune-boosting effects. When its delicate scent is inhaled, it can help to induce sleep, alleviate stress, and reduce depression and nervous tension. The oil is mild enough for use with children.

Scientific investigation of essential oils' effects when inhaled is in its infancy, but Japanese scientists recently performed one of the first such studies, on Lavender as a sedative. They found that mice that inhaled Lavender vapor for 15 minutes experienced fewer convulsions than those not exposed to the vapor. The researchers said that the anticonvulsive effect may have been due to Lavender's ability to enhance the action of certain calming neurotransmitters.

Herbalist Rosemary Gladstar, author of *Herbal Healing for Women*, says Lavender "is one of my favorite herbs for nerve stress and tension. It has a special affinity with women's spirit." She notes that it is especially useful during menopause and for menstrual discomfort.

Ylang-ylang

Ylang-ylang is a tropical Asian tree whose freshly picked flowers are used to produce a pale yellow, sweet-smelling essential oil. It is popular for use in cosmetics and perfumes. Therapeutically, Ylang-ylang is most commonly used for its calming effect. It helps reduce blood pressure, regulate heartbeat and breathing, lower adrenaline levels, and quiet the nervous system. It can offer relief from anxiety, stress-related problems, and insomnia.

Essential oils are usually sold in small bottles in natural-food stores; the oil is typically used by the drop. Essential oils are extremely concentrated substances and are generally *not* taken orally. There are a number of ways to take advantage of essential oils' relaxing properties; see "How to Use Essential Oils" in Chapter 2.

The Sedative Amino Acids

Just as amino acids can play an important role in the brain chemistry of stimulation, so can some play a role in relaxation. When compared to our use of herbs, humanity's experience with using isolated amino acid substances as calming agents is much more limited. Still, clinical experience and most of the research into amino acids over the past thirty years have indicated that amino acids are safe and nonaddictive, especially when compared to synthetic drugs used for similar purposes. Unfortunately for consumers, of the three amino-acid-based substances described below, two (tryptophan and gamma hydroxybutyrate, or GHB) are no longer available as OTC nutritional supplements, and the third, gamma-aminobutyric acid, or GABA, is in danger of also being pulled from health-food store shelves by the Food and Drug Administration (FDA). The following discussions of tryptophan and GHB are included here on the off chance that these substances do return to the market. In the meantime, you can take advantage of tryptophan's calming effects by eating certain foods.

Tryptophan

An essential amino acid, tryptophan is one of the most effective natural substances for inducing relaxation and restful sleep. Tryptophan is naturally found in a variety of foods, including dairy products, meat, fish, and some nuts and seeds. Human beings have always consumed tryptophan; average daily intake of tryptophan on the type of protein-rich diet eaten by the average American is in excess of one gram.

Tryptophan plays an important role in the production of the brain neurotransmitter serotonin and the hormone melatonin, both of which act as natural sedatives. Deficiencies of these substances have been tied to insomnia and sleep-related problems. For four decades prior to the FDA's pulling tryptophan from the market in November 1989, the amino acid had been safely used, primarily but not exclusively as a sleep aid, by millions of people. "Two percent of all American households had at least one member who swallowed tablets or capsules of L-tryptophan," notes medical writer Morton Walker. "Its use was advocated by physicians, psychologists, substance abuse centers, weight loss programs, plus health food store proprietors."

Tryptophan had passed the test not only of public acceptance but of scientific scrutiny. Researchers conducted numerous studies that confirmed the amino acid's effectiveness as a gentle sedative. Various studies found that doses of 0.5 to 4 g of tryptophan can significantly reduce the time it takes to fall asleep. Tryptophan both allows the person to fall asleep sooner and induces a normal sleep rather than the distorted sleep patterns produced by most sleeping pills. Studies have also found tryptophan to be a mild sedative when administered at any time of day. After 30 to 60 minutes the person experiences a more relaxed waking state. According to Sheldon Saul Hendler, M.D., Ph.D., author of *The Doctors' Vitamin and Mineral Encyclopedia,* "Tryptophan appears to work well as an alternative to the standard hypnotic sleeping drugs."

The FDA recalled all tryptophan supplements from stores and banned future sales of manufactured tryptophan in the U.S. when consumption was tied to a rare blood disorder called eosinophilia-myalgia syndrome (EMS) that afflicted an estimated five thousand Americans and caused some 39 deaths. Though the link between tryptophan and EMS is still being studied, medical investigators have determined that many of these adverse effects were probably caused by tryptophan supplements containing contaminants, rather than from tryptophan itself.

Despite the likely association of EMS with a contaminant in tryptophan, whether tryptophan supplements produced in the customary way are safe and deserve to be returned to the market remains controversial. Many nutritionists and supplement producers contend that the FDA has seized upon the tryptophan tragedy as an excuse to permanently ban tryptophan and eventually to regulate all amino acids as prescription drugs rather than as supplements. Although researchers have linked about 95 percent of EMS cases studied extensively with possibly contaminated tryptophan, the FDA counters that because studies have not been able to link definitively *all* cases of EMS with suspect tryptophan, a continuing ban is necessary and prudent.

Should the safety questions about tryptophan be resolved and supplements again become available, keep in mind that pregnant women should not take tryptophan supplements, nor should anyone who is taking MAO-inhibiting drugs.

When tryptophan was available in supplement form, it was frequently combined with 25 to 50 mg of vitamin B_6 and 250 to 500 mg of magnesium to promote its conversion into brain chemicals and enhance its effects.

HOW TO USE TRYPTOPHAN: Since supplemental tryptophan is currently not available in the United States, the only way that Americans can take advantage of its calming powers is through diet. The most effective strategy is to eat foods with high levels of tryptophan relative to other amino acids. Eggs, poultry, and meat are rich in tryptophan, but they also contain large amounts of other amino acids, such as L-phenylalanine, that compete with tryptophan for uptake in the brain and have a stimulating instead of calming effect on the nervous system. Among the foods with the best ratios of tryptophan to other amino acids are roasted pumpkin seeds, dried sunflower seeds, bananas, and milk. Still, you must eat relatively large amounts of these foods to approach the levels of tryptophan once widely available in supplements. For example, eating 100 grams, about 3.5 ounces, of pumpkin seeds, or drinking four cups of milk, provides a dose of about 500 mg of tryptophan. If you want to promote sleep, about an hour before bedtime eat some of these tryptophan-specific foods.

Some users of tryptophan have noticed heightened relaxing effects when the amino acid is taken with foods rich in complex carbohydrates, such as potatoes, bread, cereal, or pasta. The carbohydrates will help to raise serotonin levels in the brain gradually, and thus induce calmness and drowsiness, by promoting the secretion of insulin. Insulin helps amino acids cross from the blood into cells. Insulin has less effect, however, on tryptophan than on the other amino acids. This leaves more tryptophan in the blood to make its way to the brain and affect behavior.

GABA and GHB

GABA is a nonessential amino acid formed in the body from the amino acid glutamate, vitamin B_6, and vitamin C. In the body GABA acts as a neurotransmitter that helps to regulate nerve function in a way that induces relaxation. Instead of promoting the transmission of signals between nerve endings in the brain, as do neurotransmitters such as noradrenaline, GABA prevents nerve cells from firing too fast. It thus inhibits message transmission in the brain. This message slow-down has a calming effect and helps to relieve nervous and muscular tension. Valium and a number of the other minor tranquilizers rely for their calming effect on their ability to mimic the action of GABA.

GHB is a natural substance found in brain and other cells that is chemically related to GABA. GHB has a similar calming effect. It helps to induce a natural sleep and seems to increase dreaming.

Until a few years ago both synthetic GABA and GHB were available as nutritional supplements. GHB became popular with bodybuilders, who noticed that high doses could stimulate the pituitary to release growth hormone. Although nutritionists generally consider GHB to be safe and nonaddictive, it was recently declared to be a prescription drug by the FDA. GABA may well be next on the FDA's hit list, but as of this writing GABA supplements are sold over the counter and are available in some natural-food stores and through mail order (see "Resources").

How to use gaba: GABA is sold as a powder, in 750-mg tablets, and in capsules that go by names such as GABA Calm and GABA Plus. An average calming dosage is 500 to 750 mg, while for insomnia take 750 to 2,000 mg about an hour before bedtime. Some people find that GABA's calming effects are enhanced by taking along with it 50 to 100 mg of B-complex vitamins, mostly for the niacin and B_6.

Nutritional Supplements for Relaxation

The well-known minerals calcium and magnesium and the lesser-known hormonal substance melatonin are the two principal nutritional supplements taken for their relaxing effects. If you find it difficult to wind down at the end of a work day, you may also want to consider taking 50 to 100 mg of vitamin B complex. Thiamine, niacin, B_6, and a number of other B vitamins are important for the proper functioning of the nerves and the nervous system. Of the B vitamins, niacin has perhaps the most dramatic sedative properties when taken in megadoses, such as 500 to 1,000 mg of niacinamide, possibly because it acts to free up tryptophan in the brain for more serotonin production. If you do take more than 75 to 100 mg of niacin, make sure you take it in a form (such as niacinamide or inositol hexaniacinate) that limits niacin's normal ability to cause a dramatic but short-lived skin flush.

Melatonin

While recent research has extended melatonin's potential benefits into the fields of immunity, cancer prevention, and longevity (see Chapter 10), its most popular use today is as a mild hypnotic to induce drowsiness. A minute dose (1.5 to 3 mg) of synthetic melatonin taken orally before bedtime has a similar effect on the body as natural melatonin released by the tiny pineal gland in the center of brain. Melatonin seems to synchronize certain biological cycles, including the body's circadian (daily) rhythms. Studies have found that melatonin levels in the body have a direct effect on sleep patterns. Researchers have used supplements to treat various sleep disorders, including insomnia, disruptions in the sleep-wake cycle due to either jet lag or changing work shifts, and the condition known as delayed sleep phase disorder (characterized by an inability to fall asleep when you want to, although when you wait a few hours you fall asleep only to awaken in the morning feeling drowsy and fatigued).

Under normal circumstances, the body secretes minimal levels of melatonin during daylight hours. At the onset of darkness, the body begins to synthesize and release increased levels of melatonin, which remains at higher levels at night. Tiny amounts (0.75 to 6 mg) of melatonin taken orally are enough to support this natural cycle. Researchers who have administered large doses (40 mg) of melatonin in some studies have found decreasing sedative effects and increasing mood-altering side effects, such as depression and anxiety. Melatonin seems to be most effective when given in doses, such as those recommended below, that mirror natural bodily levels.

Most sleep studies now administer 2-to-3-mg pills. These studies are confirming that melatonin functions naturally as a sleep-inducing hormone, says Dr. Richard J. Wurtman, professor of neuroscience at the Massachusetts Institute of Technology. According to Wurtman, when he and his colleagues gave melatonin supplements to volunteers, those taking the hormone fell asleep in five or six minutes, while those on placebo took between 15 and 30 minutes. The MIT study tested melatonin on 20 young male volunteers. They were given various doses of melatonin or placebo, put in a dark room at midday, and told to close their eyes for 30 minutes. In addition to falling asleep more quickly, those on melatonin tended to sleep twice as long as those on placebo. According to Dr. Judith L. Vaitukaitis, director of the National Center for Research Resources, the MIT findings offer hope "for a natural, nonaddictive agent that could improve sleep for millions of Americans."

Wurtman contends that people should not self-medicate with melatonin, saying that safety can't be assured until the FDA has approved melatonin as a drug. The consensus, however, among the vast majority of nutritional practitioners and naturopathic doctors is that the recommended dosages of 1.5 to 3 mg of melatonin are safe and nontoxic. Taken orally, melatonin is short-lived in the body. It is rapidly absorbed into the bloodstream, metabolized, and eliminated. Clinical experience to date indicates that side effects are negligible even when taken in doses much higher than recommended. Certainly compared to conventional prescription drugs for inducing sleepiness, which are addictive and even potentially fatal in large doses, melatonin is an exceedingly safe substance. Even so, melatonin should not be taken by women who are pregnant or lactating, or by anyone suffering from kidney disease. Because it may affect growth-hormone levels, melatonin should also be avoided by anyone under the age of 20.

After taking melatonin orally, it reaches a maximum level in the blood after about an hour. How quickly melatonin causes drowsiness varies from person to person. Some people don't notice any effects for over an hour, while others experience its calming effects within 5 or 10 minutes. Thus, timing is important. To help induce sleep, many people find it works best if taken about 15 to 30 minutes before bedtime. Some insomnia sufferers prefer to take it about two hours before bedtime, or in divided doses, the first about two hours before bedtime and the second about 15 to 30 minutes before bedtime. Experiment to determine what works best for you. Generally it is best to take it at the same time every night, to avoid causing a shift in your circadian rhythms.

How to use melatonin: Melatonin comes in 750-mcg (0.75 mg) and 3-mg pills. An average daily dosage to promote better sleep is 1.5 to 2 mg; elderly people may need to take 2 to 3 mg. Start with the lower dose and increase if necessary.

Calcium and Magnesium

Calcium is widely hailed for its role in building bones and teeth, but it also plays a lesser role in transmitting nerve messages, regulating heartbeat, and stabilizing blood pressure. Magnesium also plays a role in nerve function and works in tandem with calcium to relax muscle tissue. Though studies are lacking, many people note that taking a balanced calcium-magnesium supplement an hour or so before bedtime seems to have a slight sedating effect.

How to use calcium and magnesium: Calcium and magnesium are available as freeze-dried granules, tablets, capsules, and liquids, and in some cases are combined in products with names such as Calm, Mynax, and Cal-zzz-um. To take advantage of these minerals' apparent relaxing effect, combine them in approximately a 2:1 ratio, such as 400 mg calcium and 200 mg magnesium.

Sleepytime Homeopathic Remedies

The most popular single homeopathic remedies used to relax the body, calm the mind, and relieve insomnia include *Coffea, Arsenicum,* and *Chamomilla.* Most combination homeopathic remedies for deeper sleep include these, as well as others such as *Nux vomica, Pulsatilla, Ignatia, Passionflower* or *Passiflora,* and *Hops.* Some of the popular homeopathic combination remedies for insomnia include Quiétude from Boiron, Calms and Calms Forté from Hyland's (Standard Homeopathic Company), Alpha ND from Boericke & Tafel, Sedilor Insomnia from Dolisos, Insomnia from the company Medicine From Nature, and Luyties No. 173 Sleep.

Coffea

Homeopathic *Coffea* is prepared from raw, unroasted coffee berries. It is frequently recommended for nervousness or sleeplessness due to extremes of excitement or joy, overactivity of mind or body, too much coffee or coffee withdrawal, irritability, and oversensitivity.

Arsenicum

Arsenicum is prepared from arsenic trioxide, a compound of the poisonous chemical element arsenic. In microdilute homeopathic dosages *Arsenicum* is used to treat a variety of conditions, including certain skin rashes, stomach upsets from food poisoning, and exhaustion. It is also taken for insomnia associated with anxiety or apprehension. The *Arsenicum* patient is typically anxious, restless, pale, and fearful.

Chamomilla

Chamomilla, derived from the whole fresh chamomile plant, is what most homeopaths recommend when a child is overly restless or has insomnia. It is also used to treat toothaches and childhood teething pains, colic, earaches, and fever. The *Chamomilla* patient is frequently irascible, stubborn, and inconsolable.

See "How to Use Homeopathic Remedies" in Chapter 2.

How to Choose

Sedatives share with stimulants the general rule that you should be careful about taking full doses of a number of substances at the same time. The following three natural substances, however, are probably the most popular calming remedies and can safely be taken singly or in combination.

- Valerian (1 to 2 dropperfuls of the tincture or concentrated drops, or 200 to 300 mg of the liquid or solid extract)
- Melatonin (1.5 to 2 mg)
- Calcium and magnesium (400 mg calcium and 200 mg magnesium)

Safest of the Safe

Many women who are pregnant choose to avoid sedatives of any kind, wishing to err on the side of caution. While the occasional use of average doses of the calming herbs and amino acids is not known to interfere with pregnancy, most natural practitioners agree that avoiding such sedatives during pregnancy is the safest option. The following two types of natural substances are safe calming remedies even for pregnant women.

- Calcium and magnesium (400 mg calcium and 200 mg magnesium), since they are necessary nutrients often supplemented during pregnancy
- Homeopathic remedies, which are exceedingly dilute

Beyond Herbs and Supplements

Herbs and supplements should be only a temporary or stopgap measure for relaxing or falling asleep. If you are overly nervous, or if you can't sleep because you've just had a death in your family, you've lost your job, you're moving, or you're just jetlagged, natural remedies can help you get through these tough times. If, however, you have insomnia on a regular basis, or if you're taking so many stimulants every day that by late afternoon you're a nervous wreck, you need to take more fundamental steps than merely refining your intake of relaxants. While insomnia may result from viral infections or other serious conditions, it is much more commonly a problem associated with factors relating to lifestyle, diet, or exercise. Here are some commonsensical steps that anyone who is experiencing constant nervous tension or insomnia should take.

• Cut back on consumption of caffeine-containing drinks, such as coffee, tea, and colas; foods with stimulant compounds, such as chocolate; herbal "upper" products that contain ma huang or ephedra; alcoholic beverages (alcohol is deceptive because it may make you drowsy but later in the night interferes with sound sleep); and various medications, including those for asthma that contain theophylline and pain relievers, such as Vanquish and Anacin, that contain caffeine.

• Get more aerobic exercise during the day (but not right before bed).

• Practice biofeedback, meditation, or some other method for inducing the relaxation response and reducing everyday levels of anxiety.

• Avoid eating large meals late in evening, and avoid napping late in the day.

• Make your bed and bedroom quiet and healthful.

• Consider a technique, such as psychological counseling, journal-keeping, or dream analysis, that can help you address the cause of your anxiety or nervousness.

Strengthen and Balance Your System

Many of the natural substances described in previous chapters have very specific effects: elevating mood, reducing the risk of heart attack, calming the nervous system. In terms of how they work, natural substances can mirror the actions of some conventional drugs: a specific organ or bodily system is principally affected, and bodywide actions are limited. Another class of natural substances, what has long been called tonics or tonifiers, works in a qualitatively different manner. These are herbs and nutrients that promote overall health due to their mildly strengthening and balancing effects on the entire body, including various organs and systems. Tonics act to increase energy and boost vitality. They strengthen resistance to disease and stimulate healing capacity. They can also help at work or school by improving memory and increasing your stamina for mental work. In athletes these substances tend to boost muscular strength and aerobic capacity. In short, tonics are the working class of natural substances, reliable laborers deserving of more respect.

Though the concept is ancient—many of the herbs considered tonifiers have been used for their strengthening and balancing effects for thousands of years—within recent years a new name has been applied to this class of natural substances: the *adaptogens*. In 1947 a Russian scientist, N. V. Lazarev, proposed calling a drug or other substance an adaptogen if it could help to increase "nonspecific resistance of an organism to adverse influence." Lazarev's student, the noted researcher I. I. Brekhman, M.D., expanded Lazarev's definition and proposed that a substance meet three conditions to be considered an adaptogen. It had to be:

- Safe and nontoxic—that is, it should cause no side effects or minimal side effects
- Nonspecific in its action—an adaptogen increases resistance to a wide range of biological, environmental, and other physical factors, and should boost the body's overall immune function by various means rather than by one specific action (say, an increase in immune-cell formation)
- Normalizing in the body—no matter what the disease state, an adaptogen should restore to balance all bodily systems while aggravating none

Plant-drug authority Varro E. Tyler, Ph.D., Sc.D., notes that the uses of the words *tonic* and *adaptogen* to refer to herbs that increase resistance to stress now overlap, although *adaptogen* is slowly displacing *tonic* in the herbal literature. "The Russian term [*adaptogen*] has not been widely adopted in the standard English medical and pharmaceutical literature. It is extensively used in the herbal literature."

As their name suggests, adaptogens promote the body's ability to adapt to new conditions. Today, new conditions often mean stressful conditions: a demanding boss at work, constant urban noise at home, conflicts within the family. All of these conditions put an extra burden on mind and body, and particularly on organs such as the adrenals, the liver, and the heart. Stressful conditions also especially challenge the nervous and endocrine systems. The health consequences of unrelieved stress are quite visible in the United States. According to the American Academy of Family Physicians, two out of three office visits to family doctors result from symptoms that can be tied to stress. By aiding the body in its struggle against stress, adaptogens help to prevent such harmful consequences as insomnia, fatigue, heart disease, and immune dysfunctions.

Adaptogen researcher Georg Wikman points out that "stress-busting" is a limited vision of adaptogens' capabilities. "The concept of an adaptogenic substance is still new to the West, though in Russia it has been the subject of a great deal of scientific study. There it is a branch of medicine that goes much beyond 'mental stress' to look at how substances can promote adaptation to environmental challenges, adverse situations encountered in the military, the rigors of space travel, and pressures associated with sports."

Adaptogens' ability to boost "nonspecific immunity" is increasingly important as immune-related conditions such as cancer, AIDS, lupus, chronic fatigue syndrome, and candidiasis continue to proliferate. In recent years Chinese researchers have reported success with *fu–zheng* therapy, whose name means literally "to fortify the constitution." This is a way of fighting disease by not only attacking the pathogen presumed to be causing the disease, but at the same time boosting the body's innate defense mechanisms. For example, Chinese researchers have studied astragalus and other herbs in the past two decades as adjuncts to conventional Western cancer treatments. They have demonstrated that it is possible to enhance the overall immunity of patients who are undergoing chemotherapy or radiation for various cancers. Astragalus and other herbs have been shown to act as nonspecific immune-system stimulants (see Chapter 3). Patients who combine *fu–zheng* therapy with conventional cancer therapy have increased survival rates.

Most of the studies on adaptogenic substances in recent years have been done by Russians and have focused on herbs such as ginseng, Siberian ginseng, and schisandra. It is not known which of the numerous chemical constituents found in these plants is responsible for the herbs' strengthening and balancing effects. Many of the plants contain unique compounds with complex and varied actions. Some herbs also share potentially therapeutic nutrients such as vitamins, minerals, and trace elements. In general, the adaptogens increase cells' ability to create and use energy and to process wastes. Adaptogens promote efficient oxygen use, encourage muscle building, provide nutrients crucial to bodily processes, and detoxify blood and tissues. The adaptogens smooth out swings in blood-sugar levels, hormone synthesis, and biorhythms.

In addition to considering herbs and nutrients that have a strengthening and balancing effect on the whole body, in this chapter we'll also look at substances with a potentially balancing effect on blood sugar, including vitamins (B complex), nutritional supplements (chromium), and herbs (garlic).

The Adaptogens

Many people find that tonifying, adaptogenic herbs are a better choice than nervous-system stimulants such as caffeine or ephedrine to increase daily energy levels and overcome fatigue that is not directly tied to physical exertion. Such fatigue may be caused by an underlying health problem or condition, dietary deficiencies, hormonal changes, or even abuse of caffeine or other stimulant drugs. Identifying and addressing the underlying cause is crucial, and adaptogens can often be used in conjunction with other natural substances to reenergize the body.

Harriet Beinfield, a licensed acupuncturist and coauthor of *Between Heaven and Earth: A Guide to Chinese Medicine,* notes that tonifying herbs have numerous applications. Many tonifying and adaptogenic herbs are also used to enhance athletic performance, boost immunity, and prolong longevity. She says that most people will notice only a subtle change when taking tonic herbs, adding that they are "part of a long-term strategy, and benefits accrue with consistent use." Beinfield recommends experimenting with tonic herbs, taking note of how your body reacts to each herb. She says that a knowledgeable herbalist can in many cases tailor an herbal regime for your body and your activity level.

Herbalist Ron Teeguarden, author of *Chinese Tonic Herbs* and founder of a pair of Tea Garden Emporiums in the Los Angeles area, emphasizes that Chinese tonic herbs are not for correcting ailments. According to Teeguarden, the use of Chinese tonic herbs "differs from other herbal systems in that it emphasizes the promotion of health rather than the elimination of disease." About fifty of what the Chinese call the "superior herbs" are tonics, herbs "traditionally used by the people of China to enhance vitality and lengthen life. . . . The tonics are used to promote overall well-being, to enhance the body's energy, and to regulate the bodily and psychic functioning so as to create what the Chinese call 'radiant health.' "

Teeguarden notes that in the Chinese tradition the tonic herbs are often combined and prescribed according to how they affect various organs and bodily systems. Thus, for example, energy tonics increase vitality, blood tonics promote nutrient utilization, *yin* tonics promote longevity, and *yang* tonics promote strength and sexual prowess. Practitioners of Chinese medicine can help to customize an herbal program for specific benefits, but anyone can use the most common tonic herbs for increased health.

Adaptogenic herbs are often taken every day for their long-lasting effects on health and longevity. In the West they are frequently combined with each other and with stress-reducing nutrients such as vitamin C and vitamin B complex to provide greater support for the whole body. Look for products such as Stress Arrest, Sports Adaptogen, Chinese Im-Herbs Plus, and Arko-Stress 2000.

The Top Five

These powerful adaptogens—Siberian ginseng, schisandra, ginseng, astragalus, and reishi—are among what Teeguarden calls the "superstars of Chinese tonic herbalism . . . incomparable, legendary herbal substances [that] have withstood the test of time." These five herbs also tend to be the ones with the most scientific backing for their strengthening and normalizing effects.

Siberian Ginseng

Siberian ginseng is among the most popular adaptogenic herbs on the North American market today. Many athletes, students, workers with stressful jobs, and others are now taking it on a daily basis to increase longevity, improve overall health, and balance bodily systems.

Also sold as eleuthero, this herb is related to the panax ginsengs. Interest in Siberian ginseng was stimulated in the late 1940s when the Russian scientist I. I. Brekhman, looking for strengthening, adaptogenic herbs, was frustrated by the limited, expensive supply of *Panax ginseng*. Brekhman began to study Siberian ginseng, a relatively common plant found in the wild in northern Asia. (Today it remains much less expensive than other ginsengs.)

Brekhman and other Russian scientists eventually decided that Siberian ginseng was an even more effective adaptogen than *Panax ginseng*. After studying the chemical composition of Siberian ginseng and testing the herb on animals and humans, they determined that extracts of Siberian ginseng shared many of the desirable qualities of the other ginsengs. Researchers in China, Japan, and Europe have also performed clinical trials over the past few decades, generally reporting positive results. Siberian ginseng has a positive effect on mental alertness, work quality, and athletic performance. It often increases strength and stamina and reduces the adverse effects of such stressful factors as exposure to noise and chemical pollutants. Siberian ginseng supports the adrenal glands in their efforts to balance hormones in response to stress. It has a normalizing effect on blood pressure, helping to raise it when it is too low and lower it when it is too high. It also has a regulating effect on body temperature, sleep requirements, and blood-sugar levels.

A recent double-blind German study found Siberian ginseng to be an effective "nonspecific immunostimulant." That is, it enhances the body's overall resistance to infections and immune-related ailments.

Capsulized Siberian ginseng products often specify their content of the compounds known as eleutherosides.

HOW TO USE SIBERIAN GINSENG: It is available dried and in capsules, tinctures, and extracts. An average dosage is 250 to 500 mg once or twice daily, or 1 to 2 dropperfuls of the concentrated drops two or three times daily.

Schisandra

In the Far East, everyone from Chinese emperors to family herbalists has long recognized the remarkable powers of the herb schisandra to promote longevity and increase stamina. Its strengthening effect (see Chapter 4) is combined with system-balancing properties, making it ideal for such conditions as fatigue, nervous exhaustion, and lack of energy. Schisandra is one of the most popular adaptogenic herbs in China, where it is taken to beautify the skin, strengthen the sex organs, and promote mental function. Its use has more recently spread to Russia, Scandinavia, Western Europe, and the United States.

Chinese and Japanese researchers have conducted numerous studies on schisandra and found that it deserves its reputation as a long-lasting adaptogen. Among schisandra's main chemical constituents are compounds known as lignans (such as schizandrin) that can stimulate the immune system, protect and nourish the liver, and increase the body's ability to handle stress. Scientists have also found that schisandra helps to deliver more oxygen to the body's cells and prevent damage from free radicals.

HOW TO USE SCHISANDRA: It is most commonly found in capsules, though it also comes in concentrated drops, tinctures, and extracts. An average dosage of the dried herb in capsule form is 250 to 500 mg once or twice daily.

Ginseng

People around the world use Chinese or Korean ginseng (*Panax ginseng*) and American ginseng (*Panax quinquefolius*) for the herb's tonic and balancing properties. Some Native American tribes took it for much the same reason as the Chinese did: to increase strength, energy, fertility, brain power, and appetite. Ginseng has been the subject of hundreds of scientific studies in recent years, some of which have tested the herb's power to improve a person's ability to adapt to light and dark, high and low temperatures, and other environmental conditions. Other studies have confirmed that ginseng boosts work efficiency and prevents fatigue. Ginseng also lessens the effects of stress (possibly by stimulating a part of the adrenals) and helps protect cells from damage by radiation and toxic substances. It apparently helps to regulate the body's blood-glucose levels, central nervous system, and immune system.

A traditional practice in the East has been to take daily doses of ginseng as a tonic for two weeks and then to discontinue use for two weeks. Try this cycle for a few months to see whether ginseng works for you.

HOW TO USE GINSENG: Ginseng comes in myriad forms, including as a whole root and in capsules, tablets, tea bags, tinctures, and extracts. Potency may vary considerably. An average tonic dosage of capsules standardized for 5 to 9 percent ginsenosides is 250 to 500 mg per day. An average dosage of some concentrated extracts and ginseng products with higher standardized percentages may be as low as 100 to 200 mg.

Astragalus

Astragalus is one of the most famous tonic herbs of China. Like ginseng, astragalus has long been taken in the East to strengthen and balance the entire system. Astragalus helps to energize internal organs, regulate the digestive, nervous, and hormonal systems, and protect bodily cells from heavy metals and chemical toxins. Astragalus is a good source of the essential trace mineral selenium, an antioxidant. The Chinese also take astragalus in order to assimilate nutrients better and to develop muscular strength and aerobic endurance.

Chinese herbalists say that astragalus improves the body's disease resistance and boosts overall vitality. In China it is widely taken to enhance immunity (see Chapter 3). It has been successfully tested as an adjunct to chemotherapy and radiation therapy. Studies indicate that, like vitamin C, it may reduce the number and duration of common colds and other viral infections.

HOW TO USE ASTRAGALUS: Astragalus is sold fresh or dried and in capsules, concentrated drops, tinctures, and extracts. An average tonic dose is 1 dropperful of tincture or concentrate, or 250 to 500 mg of the powdered herb in capsules, two or three times daily.

Reishi

The practitioners of the traditional medicines of China and Japan considered reishi to be among the most powerful adaptogenic and tonic herbs. They used this "mushroom of immortality" for promoting longevity, boosting overall health and immunity, and speeding recovery from illness. It is one of the traditional Chinese herbs taken to strengthen the heart and other organs and to increase muscle strength and efficiency. Chinese herbalists recommend it to improve the body's use of oxygen. It also acts as an antioxidant and immune stimulant, and can help balance the nervous and digestive systems, regulate blood sugar, and protect the body from the harmful effects of radiation and free radicals.

HOW TO USE REISHI: In the West reishi is rarely used as a food, since it is hard and bitter, but capsules, tea bags and concentrated tea granules, granulated and liquid extracts, standardized extracts, tinctures, and concentrated drops are widely available at natural-food stores. An average dosage of encapsulated powder is 500 mg two or three times daily.

Up-and-Coming Adaptogens

Other plants with notable adaptogenic effects include ashwagandha, Swedish roseroot, fo-ti, and suma. Although these are not as widely known as Siberian ginseng and the other herbs just mentioned, these up-and-coming adaptogens are worth seeking out. Tonic herbs for the nervous system, such as oats, damiana, and gotu kola (see Chapter 5), are also used as adaptogens.

Ashwagandha

Some herbalists call ashwagandha "Ayurvedic ginseng," referring to the traditional healing practice of India and the well-known tonic herb. Ayurvedic practitioners have long used ashwagandha as a general rejuvenator and as a mild sedative to reduce anxiety (see Chapter 12). Ancient Indian medical texts term ashwagandha a "vitalizer," akin to what we now call an adaptogen. In the United States ashwagandha is increasingly recognized for its ability to help strengthen the body and protect it from the adverse effects of stress.

In India ashwagandha is widely used as a tonic for a variety of ailments, including bronchitis, arthritis, and nausea. Ashwagandha or its compounds have been shown to relieve pain and inflammation, lower fever, reduce gastric ulcers, and improve cholesterol profiles. Tests done on mice show that they swim for longer durations after given ashwagandha, indicating that the herb improves how they handle stress.

Researchers S. Ghosal et al., writing in a 1989 issue of *Phytotherapy Research,* summarized their study on ashwagandha compounds and said that they "produced significant anti-stress activity in albino mice and rats and augmented learning acquisition and memory retention in young and old rats. These findings are consistent with the use of *W. somnifera,* in Ayurveda, to attenuate cerebral function deficits in the geriatric population and to provide non-specific host defense."

HOW TO USE ASHWAGANDHA: It's available primarily in capsules. An average recommended dose is 150 to 300 mg standardized for 2 to 5 mg withanolides.

Swedish Roseroot

Swedish roseroot is a Scandinavian adaptogen derived from the root of a plant (*Rhodiola rosea*) that the Vikings used centuries ago to gain extra strength for their sea journeys. Swedish roseroot eventually attracted the attention of the Chinese, who determined that it deserved to be placed among the class of "superior herbs" that includes such other strengthening, balancing herbs as ginseng. Today Swedish roseroot is among the most widely used adaptogens in Scandinavia, taken to sharpen and focus the mind, increase muscular strength, and boost stamina. Studies have found that extract of Swedish roseroot helps bodily cells to accumulate potential energy in the form of adenosine triphosphate (ATP), the chemical that provides the immediate source of energy for muscles. According to adaptogen researcher Wikman, Swedish roseroot works almost like a "smart drug" to boost the functioning of parts of the brain.

The Swedish Herbal Institute, whose U.S. headquarters is in Portsmouth, New Hampshire (see "Resources"), says that it cultivates "the only major accessible source of *Rhodiola rosea*" on a farm outside Göteborg in Sweden. In the United States the institute sells an adaptogen product called Arctic Root that contains 180 mg of a standardized extract of Swedish roseroot. It also sells Chisandra Adaptogen, a combination of schisandra and Siberian ginseng. The institute notes that it owns the registered trademark on the word *adaptogen*.

HOW TO USE SWEDISH ROSEROOT: The Swedish Herbal Institute rec-

ommends taking 1 tablet of Arctic Root per day as a dietary supplement. For special events, they suggest 2 tablets 30 minutes before a
stressful mental task or a hard physical workout.

Fo-ti

Among the Chinese this is one of the most popular tonic herbs for
greater energy and vitality. Traditional Chinese herbalists recommend
it to increase fertility and virility (see Chapter 7) and prevent premature aging (see Chapter 10). It is growing in popularity in other parts
of the world as well for its apparent ability to help lower cholesterol
levels (see Chapter 8) and to restore youthful strength and vigor.

Fo-ti is a recent American name; the Chinese refer to this herb as *he
shou wu.*

HOW TO USE FO-TI: It is sold dried and as powders, tablets, capsules,
concentrated drops, tinctures, and extracts. An average recommended
tonic dose of the concentrated drops is $1/2$ to 1 dropperful two or three
times daily.

Suma

Also known as Brazilian ginseng, suma is an herb derived from the
root of a South American plant (*Pfaffia paniculata*). For centuries, tribes
native to the area around the Amazon River and the Mato Grosso in
Brazil have used suma almost as a panacea, referring to it as *para todo,*
"for all things." Brazilian researchers are now exploring suma's potential as a treatment for cancer and diabetes.

Taking suma seems to increase a person's general sense of well-
being. The herb is gaining in popularity in North America for its
adaptogenic, strengthening, and antifatigue properties, as well as its
potential to help women suffering from symptoms associated with
menopause and hormonal imbalance. Studies have determined that
suma has relatively high levels of germanium (see below). Herbalist
Michael Tierra, author of *The Way of Herbs,* says, "As an energy tonic
adaptogen, suma is at least equal to that of Siberian ginseng and panax
ginseng in its effects. . . . I would not hesitate to recommend it to
anyone with chronic fatigue or low energy."

HOW TO USE SUMA: The herb has traditionally been used as a food
and thus can be taken in relatively large doses, such as 500 to 1,000 mg
of the dried herb two or three times daily.

Nutritional Balancers

While herbs dominate the category of adaptogens and have garnered most of the scientific attention, there are a few other natural substances that are sometimes taken for their systemwide effects, particularly organic germanium compounds, concentrated green-food supplements, and bee products.

Organic Germanium Compounds

Germanium is a trace mineral and natural element that researchers have recently developed into synthetic organic compounds with potentially dramatic medicinal effects. Chief among the new compounds is Ge-132, which has been shown to restore the normal function of immune-boosting cells and possibly prevent cancer. It also stimulates overall energy levels and is taken by some to balance bodily functions.

HOW TO USE ORGANIC GERMANIUM COMPOUNDS: These come in powders, granules, and tablets, as well as capsules ranging in size from 25 to 250 mg. An average adaptogenic dosage is 50 to 100 mg daily.

Green-Food Concentrates

Green foods refers to chlorophyll-rich supplements from sources such as microalgae (including spirulina, blue-green algae, and chlorella) and the young grasses of cereal plants (particularly barley, wheat, and alfalfa). These are among the most nutrient-dense whole foods known, containing significant amounts of protein and a diverse array of easily assimilated and naturally balanced vitamins, minerals, enzymes, and trace elements. Chlorophyll acts as an antioxidant and may have medicinal benefits against cancer and immune problems. Many people also take green-food concentrates to boost energy levels and physical and mental performance.

As whole-food concentrates, green foods are exceedingly safe even in relatively large quantities; recommended dosages are often 2 to 4 g daily.

HOW TO USE GREEN FOOD CONCENTRATES: Green foods come in powders, tablets, capsules, juices, liquid concentrates, and extracts. Follow label directions for dosage.

Bee Products

Bee products include bee pollen, propolis, and royal jelly. As nutritional substances, these are typically rich in vitamins (especially pantothenic acid and other B vitamins), minerals, flavonoids, amino acids, enzymes, certain fatty acids, and other nutrients. Many people take bee products on a daily basis basically as adaptogens: to boost overall health, increase energy and performance, and improve immunity. Though scientific backing for proponents' claims is mostly lacking, bee products may prolong youth and enhance longevity.

Allergic reactions to bee products are rare but possible. Experiment with tiny amounts before taking larger doses.

HOW TO USE BEE PRODUCTS: These come in a variety of liquids, gels, powders, tablets, and capsules. An average dosage of royal jelly is 500 to 1,000 mg; of pollen, 250 to 1,500 mg or 1 to 2 teaspoons of the granules; of propolis, 250 to 500 mg.

Blood-Sugar Regulators

Cells in the brain and throughout the body depend upon carbohydrates in the form of sugars for energy. Mostly cells need the simple sugar known as glucose. Found naturally in fruits and a few other foods, glucose is primarily derived from the digestion of carbohydrates.

Glucose levels in the blood depend upon a variety of factors, including diet and the activity of hormones secreted by the adrenal glands (adrenaline, corticosteroids) and the pancreas (insulin). These hormones can either raise or lower blood-sugar levels by stimulating the release of glucose or its uptake by cells. The body strives to keep blood-glucose levels within fairly narrow boundaries. Its ability to regulate these levels (as measured by a glucose tolerance test) is an important factor in overall health. When long-term dietary abuses, hormonal failures, or other factors allow blood-glucose levels to swing too drastically, physical and mental health suffer. When blood-sugar levels are chronically too high, diabetes may result; when too low, hypoglycemia.

Diabetes is a serious, life-threatening medical condition. It should not be self-diagnosed or self-treated. Though some of the herbs and supplements mentioned here are potentially useful in the treatment of diabetes, management of the condition should be supervised by a qualified medical practitioner. Especially if you are taking insulin for diabetes, be sure to discuss with your health provider proposed changes or additions to your treatment program.

Any attempt to treat a difficult disease such as diabetes using only drugs or only natural substances is likely to fail. Whether you have juvenile-onset, insulin-dependent (Type I) diabetes, adult-onset, non-insulin-dependent (Type II) diabetes, or just mild hypoglycemia, it is important to accompany your intake of natural substances with healthful dietary and lifestyle habits. These should include regular physical activity or exercise, a healthful, high-fiber diet rich in whole foods, grains, legumes, and fresh vegetables and fruits, and avoidance of large amounts of refined sugar and alcohol.

A number of animal studies done in the mid-1980s suggested that the trace element vanadium may help to control blood-sugar swings. In rats, high doses of vanadium work like insulin, increasing the uptake of glucose. While diabetic animals seem to benefit from taking vanadium, the supplement's potential usefulness for preventing or treating diabetes in humans has never been proven. Moreover, more-recent animal studies clearly indicate that the short-term benefits of high doses of vanadium for normalizing blood-glucose levels are canceled by the mineral's toxicity. Researchers found that vanadium and the related compound vanadyl sulfate (frequently used in bodybuilding products) accumulate in the animals' tissues and cause potentially serious long-term side effects, including suppressed immunity and even death.

Optimal daily intake of vanadium is unknown but may be not much more than the average daily requirement to prevent deficiency conditions, which some nutritionists have estimated to be between 50 and 100 mcg per day. (The federal government has not established an RDA for vanadium.) Daily doses in excess of 1 to 2 mg may have druglike effects or even be potentially harmful. Yet supplements of vanadium and vanadyl sulfate often contain 7.5 mg or even higher amounts. Until more is known about the mineral's toxicity, it is prudent to avoid any vanadium supplementation higher than 100 mcg daily.

Two herbs whose positive effects on diabetic subjects may eventually lead to wider use for regulating blood-sugar levels are fenugreek and gymnema.

Fenugreek. A legume (*Trigonella foenum-graecum*) and culinary spice that tastes somewhat like maple, fenugreek has a long heritage of use as a medicinal plant. Egyptian, Ayurvedic, Greek, and Roman healers used it as an aphrodisiac and to remedy colds and sore throats, indigestion, and other complaints. Lydia Pinkham included fenugreek in her famous nineteenth-century "Vegetable Compound" nostrum for menstrual aches. Recent studies suggest that these traditional uses may be valid. Fenugreek seeds contain mucilage, which is soothing to the mucous membranes of the respiratory and digestive tracts, and steroidal, estrogenlike chemicals that can affect female sexual functioning. In addition, the seeds contain compounds that have been shown in studies to improve cholesterol profiles and help control blood-sugar levels.

Chemical analysis of the seeds has identified a number of alkaloids, including trigonelline and coumarin, that have therapeutic potential in the treatment of diabetes. Animal and human studies indicate that fenugreek-seed powder can improve glucose tolerance and reduce sugar in urine, a marker of diabetes. Researchers use high dosages (15 to 100 g daily) of defatted fenugreek-seed powder to control non-insulin-dependent diabetes.

Fenugreek may stimulate uterine contractions, so it shouldn't be used during pregnancy.

Gymnema. Though still a relatively obscure herb in North America, this plant has a long history of medicinal use in India, where it is called gurmar. Native to India, it is derived from a tropical plant (*Gymnema sylvestre*) of the milkweed family. One of its traditional uses in India was for what herbalists there called "honey urine," which modern clinicians recognize as diabetes.

A number of human and animal studies, the first of which date back to the 1920s, have confirmed that gymnema has pronounced effects on blood sugar, at least among diabetics. Within the past two decades researchers have determined that gymnema extract may even play a role in the treatment of Type I diabetics, who typically need daily injections of insulin to control the disease. Gymnema taken orally lowers diabetics' blood-glucose levels and improves blood-fat and cholesterol profiles. A series of studies done at India's University of Madras in the early 1990s found that high doses of the dried herb (on the order of 40 g daily) or gymnema extract may actually help to repair or regenerate the pancreas's beta cells, which play a crucial role in the production and secretion of insulin. Few other substances, synthetic or natural, offer such promise for reversing beta-cell damage and at least partially reducing diabetics' need for insulin and other drugs. On the other hand, studies indicate that animals that do not have diabetes don't produce more insulin after consuming gymnema.

"Because its usefulness in diabetes was first reported almost three quarters of a century ago," says nutrition writer A. S. Gissen of Vitamin Research Products in Carson City, Nevada, "the use of *Gymnema sylvestre* as a treatment for diabetes isn't patentable. I have no doubt that if [its] effects were discovered tomorrow by a pharmaceutical company that had a patent on it, we would see it on the front page of the newspaper as it was hailed as the breakthrough of the century."

Fenugreek is sold as powders, tablets, capsules, concentrated drops, and extracts. Gymnema is not as widely available, but can be found as a single supplement and as an ingredient in weight-loss formulas (see Chapter 17). Some natural practitioners now recommend these herbs for the elderly or others who are at high risk for developing diabetes, though it remains to be proven that taking low dosages of these herbs on a regular basis helps to regulate blood sugar among basically healthy people. Diabetics should, of course, check with a medical practitioner before experimenting with these herbs or any other natural substance for controlling blood sugar.

Some of the more common supplements that generally healthy people can take every day in dosages that have been shown to help prevent wide swings in blood sugar include:

Polyphenols and flavonoids. These healthful plant compounds (see Chapter 2) tend to normalize insulin secretion. Polyphenols and flavonoids are concentrated in various vegetables, fruits, and herbs, particularly bilberry (an average dosage of an encapsulated extract product standardized for 20 to 25 percent anthocyanoside is 80 to 160 mg three times daily), ginkgo (40 mg three times daily of a standardized extract containing a minimum of 24 percent ginkgo heterosides or flavone glycosides), European coastal pine (Pycnogenol) or grape-seed extract (50 to 100 mg daily), green tea (150 to 500 mg daily of green-tea-extract capsules standardized for 15 to 50 percent polyphenols), and red wine (250 mg of red wine extract standardized to provide 40 to 60 mg of polyphenols).

Fiber. Soluble dietary fiber such as the gums and the pectins (see Chapter 8) slow the digestion of carbohydrates, thus helping to control blood-glucose levels, reduce insulin requirements, and prevent diabetes. An average intake of the supplements is a teaspoon (or 4 to 5 g in capsules or tablets) two or three times daily, taken with water.

Zinc. Zinc prevents blood-glucose imbalances due to its central role in the metabolism of insulin. When zinc is deficient, the risk of developing diabetes increases. An average daily dosage is 17 to 25 mg, taken with a meal. Taking zinc in a multimineral supplement can help prevent zinc-induced deficiencies in other minerals such as copper, selenium, and iron.

Chromium

This trace element is an essential part of glucose tolerance factor (GTF), a bodily substance necessary for proper insulin function. Chromium thus plays an important role in regulating the metabolism of carbohydrates, including glucose, and in preventing swings in blood sugar. Studies have shown that diabetics who take chromium often experience improved glucose tolerance. A number of studies indicate that even average doses (200 mcg daily) of chromium can help regulate blood-glucose levels. Chromium deficiencies may cause such symptoms as low blood sugar and high insulin levels.

Some nutritionists also recommend brewer's yeast, the dried, pulverized cells of *Saccharomyces cerevisiae,* for improved blood-sugar control because it is a concentrated source of GTF. It is also rich in trace minerals, protein, and a number of the B vitamins. Brewer's yeast is so named because it is a byproduct of beer-making and is similar to (though usually somewhat lower in nutrients than) nutritional yeast, which is grown specifically for human consumption. Brewer's yeast is a different form of yeast from that which causes yeast infections (*Candida albicans*) and is not thought to cause yeast-related conditions. Studies have found it to be useful in the prevention or treatment of hypoglycemia and diabetes. Brewer's yeast is sold in powders, flakes, tablets, and capsules. Potencies vary considerably, but a tablespoon of dried brewer's yeast contains on average about 50 to 70 mg of chromium.

Supplement manufacturers offer chromium in a number of forms and under a variety of brand names. GTF provides an organic, well-absorbed form of the element (combined with cysteine, niacin, and other nutrients), and is found naturally in brewer's yeast. Chromium is also available as chromium polynicotinate, which combines chromium and niacin, and chromium picolinate. Some chromium supplements combine GTF, chromium picolinate, and other nutrients. Chromium supplements on the market include Chromoplex, Chromium Complex, and Performance Picolinate.

HOW TO USE CHROMIUM: Chromium supplements are widely available in tablets (usually 100 to 200 mcg), capsules, and liquids. An average daily dosage for adults is 200 to 400 mcg.

Vitamin B Complex

Deficiencies or imbalances in B-complex vitamins can often cause problems with blood-sugar regulation. Various B vitamins, including niacin, thiamine, pantothenic acid, pyridoxine, and B_{12}, are needed to metabolize fats and carbohydrates, boost the effectiveness of insulin, and prevent symptoms of diabetes. Niacin is probably the most crucial B vitamin for proper blood sugar balance. Niacin is a component of glucose tolerance factor, the chromium-containing substance needed for insulin metabolism. According to nutritional expert Melvyn Werbach, M.D., "Even assuming that niacin levels are normal, it is possible that additional supplementation could still improve blood sugar regulation."

Taking individual B vitamins can cause an imbalance in other B vitamins. Many nutritionists recommend taking B vitamins as part of an insurance-level multivitamin or as B complex.

HOW TO USE B COMPLEX: It is available in liquids, tablets, and capsules. An average dosage for preventing blood sugar imbalances is 50 to 100 mg daily.

Garlic

Garlic is a frequently recommended herb for people suffering from diabetes and imbalances in blood sugar. Studies done on both people and animals have shown that garlic (as well as its relative the onion) can reduce blood-sugar levels. Scientists trace garlic's glucose-lowering effects to its sulfur compounds, which bear a resemblance to insulin in chemical structure. Naturopath Michael Murray says, "The message is clear: Diabetics and hypoglycemics should make liberal use of onions and garlic."

HOW TO USE GARLIC: Garlic supplements come in a wide variety of powders, liquids, tablets, and capsules. Many are standardized for allicin content or fresh garlic equivalent. An average daily dosage is 600 to 1,000 mg of pure or concentrated garlic or garlic extract powder, or 1,800 to 3,000 mg of fresh garlic equivalent. An average recommended dosage for allicin is 1,800 to 3,600 mcg per day.

Where to Start

Here's a two-pronged approach for taking advantage of system strengtheners and balancers. Take daily:

- Either Siberian ginseng or schisandra, 250 to 500 mg once or twice daily, singly or in combination

- Chromium (200 to 400 mcg), preferably as part of a multivitamin-multimineral supplement with optimal daily levels of other useful balancing nutrients, such as B complex and zinc

Beyond Herbs and Supplements

As herbalist Christopher Hobbs has noted, "It is certain that nature herself is our most powerful ally in our quest for health and longevity, but herbs are not the only adaptogens available. Saunas and cold water treatments can be adaptogenic in their effects, as can all forms of exercise, if practiced wisely. Also, as Norman Cousins has so eloquently said, laughing is a deeply healing activity and is, seriously, one of the greatest adaptogens."

Develop Your Senses

Humans inform themselves about the outside world by receiving sensory information. Light and sound waves, and the characteristics that give objects smells, tastes, and textures, provide us with the information we need to adapt to and control our environment. Particularly when an individual suffers from poor hearing or vision, he or she faces significant barriers to learning, achievement, and success. A young child who cannot easily hear the teacher or read words on the blackboard is more likely to fail as a student. The resulting poor self-image can set the tone for a lifetime of disappointment. The salesperson who is too embarrassed to wear a hearing aid will miss much of value during routine communications. The athlete whose vision is deteriorating with age may be forced into early retirement, even if corrective lenses restore one element (sharp acuity) of proper vision.

Unfortunately, modern medicine offers few options beyond mechanical correction to those suffering from sensory shortcomings. The usual tools are hearing aids for poor hearing and glasses, contact lenses, or surgery for poor vision. For the most part, these options are crutches for adjusting to a handicap, not remedial steps that can truly improve hearing or vision—or even halt their deterioration.

The growing awareness of and hope for better functioning of the sense organs comes at an opportune time. Hearing and vision impairments are common problems in modern society. Over half of all Americans, an estimated 140 million people, wear glasses or contact lenses. Some 60 to 80 percent of American students are nearsighted by the time they reach college. Hearing loss is also commonplace among the young and old. Problems with the organs of taste and smell are rarer but can afflict significant numbers of certain groups of people (those on kidney dialysis, for instance).

The suggestions that follow are not offered as magic bullets that will allow those who are wearing contact lenses or hearing aids to discard these tools overnight; rather, these natural substances can significantly support and improve the body's sense organs in a way that enhances their ability to function as nature intended.

Seeing Better Naturally

Conventional eye doctors contend that vision is a given, incapable of being influenced by such factors as herbs and nutritional supplements or eye exercises. Recent research and the development of new schools of thought on vision, including behavioral optometry (which uses special tools and exercises to sharpen eyesight), suggest that attempting to improve an individual's ability to see is not a quixotic pursuit.

Products in natural-food stores that contain formulas combining many of the following natural substances include See, OcuGuard Caps, Vital Vision, Vision Tone, Vizion, and Night Eyes.

The Vision Herbs

Bilberry and eyebright are the two most popular herbs taken by people who want to improve their vision. Of the two, eyebright has the longer history of use, but bilberry has more scientific backing.

Eyebright preparations are derived from a native European plant (*Euphrasia officinalis*) with flowers that resemble a bloodshot eye. Herbalists of the Middle Ages used this physical similarity of eyebright and the eye to deduce, using the "doctrine of signatures" (the idea that a plant's form suggests its function), that eyebright must improve vision. While modern herbalists recognize the doctrine of signatures as a superstition, eyebright is still sometimes included in combination herbal formulas for nourishing vision. It is also still used in the traditional way, to make an external wash for irritated, red, or swollen eyes, sometimes in combination with herbs such as goldenseal, echinacea, and fennel seeds. This external use may have a valid rationale—researchers have found that eyebright contains a tannin compound that is mildly astringent and anti-inflammatory.

Unlike bilberry, eyebright has not been the subject of any scientific studies that have demonstrated positive effects on vision. Most herbal-ists now believe that eyebright's benefits for the eyes are limited to its application as a mild topical eyewash for external redness and inflam-mation, though other herbs are more effective for even this use.

Eyebright is the source of the homeopathic remedy *Euphrasia,* often recommended for eye problems.

Bilberry

British RAF pilots during World War II claimed to have stumbled upon a surprising tactical advantage in the form of the herb bilberry. A shrub (*Vaccinium myrtillus*) that grows commonly throughout Europe, bilberry yields a blue-black berry similar to the American highbush blueberry (*V. corymbosum*). Bilberry fruit makes a tasty jam, which was eaten by the pilots prior to their night missions. The result, said the pilots, was a significant increase in their night vision and visual acuity.

After the war, stimulated by these anecdotal reports, European sci-entists performed a number of studies on bilberry, mostly on animals, though a few studies were done using limited numbers of humans. The results have tended to confirm bilberry's remarkable effects on vision. The chemical constituents of bilberry apparently responsible for its vision-boosting powers are certain flavonoids, the anthocyanosides, that can cause biochemical reactions in the eye. (Fresh bilberry fruit contains a concentration of less than one percent anthocyanosides; most studies demonstrating bilberry's effectiveness have used concen-trated herbal extracts containing 15 to 25 percent anthocyanosides.) Research indicates that anthocyanosides have a positive effect on cer-tain enzymes crucial to vision. The anthocyanosides markedly increase the eye's ability to adapt to the dark. They're also an effective, though temporary, treatment for a number of other vision problems, including chronic eye fatigue, severe nearsightedness, and day blindness. Regular consumption of bilberry may help prevent cataracts and glaucoma.

Bilberry's short-term effects are most noticeable for the first four hours or so after taking the herb. Those who might benefit from taking bilberry include not only pilots but nighttime drivers, students, computer terminal operators, and persons engaged in visually de-manding precision work. Tests have shown bilberry to be completely nontoxic even when taken in large doses for a long time.

Numerous herbal companies have formulated and released bilberry products for vision improvement in the past five years. (Species of North American blueberries, which, like bilberry, are rich in flavonoids, have not been similarly tested for therapeutic actions and currently are not used in standardized medicinal preparations.) Tablet and capsule products go by names such as Bilberry-Power, Vizion Bilberry, and Optimum Bilberry. Almost all have clearly stated anthocyanoside contents of 15 to 25 percent. Some also contain additional ingredients for boosting vision, such as bioflavonoids, vitamin A/beta carotene, and zinc.

HOW TO USE BILBERRY: Bilberry is also available in the form of tinctures and concentrated drops as well as in capsules and tablets. An average dosage of an encapsulated extract product standardized for 20 to 25 percent anthocyanoside is 80 to 160 mg two or three times daily.

Vitamins and Minerals for Improved Vision

The vision-boosting vitamins and minerals are for the most part potent antioxidants. Antioxidants are especially important for proper vision, since the eyes contain a rich abundance of nerve cells, capillaries, and other delicate body parts that can be harmed by free radicals (for more on antioxidants, see Chapter 10). When free radicals are allowed to run amok in the eye, there's an increased risk of cataracts (clouding of the lens), glaucoma (from an increase in fluid pressure within the eye), macular degeneration (a condition affecting the area on the retina where you normally experience especially sharp central focus), and other eye problems. Some ophthalmologists are finding that early supplementation with the antioxidants and other vision-boosting nutrients can improve patients' conditions so dramatically that surgery can be avoided. In some cases, people experience vision improvements of 50 percent or more.

In addition to the following, another effective antioxidant that can help maintain optimum vision is selenium (an average dosage is 100 to 200 mcg daily).

Vitamin A/Beta Carotene

In addition to boosting immunity and speeding the healing of wounds, optimal intake of vitamin A/beta carotene supports vision, especially night vision. Some of beta carotene's protective effect on vision can be traced to its role as a potent antioxidant. Ophthalmologic researchers have not found high concentrations of beta carotene in the retina, the thin screen at the back of the eyeball that transforms light into electrical signals for the brain. They have found, however, carotenoids such as lutein that, like beta carotene, can scavenge free radicals that otherwise could injure sensitive eye cells.

Vitamin A is also concentrated in the retina. A crucial step in the chemistry of vision occurs when specialized light-receiving cells in the retina, known as rods, release vitamin A upon being struck by photons. Deficiency in vitamin A often results in blurred vision (which can also result from *too much* vitamin A) and an inability to adapt to darkness. A long-term dietary study recently found that a diet rich in vitamin A/ beta carotene offers significant protection against cataracts, a condition that afflicts an estimated 20 million Americans.

Taking high doses of preformed A (such as 100,000 IU daily for months, or 500,000 to 1,000,000 IU daily for two to three weeks) can allow it to accumulate in the body and cause potentially serious adverse health effects. On the other hand, the body converts to vitamin A only as much beta carotene as it needs. Extra beta carotene is stored, but the only adverse effect of such storage is a slight orange tinge to the skin.

How to use vitamin A/beta carotene: It comes in a wide variety of tablets and capsules. An optimal daily dosage to protect vision is 5,000 to 10,000 IU of vitamin A plus 25,000 to 50,000 IU (15 to 30 mg) of beta carotene or, preferably, beta carotene plus mixed carotenoids.

Vitamin B Complex

Vision requires the assistance of more nerve cells than does any other sense, and the B-complex vitamins are crucial for proper nerve functioning. The B vitamins also help the body to deal with stress and fatigue. Not surprisingly, a deficiency in almost any of the B vitamins will usually lead to vision problems. For example, a lack of thiamine leads to burning or dry eyes, double vision, and involuntary eye movements. People who are deficient in thiamine and who suffer from glaucoma may start to recover by taking extra thiamine. A deficiency in riboflavin can cause a sensitivity to light, eye fatigue, increased cataract risk, and a worsening of acuity. Studies indicate that B_6 and other B vitamins, such as choline, inositol, pantothenic acid (B_5), and B_{12}, can also have a protective effect against various vision defects, including cataracts.

How to use vitamin B complex: B complex comes in powders, tablets (often time-release), and capsules. An optimal dosage is 25 to 50 mg once or twice daily.

Vitamin C

Widely taken to boost the immune system and reduce the symptoms of colds, vitamin C has also gained prominence recently for its role in helping to maintain sharp vision. Vitamin C strengthens blood vessels and, probably more important, neutralizes harmful free radicals that might otherwise damage the sensitive working parts of the eye. The vitamin is necessary for the formation of collagen, which is used to make the dense tissue of the sclera, the tough eye layer that, with the cornea, forms the external covering of the eye. The aqueous humor, the fluid that fills the chamber behind the cornea, has levels of vitamin C that are many times higher than those in any other bodily fluid. Studies have linked vitamin C consumption to improved visual function and a reduced risk of various eye diseases.

Separate teams of researchers in Canada and the United States have found that subjects who take vitamin C supplements are less likely to suffer from cataracts than are subjects who don't take C. One estimate is that 300 to 600 mg of vitamin C daily will reduce the average person's cataract risk by more than two thirds. Studies indicate that vitamin C is useful in the treatment of corneal burns, and in the prevention as well as the treatment of chronic glaucoma. Taking too little vitamin C tends to increase ocular pressure, while supplementing your diet with 2 to 5 g daily for as little as a week may lower this pressure.

Vitamin C is extremely safe and widely available in tablets, capsules, powders, and in combination supplements. Daily dosages of 2 to 5 g may cause loose bowels in some people.

How to use vitamin c: Optimal intake is 250 to 500 mg two or three times daily.

Vitamin E

Vitamin E, like vitamin C, is a powerful antioxidant nutrient. Although best known as a topical remedy to prevent scarring and an oral supplement to protect against heart disease, vitamin E also has positive effects on vision. The connective tissues of the eye need adequate E to remain strong and resilient. According to Richard Leviton, author of *Seven Steps to Better Vision,* vitamin E "can help improve acuity, arrest macular degeneration, reverse presbyopia [a form of farsightedness that particularly affects the elderly], and, in some instances, keep childhood myopia [nearsightedness] from getting any worse."

Some people may experience dizziness, elevated blood pressure, decreased blood coagulation, or other side effects with daily dosages of 1,200 to 1,600 IU of vitamin E.

HOW TO USE VITAMIN E: It is sold as a liquid and in dry and oil-filled capsules. An optimal supplement level is 400 to 600 IU daily, a safe and nontoxic dosage for long-term consumption.

Zinc

Zinc is a trace mineral essential for proper wound healing, male sexual potency, and numerous other bodily processes, including sense functioning. Deficiencies in zinc can lead to various eye problems, while taking supplemental zinc can halt progressive vision loss and in some cases improve visual acuity. Zinc can also be effective in the prevention or treatment of such serious eye conditions as cataracts, glaucoma, and macular degeneration. For example, one study found that, compared to people of the same age without cataracts, subjects with cataracts have lower blood levels of zinc.

Researchers believe that zinc works in concert with vitamin A to promote better vision. Low zinc levels apparently prevent efficient metabolism and absorption of vitamin A. One study showed that only when zinc was added to a vitamin A supplementation program did subjects experience improved night vision.

Zinc is frequently combined with other minerals and vitamins—taking high levels of only zinc can lead to copper, selenium, or iron deficiencies. Most people have no adverse effects from taking up to about 150 mg per day (6 to 9 times the optimal dose) of zinc; a few people experience side effects such as gastrointestinal irritation. Doses on the order of 2,000 mg are toxic enough to cause vomiting.

HOW TO USE ZINC: As an individual supplement, it comes in lozenges, tablets, and capsules. An average daily dosage for adults is 17 to 25 mg.

Chromium

Chromium is a trace element that helps to regulate energy, blood sugar levels, and protein synthesis. Researchers have shown that these key functions can play a role in vision. Chromium deficiencies can prevent the eye's ciliary muscles, which form a band around the eye and contract or relax to adjust focus, from absorbing the food energy they need for proper functioning. Sufficient chromium thus lowers the risk of vision problems, including nearsightedness and glaucoma.

Chromium is one of the safest nutritional supplements known. It does not cause side effects at dosages up to 100 times greater than the average adult dose, and can be taken on a daily basis indefinitely. Diabetics taking insulin, however, should consult with a physician before taking chromium supplements.

Chromium is often combined with cysteine, niacin, and other nutrients to make glucose tolerance factor (GTF). Another common form is chromium picolinate.

HOW TO USE CHROMIUM: It comes in tablets (usually 100 to 200 mcg), capsules, and a liquid. An optimal daily dosage for adults is 200 to 400 mcg.

Nutritional Supplements for the Eyes

The following two substances are noted for their positive impact on vision and eye health.

Bioflavonoids

A number of flavonoid plant compounds found in various fruits, vegetables, and herbs play an important role in healing and strengthening capillaries and collagen. Since the eyes are rich in capillaries and depend upon collagen for a healthy cornea, sclera, and other parts, flavonoids can have a key role in encouraging better vision. Flavonoids also help to enhance the action of vitamin C and are potent antioxidants on their own. Some studies on individual flavonoids have demonstrated healing effects on the eyes. For example, researchers recently found that most glaucoma patients given rutin for at least a month gained some benefit.

Supplement manufacturers sell a few nutrient bioflavonoids separately (particularly quercetin and rutin). More popular products are the whole bioflavonoid complex, and bioflavonoids in combination with other supplements, most often vitamin C.

Polyphenols and flavonoids are also found in high concentrations in such herbs as ginkgo (which has shown promise as a treatment for macular degeneration), hawthorn, milk thistle, green tea, European coastal pine (sold as the trademarked product Pycnogenol), red wine/ grapes and grape-seed extract, and bilberry (as mentioned above, the anthocyanosides are flavonoids that improve night vision and help prevent glaucoma and cataracts). See Chapter 2 for average dosages of these flavonoid-rich herbs.

HOW TO USE BIOFLAVONOIDS: They are typically found in tablet and capsule form. An average daily dosage of the bioflavonoid complex is 500 mg; of quercetin and rutin, 200 to 500 mg.

Taurine

Taurine is a nonessential amino acid produced by the body. It is concentrated in the brain, where it plays a central role in regulating the nerves and muscles and coordinating electrical activity. It is also found in high amounts in the retina. Studies on cats have shown that a diet low in taurine can lead to degeneration of the retina and impairment of vision. Taurine has mild antioxidant properties, and in the eye it works closely with zinc to protect against cataracts.

Taurine is found in meat, fish, and eggs, but not plant foods. Excess taurine consumption may cause depression or other adverse effects. The doses of 1 to 3 g used to treat high blood pressure, epilepsy, and certain other conditions is much higher than is necessary to ensure proper functioning of the eyes. ·

HOW TO USE TAURINE: It comes in powders, tablets, and capsules, typically 500 mg or 1,000 mg. An average dosage is 50 to 100 mg two or three times weekly.

Where to Start for Better Eyesight

An herb-nutrient combination such as the following offers the best bet for vision benefits.
- Bilberry (80 to 160 mg two or three times daily of an extract standardized for 20 to 25 percent anthocyanosides) by itself or along with other herbs rich in polyphenols and flavonoids
- Vitamin A/beta carotene (5,000 to 10,000 IU of vitamin A plus 25,000 to 50,000 IU [15 to 30 mg] of beta carotene or beta carotene plus mixed carotenoids), preferably in a multivitamin-multimineral supplement with optimal levels of the antioxidant nutrients, zinc, and chromium

Hearing Loud and Clear

Gradual hearing loss and tinnitus (a constant ringing or buzzing in the ear) are problems for increasing numbers of Americans, both because these conditions are common with advancing age and because high noise levels in city environments and elsewhere can have harmful effects on hearing. Of course, hearing problems may also result from illnesses, injuries, or even something as simple as too much ear wax. Like the eye, the ear is a delicate organ that needs to be properly nourished to accomplish its task of collecting energy waves—in this case sound—and transforming them into nerve impulses for processing by the brain.

There are several nutrients that studies indicate are closely tied to optimum functioning of the parts of the ear.

Vitamin A/beta carotene. An average dose is 5,000 to 10,000 IU of vitamin A plus 25,000 to 50,000 IU (15 to 30 mg) of beta carotene or beta carotene plus mixed carotenoids daily. The cochlea, the snail-shaped cavity located in the inner ear that converts sound into nerve impulses, has high requirements for this nutrient. Studies show that people who have low levels of the vitamin often experience hearing problems.

Vitamin D and calcium. Vitamin D is obtained from regular exposure to sunshine, or can be taken as a supplement (400 to 800 IU daily). Calcium supplements (800 to 1,500 mg daily) ensure proper levels of this nutrient in the fluid of the inner ear.

Iron (18 mg daily) and iodide (150 mcg daily). Animal studies indicate that diets deficient in these minerals can lead to hearing loss, but most nutritionists recommend that people take supplementary iron and iodide only if deficiencies in these nutrients have been clinically established.

Zinc. A dose of 17 to 25 mg daily helps prevent or treat tinnitus.

Vitamin B_{12}

Vitamin B_{12}, or cobalamin, deserves special attention. It aids in energy production from fats and carbohydrates and in the production of amino acids. It also plays a role in building and maintaining nerves, including those involved in hearing. Deficiencies in B_{12} may cause neurological problems and confusion, fatigue, depression, and memory loss. Inadequate body levels have also been tied to tinnitus and hearing problems. There is some evidence that, especially if you work in a loud environment, you should be sure to take optimum amounts of B_{12} to protect against hearing loss. For example, Israeli researchers measured B_{12} levels in 113 soldiers, 50 percent of whom suffered from either tinnitus or hearing loss. The researchers found that nearly half of the soldiers with hearing problems were deficient in B_{12}, while fewer than one in five of the soldiers with normal hearing had deficiencies. The tinnitus was most severe among those soldiers with the lowest B_{12} levels.

The U.S. RDA for B_{12} is 6 mcg. B_{12} is found in animal products such as meat, milk, and eggs. Vegetarian sources exist (principally tempeh, sea vegetables, brewer's yeast, and mushrooms) but are unreliable. Unlike the other water-soluble B vitamins, B_{12} is actually stored well in the body, so vegetarians are usually not at risk for a deficiency unless they are strict, long-term vegans (eating no dairy products or eggs). The vitamin is usually included in multivitamin formulas; as an individual supplement, it comes in tablets, capsules, and lozenges (sometimes designed to be administered sublingually, that is, under the tongue) ranging in size from 100 mcg to 2,000 mcg. Medical practitioners can also administer injectable B_{12}

HOW TO USE VITAMIN B_{12}: An optimal daily supplement level of B_{12} is 100 to 200 mcg.

The Hearing Herb: Ginkgo

Ginkgo's positive effects on hearing are remarkably wide-ranging. In China, ginkgo leaves have long been a traditional treatment for asthma and other conditions. Ginkgo's demonstrated ability to promote blood flow in the brain has made it increasingly popular in the West as a "smart herb" (see Chapter 11) and as a potential treatment or preventive remedy for conditions of aging, such as dizziness, stroke, and Alzheimer's disease. Because researchers know that ginkgo also stimulates blood flow to the inner ear and to the nerves involved in hearing, the herb has in recent years been the subject of a number of double-blind, placebo-controlled studies to test its ability to prevent or reverse acute cochlear deafness and tinnitus.

The results of these studies have confirmed ginkgo's positive effects on hearing. For example, a study done in France found that ginkgo worked even better than conventional medical therapy to reverse hearing loss due to acute cochlear deafness, both from unknown causes and from exposure to sudden loud noises. Studies have also shown that ginkgo can relieve chronic tinnitus. One study found that ginkgo completely cured tinnitus in 36 percent of the patients and improved the condition in another 15 percent. French researchers who studied ginkgo's effects on 103 chronic tinnitus sufferers who took the herb for more than a year termed ginkgo "conclusively effective" when it was shown to improve the condition in all the subjects.

Ginkgo's positive effects on the ear extend to the semicircular canals, which govern balance and orientation in space. Studies have shown that people suffering from chronic dizziness or vertigo improve when they take ginkgo. The herb may also help treat Ménière's syndrome, an inner-ear dysfunction characterized by dizziness, nausea, and hearing loss.

Ginkgo is nontoxic and can safely be taken indefinitely on a daily basis. At the average dosage below, some people experience improvements in hearing within a month, while others may take three months or longer to respond. The benefits seem to become more noticeable and the results more lasting over time.

HOW TO USE GINKGO: Ginkgo comes in tablets, capsules, concentrated drops, tinctures, and extracts. An average dosage is 40 mg three times daily of a standardized extract containing 24 percent flavoglycosides.

Heightening Your Senses of Taste and Smell

How foods and smells trigger tastes is still something of a mystery to scientists. According to Western medical researchers, the tongue, palate, and throat have specialized receptors or taste buds that allow you to experience four tastes: sweet, salty, sour, and bitter. Practitioners of the traditional medicine of China recognize a fifth taste, pungent/acrid/spicy, while practitioners of Ayurveda, the traditional medicine of India, recognize a sixth taste, astringent. Of course, variations on these themes are almost infinite, from the unique sweetness of licorice to the distinctive bitterness of roasted coffee. Smell plays a crucial role in distinguishing the tastes of various foods, beverages, herbs, and other substances. One estimate is that 80 percent of what you perceive as taste is due to smell.

Unlike vision and hearing, there are few herbs or nutritional supplements that markedly affect taste and smell. Improving these senses is primarily a function of practice, study, and observation. As connoisseurs of wine, coffee, spices, and fine foods can attest, it is possible to educate your palate to appreciate extremely fine subtleties of taste. Practitioners of aromatherapy who have experimented with many of the more than seven hundred essential oils can also confirm that the sense of smell improves with practice. Blind people by necessity often develop an acute ability to distinguish sounds and smells.

There is, however, one nutritional supplement that has been confirmed by scientific studies on humans and animals to improve the senses of smell and taste.

Zinc

In addition to playing an important role in vision and hearing, the trace element zinc is essential for taste and smell. Zinc is crucial for the process that results in your taste buds being replaced every 10 to 12 days. A long-term zinc deficiency can contribute to the loss of up to 80 percent of the taste buds among some elderly people. People who are deficient in zinc notice unpleasant taste sensations and a decreased ability to distinguish different tastes and smells. Indeed, one of the simplest clinical tests to determine whether you have adequate levels of zinc in your body involves tasting a specially formulated zinc solution. Even if you don't have any overt symptoms of a zinc deficiency, if you can't taste this solution you are probably deficient in zinc. Studies done on kidney patients on dialysis and others who are zinc-deficient have shown that taking zinc supplements can dramatically improve taste and smell. The positive effect on these senses is less dramatic but still noticeable among people with marginal zinc deficiencies. One researcher found that a few weeks of zinc supplementation can help children who are finicky eaters to increase their appreciation of different foods.

How to use zinc: Zinc is frequently balanced with copper and selenium, and combined with other minerals and vitamins. As an individual supplement, it comes in lozenges, tablets, and capsules. An optimal daily dosage for adults is 17 to 25 mg.

Beyond Herbs and Supplements

Taking the right herbs, vitamins and minerals, and various nutrients can greatly benefit your sense perception. No remedies, however, can guarantee perfect vision, hearing, taste, and smell. The same habits—regular exercise, a healthful diet, rest and relaxation—that keep the body and mind fit will also benefit the eyes, ears, nerves, brain, and other parts of the sensory systems. For example, regular activity or aerobic exercise improves circulation to all parts of the body, including to the sense organs. Likewise, the same high-fat, high-cholesterol diet that clogs the arteries of the heart can interfere with the delicate blood vessels of the sense organs. Recent studies show that elevated blood-fat levels can clog the blood vessels of the ear and slow the delivery of oxygen, thus preventing the inner ear from receiving the nourishment it needs to assist with proper hearing. People with partial deafness thus may experience restored hearing when they go on a low-fat diet. A number of studies have also demonstrated the reverse: people with low levels of blood fats and good cholesterol ratios have better hearing.

Because they are more active than the ears, the eyes benefit from both relaxation and exercise. Resting your eyes can be as simple as a few minutes of palming, in which you hold the palms lightly over the eyes to block out all light. Numerous eye exercises (see any of the books on natural vision improvement listed in "Resources") can help you to achieve better focusing, shifting, depth perception, and right eye/left eye coordination.

Another obvious step to promote sense health is to avoid the bad habits that can be most damaging to your sensory organs, such as:
- Exposing your ears to loud music and high noise levels
- Reading in inadequate light
- Staring at the TV for long periods
- Performing uninterrupted near-point work on a computer monitor
- Failing to protect the eyes when necessary from injurious objects or chemicals
- Chewing tobacco, which can cause mouth cancers and otherwise harm sensitive taste buds

Finally, recognize that although your ears are your primary organ of hearing, and your eyes the primary organ of vision, these sense organs do not work in isolation. As natural-vision proponent Richard Leviton notes, "To really understand vision, it's necessary to see it in context of not only the eyes, but the brain, the nervous system, hormonal functions, genetics, the liver, diet, behavior, work and play habits, psychoemotional states, and more. The popular perception of vision as an isolated, detached function is inconsistent with the holistic approach to health and medicine in general."

Keep Your Skin
Smooth and Supple

The largest and most exterior of the body's organs, the skin is a major protector of health—it serves as your first line of defense against microbial invaders—as well as a unique indicator of overall well-being. You need to have a series of blood tests to know whether your liver is functioning properly, but a glance in the mirror can tell you something has gone seriously wrong with your skin. In many cases, your skin problem reflects an imbalance in some other bodily function as well. Diseases, nutrient deficiencies, allergic reactions, and a whole host of other medical problems often show up prominently on the skin, causing it to redden, become inflamed, or blister.

The skin has close links to a variety of the body's other organs and systems. The skin's connection to the nervous system is evidenced by the immediate and dramatic effects such emotions as fear, shame, and panic have on the skin. Since the skin governs touch and is closely allied with physical appearance (as any teenager cursed with acne can attest), its role in sexuality should come as no surprise. Because the skin contains one third of the body's supply of blood, its effects on circulation and thus regulation of body temperature are considerable. The connections between mind, immunity, and the skin are wondrous. One recent study found, in effect, that subjects rubbed with a tea leaf they believed to be poison ivy would have an allergic reaction, while those rubbed with poison ivy leaves, if convinced they were tea leaves, would not get the characteristic rash.

There are also crucial links between skin health, physical appearance, and self-esteem. Skin that is in optimal health is a joy to have and to behold. Healthy skin is elastic yet firm, soft yet toned, pliable yet sturdy. It is smooth, supple, and evenly colored. A person in possession of excellent skin is said to be radiant, as if her skin is emanating a vital energy from her very core. Another may be described as having a ruddy glow, again indicating inner health emanating outward.

Skin-Deep Health

The skin is a complex organ that plays a central role in many bodily functions, and keeping it performing optimally is vital to overall health. The 3,000-plus square inches of skin on the average person help to:
* Shield the body from toxins
* Eliminate wastes
* Regulate body temperature
* Conserve moisture
* Protect other organs from injury and infection
* Provide the sensations of touch, hot and cold, pleasure and pain
* Manufacture vitamin D

How does an organ that is a mere one to three millimeters thick accomplish this remarkable range of functions? Let's take a look at its two main layers, the epidermis and the dermis, in more detail.

The epidermis is the skin's tough outer layer. Dead and dying skin cells at the topmost part of the epidermis are continuously being shed, while new cells generated in lower sections of the epidermis are pushed up from below. The epidermis lacks blood vessels but has plenty of fine nerves to collect and relay messages to the brain about the body's immediate surroundings. Carbon dioxide and other forms of waste are eliminated through the epidermis.

Most of the epidermis's important biological supplies are provided by the skin's thicker dermis and the subcutaneous fatty-tissue layer. The system of blood vessels and capillaries in the dermis can contract to conserve bodily heat and expand to give off heat. The dermis also contains a rich network of nerves to transmit sensations of pain and pleasure, sweat glands to cool the body, and sebaceous glands to provide the naturally oily, waxy substance (sebum) that keeps the skin lubricated and supple. Hair follicles are embedded in the deepest part of the dermis. Bundles of fibrous proteins, known as collagen and elastin, in the dermis are crucial to overall skin structure and appearance. The effects of sun, aging, and free radicals can cause these proteins to degrade, becoming stiff and cross-linked with each other. This eventually leads to coarse, wrinkled, leathery skin.

As an external organ intimately bound up with the nervous, immune, and circulatory systems, it is no surprise that the skin frequently shows signs of malfunctioning. Some of the most common skin conditions include acne (due to sebum collecting on the surface of the skin and blocking the pores and hair follicles, thus allowing bacteria and other foreign bodies to gather there and cause the red, inflamed bump known as a pimple); ringworm and athlete's foot (fungal infections resulting in scaling, dryness, itching, and cracking); eczema (an inflammation of the skin that often causes itching and blistering); the rash of poison ivy (an allergic reaction of the skin to a toxic oil produced by the poison ivy, poison oak, or poison sumac plants); and psoriasis (a skin disease characterized by thickened patches of red, inflamed skin, due to new skin cells forming too fast and old cells not being shed quickly enough).

The direct causes of some of these conditions (particularly psoriasis and eczema) are not always known. However, skin problems commonly result from hormone imbalances, poor diet (particularly eating too much saturated fat), allergic responses and immune-system dysfunctions, and poor personal hygiene. Humans have also devised a variety of ways to abuse the skin and prevent it from accomplishing its natural functions:

Cosmetics. Heavy layers of makeup, deodorants, and other products present two drawbacks. One, they block the release of sebum and work in other ways to prevent the skin from performing its natural functions. Two, body-care products may contain a wide variety of petrochemicals, coal-tar dyes, and other substances with potentially toxic effects.

Soaps and detergents. The natural oils secreted by the skin help to keep it moist, supple, and free of bacteria. Frequent washing can sweep away these protective substances; it can also change the natural balance of acidity/alkalinity (pH) on the skin's surface. Chemicals in soaps and detergents can also be irritating or drying to the skin.

Sunlight. Getting frequent sunburns is one of the most damaging things that you can do to your skin. Among other adverse effects, it substantially increases the risk of skin cancer. Sunlight has become more problematic in recent years because of the ongoing depletion of the atmosphere's ozone layer. This increases the ultraviolet exposure at the earth's surface for all living organisms, including humans.

Heat and humidity. Some types of heating, especially forced-air systems, and air-conditioning can make the home or workplace very drying to the skin. Extremely high humidity, such as is found in some tropical climates and in indoor pools, can have the opposite effect, leaving your skin so moist that it is more susceptible to bacterial and fungal infections.

"What your skin needs is based on how your skin works," states skin-care authority Aubrey Hampton, author of *Natural Organic Hair and Skin Care*. The corollary to this premise is that natural substances, by promoting rather than suppressing the skin's vital functions, work with it to keep it smooth and supple.

Topically Speaking

Drugstores' shelves are overflowing with topical skin-care products, including baby lotions, bar soaps, facial toners, beauty masks, lip balms, moisturizers, shaving creams, and sunscreens. Moreover, if you take the time to read the ingredient lists on product labels, you quickly notice that conventional body-care producers make use of hundreds, if not thousands, of synthetic chemical compounds. Depending upon the type of product, these compounds perform various and often overlapping functions. There are binders to maintain the product's consistency, colors for dyeing it, emulsifiers to hold liquids together, fragrances to add odors and fixatives to prevent the odor from vaporizing, humectants to keep it moist, preservatives to prevent it from spoiling, thickeners to add body, and surfactants to help it spread out and penetrate the skin more thoroughly.

Entire volumes have been devoted to explaining the production, function, and safety of the chemical compounds used in cosmetic products (see "Resources"), and it is not within the scope of this chapter to examine fully even the most commonly used substances and compounds. For health-conscious people, safety is often a primary concern. While it is true that some compounds are found in both conventional and natural body-care products, in general the conventional products are much more likely to make extensive use of various petrochemicals, formaldehyde compounds, artificial colors, and other synthetic chemicals that many people would prefer not to be exposed to. Keep in mind that the body absorbs as much as 50 percent of some substances applied to the skin. Nontoxic alternatives are readily available that are just as effective as the synthetic products at softening and moisturizing skin, promoting new cell growth, reducing free-radical damage, and stimulating circulation.

To begin with, let's take a look at a half dozen or so of the plant- and nutrient-based substances with the most dramatic healing and nourishing effects on the skin, and then look at some specific types of body-care products and the different approaches taken in formulating them by the conventional and natural body-care companies.

All-Purpose Skin Healers

Some of the herbs and nutritional substances that are often included in skin-care products for their healing, moisturizing, or toning effects include vitamins D and E, the compound allantoin, and the herbs aloe and chamomile. Aloe stands on its own among these since it is not only a prominent ingredient in skin-care products but is also sold as a whole gel or lotion for the skin.

Vitamin D. This vitamin is closely allied with the skin, since the body manufactures it in the skin with the aid of sunlight. Many people are now so afraid of sunlight that they avoid all exposure, but some sunshine is beneficial. Studies have linked higher vitamin D levels with a reduced risk of various cancers, including skin cancer.

Pharmaceutical companies have developed creams based on vitamin D, but they're primarily prescription remedies to treat conditions such as psoriasis. Psoriasis sufferers have also noticed that having a slight tan —a vitamin-D-related process—may help alleviate the condition.

Oral vitamin D supplements should be used with caution. Vitamin D is one of the fat-soluble vitamins capable of building up to toxic levels in the body. People who live in cold climates or who get little regular sun exposure may benefit from 400 to 800 IU daily in supplements. Topical vitamin D products present a lower risk of side effects; the amount of vitamin D found in OTC body-care products is very safe.

Vitamin E. Along with the other antioxidant nutrients (especially vitamins A and C, and the mineral selenium), vitamin E is often included in topical creams for its antioxidant effects. Free radicals formed in skin tissues by sunlight and industrial pollutants can have harmful effects, possibly even triggering cancer. How much free-radical-bashing topical antioxidants do is somewhat controversial, though there is some evidence that they help protect against skin cancer. Vitamin E may also play a role in preventing acne and improving skin circulation.

Vitamin E oil applied to the skin seems to accelerate the healing of burns and prevent scars from forming. Definitive studies are lacking, but many alternative practitioners have seen positive results among their patients from using E on burns. Vitamin E oil can also be applied to canker sores and to nipples that are sore and cracked from breast-feeding.

Vitamin E oil is very viscous (and expensive) for application to large areas of the body. Vitamin E oils sold as beauty products are combinations of E and vegetable oils, such as those from sunflowers, almonds, and wheat germ. These products are not for internal use.

Allantoin. Allantoin is a crystalline substance that may be derived from animal or plant sources. The principal plant source is the herb comfrey, a hardy perennial (*Symphytum officinale*) with small purple flowers. Because comfrey contains other compounds, the pyrrolizidine alkaloids, that are potentially toxic to the liver, comfrey itself is of questionable safety as an external remedy. Comfrey-derived allantoin is safe and nontoxic. It is used in skin lotions and creams, lip balms, sunscreens, and shampoos as a moisturizer and for its healing effects on the skin. Allantoin both promotes cell regeneration and helps relieve inflammation.

Chamomile. This ancient herb has long been used as an oral remedy for insomnia (see Chapter 12), digestive problems, and fevers. Chamomile is still taken internally for these problems and has also enjoyed widespread use externally to spur the healing of cuts and scrapes, rashes, and burns. Its soothing, softening effect on the skin has prompted body-care companies to include it in a wide variety of skin creams, facial treatments, and body lotions.

Chamomile contains a complex mixture of chemical constituents that is still being analyzed. Researchers suspect that a key compound in chamomile is azulene, derived from the flowers' distinctive blue essential oil. Azulene is also found in the herb yarrow. Azulene helps to reduce inflammation, relieve local pain, improve tissue regeneration, and stimulate the immune-boosting activity of white blood cells.

In general, topical chamomile products are minimally toxic and are gentle enough for use on children. Natural-food stores carry a variety of chamomile-based skin care products, including the popular Camo-Care line of creams and lotions. You can also brew a strong infusion and apply it as a compress or herbal wash to irritated skin.

Aloe

Aloe preparations are derived from the leaf gel and juice of a cactus-like member of the lily family with some three hundred species, among them the popular *Aloe vera.* Ancient Egyptian and Greek herb-alists knew of aloe's benefits as a topical healer, often applying the transparent gel from the inner leaf on burns, wounds, and skin irrita-tions. Diverse cultures around the world have incorporated aloe into their medical practices. Today aloe is widely grown in arid parts of Africa, the Mediterranean, and other regions.

The semisolid, transparent gel obtained from the innermost layers of the plant's fleshy leaves contains a number of therapeutically active compounds, including glycosides (a sugar derivative), polysaccharides (complex carbohydrate molecules), resinous material, and volatile oil. Other compounds that may account for aloe's healing, softening, and moisturizing effects on skin include vitamins C and E and the mineral zinc.

Studies confirm aloe's antibacterial, burn-soothing, and wound-healing effects. The gel is a common ingredient in first-aid skin creams, shampoos, and natural and conventional body-care products. (The plant's juice, or latex, is used to make herbal remedies that are sometimes taken internally. Oral aloe remedies act as potent laxatives, though most herbalists recommend milder herbs for this purpose.)

Natural body-care companies market various products with aloe as a main ingredient, including lotions and creams. Quality juice or gel products are usually 96 to 100 percent pure aloe. Bottled and "stabi-lized" aloe that is produced by harsh solvent extraction methods may contain little of the healing ingredients of fresh aloe. Also look for aloe products that haven't been preserved with alcohol, which will neutral-ize aloe's skin-healing properties, and don't contain mineral oil, paraf-fin waxes, or coloring.

Essential Oils for Better Skin

"Skin problems are often the surface manifestation of a deeper con-dition, such as a build-up of toxins in the blood, hormonal imbalance, or nervous and emotional difficulties," notes Julia Lawless, author of *The Encyclopaedia of Essential Oils.* "In this area the versatility of essen-tial oils is particularly valuable because they are able to combat such complaints on a variety of levels. Since essential oils are soluble in oil and alcohol and impart their scent to water, they provide the ideal ingredient for cosmetics and general skin care as well as for the treat-ment of specific diseases."

Essential oils are widely used in skin-care products, as are essential-oil-derived compounds such as menthol, eugenol (a colorless, aromatic liquid derived principally from the essential oil of Clove), and camphors (derived from the essential oil found in the wood of an evergreen tree native to Asia). Essential oils are used as preservatives, skin fresheners, and antibacterial agents in skin creams. Two of the most commonly used essential oils for skin health are Tea Tree and Chamomile.

Tea Tree is derived from the leaves of an Australian tree (*Melaleuca alternifolia*) of the myrtle family. Tea Tree is recognized as one of the premier essential oils for first aid, widely used for treating burns, cuts, scrapes, bites, stings, and various types of skin irritations. Chamomile, the source of azulene, is also widely used to soothe problem skin.

Lavender

Perhaps the most versatile of the essential oils for use on the skin is Lavender. The leaves and blue flowers of this Mediterranean shrub have been used since ancient times for skin complaints. Today the exquisitely scented essential oil is prevalent in various body-care products, including lotions, perfumes, soaps, and cosmetics. Topically, the oil is a wound healer, promoting cell rejuvenation and stimulating the immune system. Lavender reduces skin inflammation and counters fungal infections such as athlete's foot. It also has antiseptic effects. Lavender is mild enough to be applied full-strength to treat various types of skin conditions, from burns, cuts, scrapes, and insect bites to dermatitis, eczema, and psoriasis.

Lavender and other essential oils are popular ingredients in skin creams and other body care products. The most common ways to use essential oils for better skin health include massage, baths, and compresses. See "How to Use Essential Oils" in Chapter 2.

Saving Face

Four of the most common types of skin products are moisturizing creams and lotions, abrasives and exfoliants, cleansers, and fresheners and toners. Let's take a look at what these do, what kind of chemicals most conventional products use, and what types of natural alternatives there are from the plant and nutrient fields.

Moisturizers

These moisten the skin by increasing the amount of water in the uppermost skin layers. This serves to soften and soothe the skin, and to some extent plump it up and erase fine wrinkles. Moisturizers are used to prevent and relieve dry, rough, and flaky skin as well as wrinkles. Moisturizers work best when applied while skin is slightly damp.

Most moisturizing products are lotions or creams whose main ingredients are water, glycerin (a sweet, syrupy, colorless, nontoxic liquid that can be produced synthetically from petrochemicals or derived naturally from vegetable fats and oils), and oil. Glycerin acts to capture moisture from the skin and surrounding air. Some commercial moisturizers also contain substances to block moisture loss from the skin, though they tend to clog pores as well. These moisture blockers include mineral oil (a colorless liquid mixture of refined hydrocarbons derived from petroleum), lanolin (a natural fatty substance derived from the oil glands of sheep), and petrolatum (also known as petroleum jelly and Vaseline, a yellowish, greasy, jellylike mixture of semisolid hydrocarbons derived from petroleum). Commercial moisturizing products may also contain various synthetic additives for color, fragrance, binding, and so forth.

Natural products usually moisturize with glycerine as well as oil from such sources as almonds, wheat germ, vitamin E, jojoba (a desert shrub), avocados, sunflowers, peanuts, or olives. Other ingredients may include aloe, cocoa butter (a natural fat expressed from the roasted seeds of the tropical cacao tree), allantoin, and honey. Another natural moisturizer is squalene, a compound found in oil derived from certain plants (wheat, rice, olives) and the liver of a rare species of shark. Squalene is popular in Japan and elsewhere both as a topical moisturizer and as a food supplement (it is said to boost the immune system). Herbs for soothing and healing effects often used in natural moisturizers include calendula, rosemary, chamomile, lavender, marigold, sage, and yarrow.

An unusual moisturizing product is colloidal oatmeal. This powdered form of oatmeal turns into a slippery mass when mixed with water. Added to a bath, it disperses throughout the water and forms a thin gel that coats your skin, holding moisture in and providing relief from itching. Regular oatmeal is too coarsely ground to bind with water and have this soothing effect; either grind your own oats down to a flour-like powder, or look for the popular commercial colloidal oatmeal product Aveeno in your local pharmacy. Add 1 to 2 ounces of colloidal oatmeal to the bath water.

Abrasives and Exfoliants

Abrasives and exfoliants are agents used for cleaning and scrubbing the skin. Abrasives are found in heavy-duty bar soaps for removing grease and dirt. Exfoliants work more gently by peeling or flaking off the surface scales of the skin. Abrasives and exfoliants need to be effective but not so harsh that they scratch the skin.

Conventional skin scrubs often use pumice (a rough and porous powder derived from volcanic rock) or the mineral feldspar as abrasives. Natural body-care companies also use these as well as various powdered herbs, vegetable or almond meal (pulverized blanched almonds or the residue that remains after the almond oil has been expressed), clay, or bran.

Popular natural exfoliants include apricot kernels and citrus fruit and green papaya extracts or concentrates (for their enzyme action). Two of the hottest natural skin care ingredients of recent years—vitamin A derivatives and the alpha hydroxy acids—are basically exfoliants.

Vitamin A derivatives. There are several retinoids—compounds derived from vitamin A—with the most widely known one being tretinoin (Retin-A, Renova). Retin-A has an exfoliating effect and may also nourish collagen. Developed to alleviate severe acne, Retin-A became popular in the late 1980s as a prescription-only "miracle skin cream" to erase wrinkles and spots and restore a youthful appearance to sun-damaged skin. After the initial enthusiasm and media-backed hoopla, however, it became apparent that the drug was not for everyone. Retin-A's ability to (eventually) smooth out some surface wrinkles was accompanied by some rather harsh potential side effects, including skin that became dried out, irritated, or even burned. Retin-A can also cause the skin to become more sensitive to sunlight.

Alpha hydroxy acids. Also known as fruit acids and glycolic acids, alpha hydroxy acids (AHAs) are natural substances derived from various fruits, most commonly grapes, apples, and citrus; milk (the source of lactic acid); and sugar cane (the source of glycolic acids). AHA products have been around for almost twenty years—an AHA patent was filed in 1976. In high concentrations (30 percent and above), AHAs have important therapeutic uses. For example, dermatologists and surgeons use prescription AHA products to help remove dead cells from the skin's surface, thereby erasing large age spots or reducing scar tissue.

Within recent years the cosmetic industry realized that lower concentrations of AHAs could enhance a wide range of over-the-counter body-care products. Lower concentrations (between 4 and 10 percent) of AHAs are now widely used in both conventional and natural body-care products. The mild exfoliating effect they have is accompanied by moisturizing and antiaging effects. Many people have found that AHAs help to erase age spots and fine lines and also improve the skin's texture and tone, creating a complexion that is smooth and supple. Studies have shown that AHAs can alleviate dry skin and help reduce acne as well.

Though available in OTC products, alpha hydroxy acids have effects somewhat similar to prescription-only Retin-A. In moderate concentrations (6 percent, according to the FDA), AHAs are much less likely than Retin-A to cause side effects. AHA concentrations in OTC products have, however, begun to creep up in the past few years. Some formulas sold in drugstores and natural-food stores now provide 10 to 12.5 percent AHAs or even more. Such concentrations increase the risk of skin irritation or even burning, especially if the products are left on the skin for longer than the usual 15 to 20 minutes. Products are also becoming more specialized, with lower concentrations in those that are for use on areas of sensitive skin, such as the eyes. AHA products often need to be used for 6 to 8 weeks before their full effects are noticed. Body-care companies are also developing products that combine AHAs and Retin-A.

Skin Cleansers

Bar soaps are cleansers formulated by mixing mineral salts (usually sodium or potassium salts) with some type of fatty acid. Conventional bar soaps often contain compounds derived from tallow (fat from the fatty tissue of animals such as cattle and sheep), such as sodium tallowate, and/or fatty compounds in coconut or palm kernels. For instance, magnesium cocoate is a coconut-fat-derived sudsing and cleansing agent, and palm kernelate and palm kernel acid are fatty compounds from palm kernel oil. Conventional bar soaps may also contain ammonium compounds such as detergents, synthetic preservatives such as BHA or BHT, artificial colors such as titanium dioxide, and sudsing agents such as dioctyl sodium sulfosuccinate. Deodorant soaps often contain strong topical antibacterials—triclosan, for example. Most conventional bar soaps are heavily scented with synthetic fragrances and also contain fixatives.

Natural bar soaps avoid animal fats by substituting cocoa butter or plant-derived oils from almonds, coconuts, or olives. Natural glycerin is often used as an emulsifier and moisturizer. Herbs such as lavender, calendula, aloe, rosemary, and rose may be used for skin soothing, astringency, and fragrance, and oatmeal may be included for its soothing and exfoliating effects. Other ingredients may include citric acid (as a preservative) and essential oils such as Lemon and Cinnamon for fragrance or antibacterial action.

Fresheners and Toners

Fresheners are agents that have an astringent effect, contracting body tissue, while toners (typically applied to the face with a cotton pad) add to this astringent effect mild exfoliation. Astringents tighten and close the pores of the skin, help to clean oily skin, and remove cleanser residues left on the skin. Fresheners and toners generally leave the skin feeling cool or tingling.

Producers of conventional cosmetics who want an astringent effect typically use synthetic chemicals that contain alcohol, which do tighten the skin but are also fairly drying. Freshener and toner products may also contain other chemicals such as acetone (a synthetically derived volatile liquid commonly used as a solvent in commercial cosmetics), boric acid (a crystalline compound of an alkaline salt, borax), or alum (a solid, sulfated compound of ammonium, sodium or potassium, and a metal such as aluminum).

Milder, less toxic astringents that are widely used in natural cosmetics include those made from menthol (a crystalline alcohol that may be synthetically derived or obtained from the essential oil of mint plants), herbs (such as witch hazel, chamomile, lavender, yarrow, and calendula), rose water (a watery solution made by distilling fresh rose petals), almond meal, or vinegar.

Natural facial toners may make use of green papaya concentrate, apricot kernels, or citrus-oil extracts as exfoliants, cleansers, and abrasives; glycerin, sunflower oil, or honey as moisturizing agents; vitamin E as an antioxidant; jojoba, apricot, or almond oil as lubricants and fragrances; and astringent or skin-healing compounds such as allantoin, sea kelp and other seaweeds, and herbs including aloe, comfrey, calendula, witch hazel, and nettle.

Cosmetic clay is another popular natural substance with skin-contracting, cleansing, and drying effects. *Clay* is the generic term for any finely grained decomposed rock or volcanic ash that can be used both topically (to relieve insect bites, rashes, poison ivy, and other minor skin irritations) or internally (to relieve digestive complaints, for example; see Chapter 16). Green clay and other cosmetic clays have also been used for thousands of years to beautify the skin. Clay is excellent for mud baths and beauty masks, in which the powder is mixed with water into a paste, applied to the skin, left on until it is dry, and washed off. A cosmetic clay widely used in beauty masks is kaolin, a fine white powder also used in porcelain making.

Oral Supplements for Better Skin

Nutritional deficiencies are often first noticed because of their effects on the skin, ranging from acne to eczema. In many cases studies have also confirmed therapeutic uses for nutrients in the treatment of skin conditions. Taking optimal levels of various nutritional substances should help to keep your skin smooth and blemish-free.

Supplement makers offer various products for better skin health. Some are formulated especially for the skin; others target the hair, skin, and nails. Look for products such as Elements for Skin, SHN, 30-Day Beauty Secret, and Skin Support. Most of these are combinations of minerals such as the following as well as vitamins, essential fatty acids, and other nutrients tied to better skin health.

Selenium. This mineral antioxidant may help to reduce the risk of skin cancer. Few studies have been done on its effects on skin, but there is some evidence that therapeutic doses (400 mcg) can improve acne and other skin conditions, and average doses lead to healthier, better-looking skin. Shampoo makers use selenium compounds for dandruff control (the *sel-* in *Selsun* refers to selenium). Selenium is widely available in tablets and capsules ranging in size from 50 to 200 mcg. An average daily dosage is 100 to 200 mcg.

Calcium. Calcium may enhance the action of an enzyme in skin that slows the effects of aging and keeps skin soft and smooth. An optimal supplement level is 800 to 1,500 mg daily. (Many nutritionists recommend combining supplemental calcium and magnesium in approximately a 2:1 ratio, as in 750 mg calcium and 375 mg magnesium.)

Zinc and copper. Zinc aids in skin repair and wound healing; a deficiency may lead to acne, eczema, and other skin problems. Topical zinc preparations may cause the skin to secrete less oil and may thus help control acne. Copper plays a role in producing the important skin proteins collagen and elastin, as well as the skin pigment melanin. An average daily dosage to maintain healthy skin is 17 to 25 mg of zinc and 2 to 4 mg of copper.

Silicon. Abundant in the earth's crust, silicon is a mineral found in plant fiber and most hard water. Many nutritionists consider silicon to be essential, though it has only recently begun to gain scientific recognition for its role in health. Silicon is necessary for optimal skin health, providing skin with resilience and protecting it from the effects of aging. Silicon is also needed to form bones, teeth, nails, cartilage, and connective tissue. Along with the skin, these are the tissues where the highest levels in the body are found.

The most common dietary sources of silicon include whole-grain breads and cereals, vegetables, dried beans and peas, and seafood. It is also found in high concentrations in the herbs horsetail, nettle, and alfalfa. Some researchers believe that the overprocessing of industrialized nations' food supplies has led to a general deficiency of this trace mineral. The FDA has not established a U.S. RDA, although it admits there is "substantial evidence" that silicon is essential to health. Though toxic if inhaled (as silica dust, a byproduct of semiconductor production), no adverse effects have been reported from consuming silicon supplements. Few supplement makers offer silicon tablets, but silicon is frequently combined with other nutrients in formulas for hair, skin, and nails. A popular silicon-rich horsetail extract supplement is Alta Sil-X Silica (an average dosage is 500 mg of extract). Silicon (20 to 30 mg) is sometimes included in insurance-level multivitamin-multimineral supplements.

Vitamin A/Beta Carotene

One of the supplements sometimes taken on its own to support skin health is Vitamin A/beta carotene. Preformed, animal-derived vitamin A or its plant-based precursor beta carotene are key nutrients for better skin health, as they promote regeneration of skin cells, faster healing of wounds, and resistance against infections and cancer. A deficiency in vitamin A/beta carotene often leads to skin that is dry, rough, and old-looking. Optimal intake of the nutrient protects the skin from damage by free radicals and helps to keep it smooth and moisturized.

In addition to the aforementioned topical drug Retin-A, vitamin A is the source of a number of oral prescription drugs used to treat skin conditions. Most of these vitamin-A-derived drugs, such as isotretinoin (Accutane), an oral remedy for acne, psoriasis, and other skin conditions, share the same advantages and disadvantages of preformed vitamin A itself: They are effective against severe conditions, but must be taken at dosages that can be accompanied by unwanted side effects. Beta carotene is nontoxic, and in some cases large doses (100,000 IU) can also help to reverse psoriasis and other skin conditions.

Taking high doses of preformed A (such as 100,000 IU daily for months, or 500,000 to 1,000,000 IU daily for two to three weeks) can allow it to accumulate in the body and cause potentially serious adverse health effects. On the other hand, the body converts to vitamin A only as much beta carotene as it needs. Extra beta carotene is stored, but the only adverse effect of such storage is a slight orange tinge to the skin.

HOW TO USE VITAMIN A/BETA CAROTENE: It comes in a wide variety of tablets and capsules. An optimal daily dosage for better skin health is 5,000 to 10,000 IU of vitamin A plus 25,000 to 50,000 IU (15 to 30 mg) of beta carotene or beta carotene plus mixed carotenoids.

Vitamin B Complex

Almost all of the B vitamins have some healthful impact on the skin, and deficiency in almost any of them will cause skin problems. For example, cracked lips are a common symptom of riboflavin deficiency, and dry skin may be due to a B_6 deficiency. Vitamin B_6 supplementation has been known to clear up cases of acne, and a topical B_6-based cream has shown promise as an aid in treating the deadly skin cancer melanoma. Niacin's importance to skin is evident in the word *pellagra,* the niacin-deficiency condition named from the Italian for "sour" or "rough" skin. The skin-relevant B vitamins include not only these principal ones but a few of the "minor" B vitamins, such as biotin and para-aminobenzoic acid (PABA). Signs of a biotin deficiency include dry, flaky skin and loss of hair. PABA is well known as a topical sunscreen and may have some healthful effects on the skin when taken orally as well.

Taking individual B vitamins can cause an imbalance in other B vitamins. Many nutritionists recommend taking them as part of an insurance-level multivitamin or as B complex.

HOW TO USE B COMPLEX: It is available in liquids, tablets, and capsules. An average dosage for better skin is 25 to 50 mg one or two times daily.

Vitamin C

This vitamin's importance to the healing of skin wounds and bruises is well established. Oral doses and possibly even topical applications of vitamin C enhance the production of collagen and protect fragile capillaries from breakage, promoting younger-looking, better-toned skin. Vitamin C may also help prevent acne and skin allergies.

Vitamin C is safe at many times the optimal dosage; daily consumption of 2 to 5 g may cause loose stools in some people.

HOW TO USE VITAMIN C: It comes in a wide variety of powders, tablets, and capsules. An optimal dosage for skin health is 250 to 500 mg two or three times daily.

Essential Fatty Acids

The omega-3 essential fatty acids (primarily from cold-water fish) and the omega-6 EFAs (mostly from a few plant-seed oils) seem to soothe, nourish, and heal the skin. In general, studies have found that EFAs do offer some relief when taken at high dosages to relieve skin conditions such as eczema and psoriasis. Frequently taken for their anti-inflammatory effects, EFAs also reduce itching, slow the skin's aging process, promote moisturizing, and protect against harmful ultraviolet rays. Positive results may take two months or more to become evident.

HOW TO USE ESSENTIAL FATTY ACIDS: They're typically sold as liquids or oil-filled capsules (supplements may need to be refrigerated). An average daily dose of fish-oil or plant-oil capsules is 500 to 1,000 mg daily.

Brewer's Yeast

Brewer's yeast is often taken to keep skin smooth and soft. It is a concentrated source of various B vitamins and trace minerals necessary for skin health, including B_6, biotin, and selenium. Researchers have also isolated other skin-enhancing substances from brewer's yeast, including a polysaccharide (glucan) and a chemically mysterious derivative known as skin respiratory factor (SRF). These brewer's-yeast compounds have been shown to help form collagen, connective tissue, and capillaries in the skin, thus promoting skin repair. Animal studies and clinical trials indicate that SRF speeds the healing of burns and skin wounds. SRF is the "live yeast cell derivative" that is the active ingredient in Preparation H, which many people have found is useful not only for healing hemorrhoids but also for treating dry skin.

How to use brewer's yeast: Brewer's yeast is sold in powders, flakes, tablets, and capsules. An average dosage is $^{1}/_{2}$ to 1 tablespoon two or three times daily.

Where to Start

Taking the following nutritional supplements can help keep your skin looking young and healthy.

- An insurance-level multivitamin-multimineral supplement, especially one providing optimal daily levels of vitamins A/beta carotene, B complex, and C, and the minerals selenium, calcium, magnesium, zinc, copper, silicon, and chromium
- Essential fatty acids (500 to 1,000 mg daily)

Beyond Herbs and Supplements

One of the most important nutrients for your skin is a very simple compound: water. With its large reservoirs of blood, oils, and other fluids, the skin is one of the first tissues to suffer from dehydration. Thus, drinking adequate amounts of fluid is essential for optimal skin health. Depending upon individual factors such as body size, weather, and activity level, most people should be drinking at least one to two quarts of water, herbal teas, and fruit juices every day. Foods that are high in water content, such as fresh fruits and vegetables, are some of the best for skin health as well.

Following are a few other steps to take to keep your skin soft and supple.

- Avoid those activities that tend to undermine skin health, including smoking, excessive alcohol consumption, frequent use of broad-spectrum antibiotics and other potent pharmaceutical drugs, exposure to radiation, and a high-fat, high-sugar diet.
- If someone in your family suffers from a skin infection, particularly a viral or fungal one, avoid touching the area, or wash your hands afterward. Don't share personal items such as towels, clothing, combs, toothbrushes, and eating utensils. Herpes in particular is highly contagious, and easily spread, both to other people and to other parts of the body, especially the eyes, by kissing or touching.
- Take an occasional sauna to improve circulation and eliminate toxins.

• Never expose the skin to ultraviolet light long enough for it to cause a burn.

• Get a whole-body massage every once in a while. A vigorous massage has the dual benefit of increasing circulation and the vitality of skin tissues while alleviating harmful mental stress that can lead to premature aging of the skin.

Revitalize Your Digestive System

The 30-foot-long digestive system in the human body is something of an unappreciated marvel, almost miraculous in its intricacies, checks and balances, and well-coordinated functions. The process of breaking down food into its component parts so that the body is able to process and absorb them is accomplished without conscious intent, muscle fatigue, or vast expenditures of energy. The digestive system separates wastes from potential nutrients with the efficiency of a computer and the subtlety of a chemical genius, absorbing some nutrients here and others there, some now and others later. Scientists have noted that you would have to boil food in strong acids to begin to break it down the way the digestive system manages to do at a normal body temperature of 98.6°. The digestive system takes an apple or a cracker and some-how transforms it into our own life-giving fluid: blood.

The stomach garners most of the attention directed at the digestive system, yet it is only one element of the miracle. Proper digestion requires the finely tuned and well-coordinated actions of a half-dozen major organs, numerous ducts and gateways between them, and vari-ous hormones, enzymes, and acids. Eons of time has allowed evolution to craft a system with mechanical, chemical, and informational ele-ments that can somehow automatically recognize what to do with whatever foods, liquids, or drugs it is subjected to, even if you're a Greenlander experiencing your first taste of South American tamarillo.

Digestion begins at the mouth, where the teeth crush food and saliva moistens it. The enzyme amylase in saliva begins the digestion of carbohydrates. The expansion and contraction of muscles in the esophagus then force food down the esophagus, with no help needed from gravity (luckily for astronauts). Food passes through a special muscle, or sphincter, at the end of the esophagus, and goes into the stomach.

The stomach mechanically kneads food. It also contains impressively potent acids and enzymes to continue the chemical breakdown. The enzyme pepsin begins the digestion of proteins, and gastric juices, including hydrochloric acid, go to work on whatever they encounter. As important as the stomach's actions are to digestion, it plays a limited role in the digestion of carbohydrates and fats and is principally a storage tank. More dramatic digestion occurs at the next stop, the small and large intestines.

From the stomach, food enters the duodenum, the short first section of the small intestine and the site of the body's most powerful digestive enzymes. The duodenum neutralizes any stomach acid that has entered and provides new enzymes to start the chemical reactions that break down the food particles. The small intestine, with help from the secretions of the gallbladder, liver, and pancreas, digests fats and oils, proteins, and carbohydrates. Nutrients are separated from wastes and absorbed. It is mostly waste matter and indigestible ingredients, such as cellulose from raw vegetables, that reach the large intestine (or colon) and are excreted from the rectum.

Most people give nary a thought to their digestive systems—until the abuses inflicted (such as a lifetime of pepperoni pizzas washed down by black coffee) finally prevent digestion from working as it should. Remarkably self-repairing, the digestive system nevertheless benefits from our regular attention and concern. With a minimum of care, most people's digestive systems will prove to be tough, hard-working, and smart.

When the Miracle Fails

A variety of factors can interfere with this complex flow of nutrients, enzymes, acids, and wastes, resulting in common digestive problems.

Heartburn. Also known as acid indigestion, this condition results from conditions such as hiatal hernia and from such dietary habits as eating too quickly, not chewing food thoroughly, and overeating. These actions can fill the stomach beyond its normal capacity and allow stomach acid to flow up through the sphincter that separates the stomach from the lower esophagus. Since the esophagus lacks the mucous lining that protects the stomach from its own acids, the acid causes a burning pain that sometimes extends up the chest. In addition to the immediate discomfort, food gets only partially digested, leading to gas and a bloated feeling in the gut. In particular, consuming too much fatty and greasy foods often triggers heartburn because these foods require more time, and stomach acid, to digest than do fresh vegetables, for instance.

Antacids and other over-the-counter (OTC) digestive remedies are a multibillion-dollar market in the United States today. Drugs that neutralize some of the stomach's acid are the most widely prescribed category of drugs in the world. An estimated one in ten Americans suffers from daily bouts of heartburn, while almost one in three has it occasionally.

Although antacids are widely taken to relieve temporarily the discomfort of heartburn, they should not be used regularly. Overuse can disturb the body's acid/alkaline balance. And since antacids neutralize some of the stomach's acids and enzymes, by definition they partially prevent these substances from performing a necessary function: breaking down and beginning to digest food constituents, particularly protein. Some conventional drugs neutralize stomach acid, including over-the-counter favorites like Mylanta and Maalox, contain aluminum compounds. Excess aluminum from antacids, food additives, and other sources can accumulate in the body. A number of studies suggest prolonged aluminum consumption has an adverse effect on brain and kidney function and can lead to weakness, tiredness, and possibly dementia. Calcium-based OTC antacids such as Rolaids and Tums (or even calcium citrate supplements) are just as effective at neutralizing acid. Although calcium is an essential nutrient while aluminum probably is not, prolonged overconsumption of calcium-based antacids can increase the risk of kidney stones. Some doctors also prescribe potent prescription drugs such as cimetidine (Tagamet) and ranitidine (Zantac) to neutralize stomach acid. Potential side effects include diarrhea, constipation, nausea, and even mental confusion.

Constipation. Difficulty or straining while moving the bowels is almost unheard of in developing countries where people still follow a traditional diet, since a primary cause of such problems is insufficient fiber in the diet. Fiber absorbs water in the intestines, thereby bulking up the stool, lubricating it, and making it softer and easier to expel. Constipation may also be due to colon problems, pregnancy, prescription drugs, dehydration, or a lack of exercise. It can lead to hemorrhoids, fatigue, irritable bowel syndrome, and other health problems if it becomes chronic.

Many people rely on stimulant laxatives to treat chronic constipation. Stimulant laxatives, such as the crystalline powder phenolphthalein (Alophen, Ex-Lax) and the plant concentrate senna (Senokot), cause bowel contractions by irritating the lining of the intestines. Unfortunately, side effects such as severe cramping are common, and the benefits are short-term. Whether conventional or natural, stimulant laxatives eventually cause the colon to become lazy, possibly leading to a cycle of relying on stronger and stronger remedies. Fiber-bulking laxatives, such as the psyllium-based Metamucil, are very effective and, as an FDA panel found, "are among the safest of laxatives."

Long-term solutions to constipation involve getting more exercise (especially walking), eating a high-fiber diet and taking meals at the same time each day, drinking plenty of fluids, and reducing anxiety.

Flatulence. Flatulence is gas generated in the stomach and intestines and then expelled from the anus. It may be caused by taking in air while eating (by talking while eating, for instance), insufficient chewing, or eating while feeling anxious. More commonly it is the result of dietary choices. Food that isn't fully digested in the intestines tends to ferment from bacterial action and form methane and other gases. Some people don't have the right digestive enzymes for certain foods, particularly dairy foods. Also, because of compounds such as raffinose in beans, some foods are especially gas-producing in almost all people. (In the case of beans, soaking them overnight before cooking may allow them to be more easily digested.) In addition to beans, cucumbers and cabbage are common culprits. Excess flatulence (two dozen or so episodes a day is considered normal) may also result from taking too many bran or vitamin C supplements.

Natural remedies can often reduce flatulence, but should be used in conjunction with long-term changes in diet or eating patterns to address the underlying causes.

Diarrhea. Diarrhea may be either chronic or acute, depending upon the cause. Diarrhea often results from stress, a laxative habit, drugs (especially broad-spectrum antibiotics), poor diet, intestinal parasites such as *Giardia,* flu viruses, and food poisoning. Diarrhea in infants or children may be due to a food allergy or formula problem. Warning signs that diarrhea is a symptom of a more serious underlying condition include fever, severe cramps, and blood in the stool.

Diarrhea that is chronic may present a serious health risk, since it can cause a loss of nutrients via the stool and can also lead to dehydration. (A sign of dehydration is dark, scanty urine.) Dehydration from diarrhea is a particular danger for infants. Consult with a health practitioner for any infant diarrhea that lasts longer than one day. Acute diarrhea in adults that lasts for only a few days is often a sign of a "bug" or a toxin in the system.

Diarrhea sometimes results from dietary factors such as overeating (especially too much raw or dried fruit or spicy foods), food allergies (including lactose intolerance), caffeine addiction, and overuse of sugar-alcohol-based artificial sweeteners such as sorbitol and mannitol. It may also result from consuming too many vitamin C supplements (though most people don't notice any effects from taking 2 to 5 g in divided doses daily). In addition to drinking plenty of liquids to prevent dehydration, eating foods such as bananas, miso soup, and yogurt can sometimes help restore normalcy to the colon.

Over-the-counter diarrhea drugs such as loperamide (Imodium A-D) are taken to reduce intestinal contractions and limit fluid loss. Constipation, nausea, and drowsiness are potential side effects. Such drugs are probably used much more frequently than they should be, since many cases of diarrhea are self-limiting. Antidiarrheals can actually prolong some cases of diarrhea by interfering with the body's efforts to eliminate an infective agent. Fiber-bulking diarrhea drugs such as polycarbophil (Equalactin) have fewer side effects and more potential benefits.

Peptic ulcers. These are erosions in the inner walls of digestive organs, most commonly in the lower stomach or the upper duodenum. Peptic ulcers result when too much stomach acid breaks down these organs' protective lining. An estimated one in ten Americans suffers from peptic ulcers at some time in their life. Psychosomatic causes are common; studies indicate that peptic ulcers are most common in sedentary workers who face frequent deadline pressure and adopt irregular eating habits. Aspirin, alcohol, nicotine, and caffeine consumption may also be factors. Milk was once a popular remedy, but no longer—studies have shown that it briefly neutralizes stomach acid only to cause it to increase later to higher levels, thus worsening the condition.

Until about fifteen years ago, high doses of antacids were the most commonly recommended drugs for peptic ulcers. A number of extremely successful (and expensive) prescription drugs for ulcers have been released in the past two decades, such as the aforementioned Tagamet and Zantac (each of these now garners sales in excess of a billion dollars annually). These alleviate ulcer pain by reducing hydrochloric acid production in the stomach. In about one third of patients they need to be taken for extended periods of time, increasing the risk of adverse effects. While neutralizing or reducing the secretion of stomach acids can give the ulcer time to heal, unless drug-taking is accompanied by changes in diet and lifestyle, the condition is likely to return within a year or two.

Herbs and nutritional supplements can often be used to help treat digestive complaints. More importantly for long-term health, herbs and nutritional supplements can play a role in regulating and strengthening the digestive system, allowing it to function as it should without the need for continuous drug-induced interventions and adjustments.

Herbs for the Digestive System

Herbs can affect the digestive system in a number of positive ways. Different herbs can stimulate the secretion or release of digestive enzymes, relax the muscles and organs of the digestive system, and coat or soothe the mucous membranes that line the intestines. The so-called carminative herbs, often used to relieve flatulence, help to relax the stomach and expel gas. The herb licorice (*Glycyrrhiza glabra*) has traditionally been used to treat peptic ulcers, and studies of a licorice extract confirm it has a powerful healing effect on ulcers. The bioflavonoid quercetin and green-tea extracts may also help relieve peptic ulcers.

There are also numerous herbal stimulant laxatives, and some of these may be less harsh than conventional over-the-counter products. These herbs are, however, still strong enough to cause possible intestinal cramps. And even herbal preparations should not be used habitually, since they too can lead to a laxative dependency. Herbal stimulant laxatives, which can be taken in capsules (a typical dosage is 1 to 3 capsules daily), tinctures, and other oral forms for a day or two, include aloe, buckthorn, senna, castor oil (which can be taken internally or massaged into the abdomen), and cascara sagrada. More gentle herbal laxatives that work by stimulating the secretion of digestive juices or adding extra bulk to the stool are discussed below.

Some of the most commonly used herbs for digestive complaints include those that follow.

Ginger. The dried root of this native Asian plant has long been recognized as a prominent digestive remedy. Ginger works to reduce intestinal gas, prevent nausea, and relax the smooth muscles of the intestines. As a flatulence remedy or nausea preventive, take 500 to

1,000 mg of the powdered herb or 1 to 2 dropperfuls of tincture or concentrated drops three times daily.

Peppermint. The leaves of this mint plant contain essential oils rich in menthol, a crystalline alcohol that has been shown in studies to calm the smooth muscles of the digestive tract. Peppermint may also stimulate the liver to secrete bile, a bodily fluid that helps break down fats. To soothe stomach cramps or alleviate flatulence, try a cup of peppermint-leaf tea or take 1 dropperful of tincture or concentrated drops.

Garlic. This all-purpose herb helps to destroy harmful microorganisms in the intestines and promotes digestive activity. It is often used for digestive complaints such as diarrhea, flatulence, and indigestion. A few individuals, however, find that garlic irritates the digestive tract; in high doses (five cloves daily) it can actually cause flatulence. An average daily dosage is 600 to 1,000 mg of pure or concentrated garlic or garlic extract powder, or 1,800 to 3,000 mg of fresh garlic equivalent. An average recommended dosage for allicin is 1,800 to 3,600 mcg per day.

Valerian. This European plant with a strong-smelling root is the preeminent herbal sedative (see Chapter 12), but it also has some digestive applications. Herbalists recommend its relaxing properties for when indigestion is due to nervous tension or when constipation can be traced to tense bowels. An average dose for such conditions is 1 to 2 dropperfuls of tincture or concentrated drops two or three times daily. (For a milder effect, another calming herb that is great for indigestion is chamomile.)

Slippery elm. These preparations are derived from the ground inner bark of an embattled tree (*Ulmus rubra, U. fulva*) recently ravaged in the United States by Dutch elm disease. Slippery elm was once a medicinal food eaten for its beneficial effects on the digestive system. Even the FDA calls it an "excellent demulcent," or soothing agent. To soothe and protect irritated mucous membranes in the intestines or to treat diarrhea, eat it as a gruel. Mix one tablespoon of the powder with one tablespoon of sugar and one cup of boiling water.

Goldenseal and barberry. These healing herbs (*Hydrastis canadensis* and *Berberis vulgaris*) contain potent alkaloids, such as berberine, that have been shown to kill a wide variety of harmful bacterial and fungal invaders. Goldenseal and barberry are often used to help treat diarrhea from food poisoning or intestinal parasites, and constipation due to weak muscular activity in the gut. An average healing dosage is 1 dropperful of tincture or concentrate three times daily. Some herbal enthusiasts also take goldenseal or barberry from the week before to the week after traveling to a foreign country. This can help prevent traveler's diarrhea. A common such tonic dosage is 1 dropperful of the tincture or concentrated drops once or twice daily. (Children under two years old and pregnant women should not use berberine-containing herbs.)

Treating Minor Ailments

• For chronic constipation, ginger, barberry, and dandelion are better than stronger herbs such as buckthorn. Valerian also relieves some forms of constipation.

• For flatulence, try either of the carminatives ginger and peppermint.

• Slippery elm, goldenseal, and barberry can alleviate many cases of diarrhea.

• To help a digestive system that has been racked by food poisoning return to normal, try garlic, goldenseal, or barberry.

The Herbal Bitters

Herbal bitters are single herbs or combinations of herbs whose pungent taste helps to stimulate appetite and promote complete digestion. They are taken regularly to strengthen the digestive system and promote better overall intestinal health. Bitters have been used as appetizers and digestive tonics for thousands of years. "In the springtime, traditional peoples commonly forage the first shoots of bitter young greens to revitalize their digestive systems after a long winter of consuming heavy, rich foods," notes herbalist Brigitte Mars. "Even in the animal kingdom, many species instinctively seek out bitter plants to cure digestive ailments."

The most prominent bitter herbs include angelica, dandelion, gentian, rue, rhubarb, yellow dock, barberry, and goldenseal. Bitters are made by steeping these herbs in alcohol or vinegar. A number of clinical studies have confirmed that bitter herbs are effective at relieving digestive problems such as flatulence and heartburn. Exactly how bitters promote digestion is not clear, but a popular explanation is that these herbs activate the bitter-taste receptors on the back of the tongue. This encourages salivation and increases secretion of digestive juices, thus promoting the functions of the stomach, small intestine, and gall bladder. Bitters are thought to assist in naturally cleansing the liver, intestines, and other organs.

Natural-food stores offer a number of brands of combination herbal bitters. Look for products such as Swedish Bitters. Bitter herbs may also be included in herbal products promoted as intestinal cleansers, colon tonics, and natural detoxifiers. In such products the bitter herbs may be combined with fiber sources, clay, and beneficial live bacteria.

Bitter tonics are safe to take indefinitely; many people find they work best when used for an extended period of time.

HOW TO USE HERBAL BITTERS: Though some proponents claim that bitters work best when the sense of taste is activated, they're available in capsules as well as the more common liquid form. Bitters are usually most effective when taken 15 to 30 minutes before a meal. To promote complete digestion, relieve flatulence, and revitalize the digestive system, take 1 teaspoon three times a day, either undiluted or mixed with ¼ cup of warm water, carbonated spring water, or herbal tea. Obliterating the bitter taste in a sweet juice is difficult and possibly countereffective. Some people use a dropper to place the liquid on the tongue.

Angelica

Angelica preparations are derived from the leaves, roots, or seeds of a tall, celerylike plant in the parsley family. It is also called American angelica, to distinguish it from dong quai, which is the Chinese species of angelica more known for its effects on menopause and other female conditions (see Chapter 7). Angelica is a popular folk remedy taken to alleviate respiratory complaints, including colds and the flu, as well as digestive problems. Studies confirm that it has chemical compounds that can relax the smooth muscles of the windpipe and intestines and thus may be beneficial for bronchitis, asthma, indigestion, flatulence, and heartburn.

Angelica exhibits low toxicity, though in some people it can make the skin more sensitive to the effects of sunlight.

HOW TO USE ANGELICA: The roots are sold dried, since the fresh root is poisonous. It is also sold in capsules, concentrated drops, extracts, and tinctures. For digestive complaints, take 1 dropperful of the tincture or concentrated drops diluted in ½ cup of tea or water two or three times daily. To stimulate digestion, take 1 dropperful daily.

Dandelion

Dandelion is a bitter but nutritious herb prepared from the roots, leaves, and other parts of the well-known, widely distributed, yellow-flowered weed that is the bane of many suburban lawn-tenders. Herbalists have long relied upon dandelion to relieve inflammation of the liver and gallbladder and treat conditions such as congestive jaundice. It is also a favorite herb for cleansing the blood, stimulating the flow of urine (another name for dandelion is piss-in-bed), and promoting weight loss. Dandelion may help lower blood-cholesterol levels, reduce high blood pressure, and prevent heart disease.

Dandelion has also long been relied upon by the Chinese and others as a digestive tonic and a mild laxative. Studies have shown that dandelion promotes bile availability in the small intestine, where the liquid helps break down fats. Dandelion both enhances the liver's secretion of bile and stimulates the gallbladder's release of it into the small intestines (the gallbladder stores bile produced by the liver). The fresh leaves are high in nutrients, including beta carotene, vitamin C, and potassium. They are also rich in dietary fiber and inulin, a type of complex carbohydrate that has been tied to improved digestive function.

Dandelion is safe and nontoxic for regular use. Drink plenty of fluids to replace those lost through its diuretic effect.

HOW TO USE DANDELION: It is sold as tablets, capsules, concentrated drops, tinctures, and extracts. An average daily dosage for chronic constipation or other digestive problems is 1 to 2 dropperfuls of concentrated drops two or three times daily, or 500 to 1,000 mg of the powdered extract. As a daily tonic for better digestive function, take 1 dropperful of the concentrated drops twice daily or 250 to 500 mg of the powdered solid extract.

Supplements for Better Digestion

Vitamin and mineral supplementation doesn't play as direct a role in regulating the digestive system as it does in other aspects of bodily function. The principal vitamins essential for a healthy digestive tract are a few of the B vitamins, particularly pantothenic acid and folic acid. Deficiencies in these may lead to constipation, diarrhea, or other digestive complaints. An average dosage of vitamin B complex is 25 to 50 mg twice daily.

A number of natural substances are generally not taken on a regular basis but can often help relieve some specific digestive problems.

Pancreatic enzymes. The pancreas produces the digestive enzymes lipase, protease, and amylase, and secretes them into the duodenum to help break down fat, protein, and carbohydrates. Because of genetic problems, diseases such as cystic fibrosis, excessive consumption of alcohol, and other factors, some people don't secrete enough of one or more of the pancreatic enzymes to fully digest their food. The result may be indigestion and chronic nutrient deficiencies. Supplements sold in natural-food stores contain pancreatic enzymes such as pancreatin, derived from the pancreases of hogs. Many natural health practitioners recommend using animal-based digestive enzymes only under the supervision of a knowledgeable practitioner. Look for products such as Pancreatin 1300, Lipanase, Aler-gest, Enzyme Caps, and Pancrea-Lind. Some contain additional digestive ingredients, from ox bile extract to papain.

Hydrochloric acid. This is the major digestive juice of the stomach. When the stomach secretes excessive amounts of it, often in response to eating fatty, high-protein foods or experiencing extreme stress, most people respond by reaching for Rolaids and other neutralizing antacids. In older people (gastric acid secretion falls with age) and some others, however, digestion is sometimes hampered by a deficiency of hydrochloric acid (HCl). These people can benefit from taking supplemental hydrochloric acid, often prepared in a sweet-tasting betaine (from beets, or synthetically derived) base. Combination HCl products sometimes include pepsin, a protein-digesting stomach enzyme derived from pigs or other animals.

Before you conclude you have insufficient HCl and need to take a supplement, you should see a health practitioner who can arrange for a special stomach acid test. One test uses an acid-measuring, radio-transmitting capsule attached to a string. The capsule is swallowed and kept in the stomach while it measures levels of HCl. Without a proper diagnosis, you risk seriously irritating the stomach by taking unnecessary HCl supplements. HCl shouldn't be taken in conjunction with aspirin, ibuprofen, and certain other drugs that may increase the risk of gastrointestinal bleeding.

Activated charcoal. This is pure carbon processed in a special way to make it highly absorbent of particles and gases in the body's digestive system. Activated charcoal slides through the intestines without itself being absorbed. It is taken internally to relieve gas pains, reduce flatulence, and absorb and excrete from the body gases and toxins. A number of double-blind studies have shown that activated charcoal works better than the conventional OTC drug simethicone (Gas-X) for reducing flatulence. Activated charcoal may also lower blood cholesterol levels (see Chapter 8).

Avoid taking activated charcoal within 60 to 90 minutes of taking nutritional supplements, since the charcoal can eliminate such potentially healthful substances from the intestines as well. Megadoses in excess of 20 g daily (to lower cholesterol levels, for example) may interfere with nutrient absorption, but otherwise activated charcoal is safe and nontoxic. It is available in powder, tablet, capsule, and liquid forms. Look for products such as Charcocaps. An average dose for indigestion, flatulence, or other digestive problems is 500 mg at the first sign of discomfort (or to prevent expected discomfort) and another 500 to 1,000 mg every two hours as needed.

Bromelain and papain. These are naturally occurring enzymes derived from pineapples and unripe papayas, respectively. Papain is the ingredient in meat tenderizers that softens meat by breaking down muscle tissue. As nutritional supplements, bromelain and papain are widely used to assist in the digestion of protein. They help the intestines to break down food more completely, thus reducing the likelihood of uncomfortable intestinal fermentation. Nutritionists also recommend bromelain and papain for diarrhea due to digestive enzyme deficiency. Bromelain has also become a popular sports injury medicine, taken internally to reduce bruising, relieve pain and swelling, and promote wound healing. Typically bromelain and papain are taken with meals when they are used as digestive aids. They come in tablets. An average dosage for indigestion is to chew 2 to 4 tablets after each meal.

Food-grade clay. This is clay that is formulated to meet special standards, ensuring that it is safe to be taken internally. It is used to cleanse the intestines and absorb toxins after food or chemical poisoning. Clay (and originally, though no longer, pectin) is the active ingredient in the OTC diarrhea remedy Kaopectate, which absorbs and binds material in the intestines. Some popular forms of clay that may be food-grade (read labels closely) include cosmetic clay, green clay, and bentonite. It is sold as a powder or liquid. An average dosage is 1 teaspoon with 8 ounces of juice or water. Clay is also found as an ingredient in products such as Colon Cleanse.

Supplement manufacturers offer various combinations of many of these digestive substances. For example, supplements might contain pancreatin, papain and bromelain, and peppermint leaves; or psyllium husks, activated charcoal, and acidophilus; or hydrochloric acid, pepsin, and gentian. Look for products such as Super Digestaway, GastroCleanse, and Maxigest.

Beneficial Live Bacteria

Some natural substances are taken on a regular basis for better digestive function and to prevent gastrointestinal illnesses. Beneficial live bacteria are one of them.

Many bacteria are disease-causing, yet some live bacteria are not only useful but essential for proper human health (see Chapter 2). Without them, your gastrointestinal system won't function as it should. Some "friendly" bacteria in the human gut play crucial roles in food digestion, the production of certain vitamins, and the establishment of your body's natural defenses against harmful microorganisms. These beneficial live bacteria are also necessary to help prevent indigestion, flatulence, diarrhea, and constipation.

Hundreds of different bacteria, some healthful and some potentially harmful, can inhabit the intestines at the same time. There are many strains of friendly bacteria besides *L. acidophilus* and *B. bifidum,* such as *L. casei, L. plantarum,* and *L. fermentum.* A species of streptococcus bacteria, *Streptococcus thermophilus,* is also beneficial and is normally found residing in healthy intestines. (Some forms of beneficial bacteria are more appropriate for children up to the age of five than for adults. Look for products with names like Primadophilus Junior, Babylife, and Life Start.) *L. bulgaricus* is a beneficial bacteria often found in yogurt cultures and some live bacteria products. Unlike acidophilus and bifidus, it is a transient that passes through the intestines rather than a resident that colonizes them.

Live bacteria products are nontoxic and safe (though expensive) to take indefinitely. A high-fiber, whole-foods diet can complement their positive effect on intestinal flora. Follow label instructions for the live bacteria products; avoid taking them within two hours of taking antibiotics.

Acidophilus

Acidophilus has become the generic term for various types of naturally occurring live bacteria that are increasingly popular as dietary supplements. Technically acidophilus is the strain *L. acidophilus,* though products sold as acidophilus may also contain *B. bifidum, L. bulgaricus,* and other strains of bacteria.

L. acidophilus is the primary beneficial bacteria in the small intestine. Healthy colonies of *L. acidophilus* prevent food-borne pathogens, including species of salmonella, klebsiella, and staphylococcus, and fungi including *Candida albicans,* from multiplying and impairing the function of the small intestine.

Acidophilus also protects against traveler's diarrhea and counters some of the ill effects of broad-spectrum antibiotics and birth control pills. "When a person requires oral antimicrobial treatment for an illness," according to nutritional biochemist Jerzy Meduski, M.D., Ph.D., "certain drugs used can suppress many probiotic flora in the intestine and allow drug-resistant microbial strains and yeast-like organisms to predominate. This, in turn, allows the drug-resistant bacteria to produce toxins and gases, and causes the loss of the benefits derived from healthy bacterial activity; for instance, the intestinal synthesis of certain vitamins, particularly vitamin K and certain members of the B complex. *L. acidophilus* has been shown to counterbalance the disturbed intestinal flora after antibiotic therapy, sulfonamide therapy, or irradiation." Vitamin K is necessary for proper blood coagulation and bone development; a deficiency of K is not uncommon among people on prolonged antibiotic therapy.

Live acidophilus bacteria may also be found in fermented milk products such as yogurt and kefir. Check labels closely to see what strains of live bacteria (if any) are included. Levels in such food products are high enough to be helpful in maintaining healthy intestines, though most nutritionists agree they are not high enough to replenish the intestinal flora wiped out by antibiotics or an illness. Much higher concentrations of acidophilus are available in the supplements sold in most natural-food stores.

Many acidophilus supplements are milk-based, but nondairy products are now widely available. Products include Floradophilus, Maxi Dophilus, Neo-Flora, Bio-dophilus, Primadophilus, and Mega Dophilus. They may need to be refrigerated. Supplement manufacturers are also beginning to combine acidophilus with herbs or nutrients (cranberry extract and acidophilus capsules, for example).

HOW TO USE ACIDOPHILUS: It comes in tablets, powders, capsules, and liquids. An average daily dosage to replenish intestinal flora is 10 billion viable organisms daily. To maintain a healthy gastrointestinal tract, take $1/2$ to 1 teaspoon of powder or liquid daily, or capsules containing 2 to 3 billion viable organisms.

Bifidus

Bifidus, the common name for *B. bifidum, B. breve, B. longum,* and other bifidobacteria, are the most prominent helpful bacteria of the large intestine, and should exist in greater quantities than any other intestinal microorganism. In proper balance with *L. acidophilus,* they help to inhibit harmful organisms and improve bowel function. Natural-health practitioners recommend taking both acidophilus and bifidus supplements after finishing a regimen of broad-spectrum antibiotics or while taking birth control pills.

Many producers sell only separate strains, maintaining that multiple types of bacteria in the same product will compete for nutrients and are not compatible with guaranteeing a specific minimum potency at the expiration date. Some manufacturers, however, do combine acidophilus and bifidus strains in a single product; look for products such as GIFlora, Multidophilus, Spiradophilus, and BioPRO, though check to see whether potency is guaranteed at time of manufacture or product expiration date. Natren, of Westlake Village, California (see "Resources"), which specializes in probiotic products, says that for its multiple-strain Bio-Flor product, it developed a special "micro-enrobing" encapsulating technology that keeps combined strains separate. Bifidus products include Maxi Bifidus, BifidoBiotics, and Bifido Factor. Like acidophilus, they may need to be refrigerated.

HOW TO USE BIFIDUS: It comes in tablets, powders, capsules, and liquids. An average daily dosage to replenish intestinal flora is 10 billion viable organisms daily. To maintain a healthy gastrointestinal tract, take $1/2$ to 1 teaspoon of powder or liquid daily, or capsules containing 2 to 3 billion viable organisms.

Other Digestive Enhancers

Two additional natural substances are worth considering for their ability to promote healthy intestinal fauna or otherwise enhance the digestive process.

Inulin/Fructooligosaccharide

This is a complex carbohydrate found in small amounts in fruits, vegetables, and grains. Technically inulin is a white, starchlike polysaccharide also known as fructooligosaccharide (FOS) because it is converted into fructose when it reacts chemically with certain agents. Bananas, onions, garlic, barley, and tomatoes are natural sources of small amounts of inulin. Many members of the large Compositae plant family, which includes artichoke, daisy, elecampane, dandelion, and echinacea, are rich in inulin/FOS. The tubers of two plants in the

Compositae family, Jerusalem artichoke and dahlia, are concentrated sources of inulin/FOS.

A number of human studies done in Japan and elsewhere have shown that supplemental inulin/FOS can help promote up to a tenfold increase in the growth of beneficial bacteria in the gut, particularly bifidobacteria in the large intestine. In a manner similar to taking supplemental live bacteria, this can restore a healthy colonic ecology and prevent the adverse health effects associated with an overabundance of such pathogenic microorganisms as clostridium and candida. In addition to helping to prevent digestive ailments such as constipation and diarrhea, inulin/FOS may also benefit diabetics by discouraging swings in blood sugar.

Among the best dietary sources of inulin/FOS is the potatolike edible tuber of Jerusalem artichoke (*Helianthus tuberosus*), a tall, yellow-flowering relative of sunflower. (This native North American plant is not from Jerusalem and is not an artichoke (*Cynara scolymus*), but it is in the same plant family.) Jerusalem artichoke is also rich in potassium and fiber. A favorite remedy among those who follow the teachings of the late psychic Edgar Cayce, it is now sold as a flour and in tablets that are frequently taken to help maintain a healthy colon. The powder has a slightly nutty taste and can be sprinkled on cereal, dissolved in liquids, or added to other flours for use in baking (up to about 10 percent of total flour content).

Inulin/FOS is most commonly sold as fructooligosaccharide in products such as NutraFlora and Garlic Plus FOS. It comes in a mildly sweet, sugarlike powder and has half the calories of sugar. It does not need to be refrigerated. Supplement manufacturers are now also including inulin/FOS in combination live bacteria–FOS products such as BioPRO and SymBiotics with FOS.

How to use inulin/fos: An average dosage for better intestinal health is 500 to 1,000 mg of Jerusalem artichoke tablets or ½ to 1 level teaspoon (1.25 to 2.5 g) of FOS powder two or three times daily.

Fiber Supplements

As a rule insoluble fiber, found mostly in wheat bran, rice bran, oats, and psyllium, is more important than soluble fiber (from gums and pectins) for maintaining gastrointestinal health. Insoluble fiber can help treat diarrhea by adding bulk to stools and absorbing fluid in the intestines. Surprisingly, insoluble fiber also has a positive effect on constipation, since by adding bulk to stools they help to trigger the contractions that lead to defecation, and by absorbing water they lubricate bowel movements. Insoluble fiber may help prevent and treat intestinal diseases such as irritable bowel syndrome and diverticulosis, as well as such conditions as hemorrhoids. There is also some evidence that they help prevent cancers of the colon and rectum.

Population studies have shown that the traditional diets of nonindustrialized peoples tend to be high in diverse dietary fibers (50 g or more per day). As a result, compared to the average low-fiber diet found in the industrialized world (20 g daily), food is more quickly moved through the digestive system, allowing the body to absorb nutrients without taking so long that putrefaction occurs. Stools are larger and more regular. The intestinal balance of beneficial live bacteria is improved. Bacterial fermentation of certain fibers in the intestines results in the production of some healthful fatty acids. Over time, disease rates are markedly lowered.

Psyllium is especially popular as a source of both soluble and insoluble fiber. It is derived from the seeds or husks of various plantain plants, including those known as fleawort and fleaseed. Psyllium promotes intestinal function and elimination and is often used in laxatives (such as Metamucil) to treat constipation because it speeds transit time and eases bowel movements. Psyllium also adds bulk to stools and treats diarrhea. The mucilage in the seed husks absorbs water and makes the stomach feel full, thus reducing appetite and aiding in the treatment of obesity. Finally, psyllium may aid in preventing diabetes and lowering blood cholesterol levels. The whole seeds or husks should always be taken with liquid.

Many supplement companies offer products combining soluble and insoluble fiber from various sources. Look for products such as Fiber-Plex, Fiber Plus, and Super Fiber.

The best way to increase your dietary fiber is to eat plenty of whole grains, fresh vegetables, fruits, and legumes. Though supplements can also help, they shouldn't be consumed as a substitute for healthful foods.

Don't overdo supplemental fiber. Start with up to 4 to 5 grams per day and gradually increase your intake if necessary as your body adjusts. Some people who take excessive levels of supplementary fiber (usually over 30 g per day) may experience mineral deficiencies due to impaired absorption of nutrients. You should also drink healthy amounts of water (6 to 8 glasses per day) to prevent fiber supplements from leading to constipation.

How to use fiber supplements: Psyllium and other fibers come in powders, tablets, capsules, and liquids. For indigestion or constipation, an average dose is 1 to 2 teaspoons in a glass of water, followed by more water, three times daily, with meals. A beginning dosage to try for overall digestive health is 1 teaspoon (or 4 to 5 g in capsules or tablets) once or twice daily with water.

Homeopathic Remedies for Digestive Complaints

Homeopathic remedies are generally taken to address specific conditions rather than as daily supplements to strengthen bodily systems. Many people find them beneficial for treating digestive complaints, and homeopathic producers offer a limited number of combination remedies for flatulence, indigestion, and diarrhea. Two of the most popular single homeopathic remedies for digestive complaints are *Nux vomica* and *Carbo vegetabilis*. Other single remedies sometimes used include *Chamomilla* (for childhood diarrhea, especially if the child is irritable and oversensitive), *Arsenicum* (for diarrhea with nausea, extreme thirst, and weakness), *Sulphur* (for diarrhea in the morning), and *Pulsatilla* (for changeable stools or rumbling stomach).

Nux vomica

Nux vomica is derived from the toxic, strychnine-containing seeds of the poison nut tree (*Strychnos nux vomica*). Homeopathically diluted, it can help to relieve back pain, fight cold and flu, and boost energy and treat fatigue (see Chapter 5). More frequently, homeopaths recommend it to treat nausea and vomiting, especially from ailments due to overeating, excessive drinking, or motion sickness. The remedy may be beneficial for flatulence (particularly when there is a sense of heaviness in the stomach), constipation, or indigestion due to eating rich, fatty foods. Some homeopaths recommend *Nux vomica* to break an existing laxative habit.

Carbo vegetabilis

This remedy is derived from wood (often birch or poplar) charcoal. It is the homeopathic analogue of activated charcoal, used predominantly to absorb gases, remove excess mucus from the digestive system, and treat digestive problems related to various ill-advised eating habits. Specific complaints it treats include flatulence accompanied by belching, slow digestion, headaches after overeating, and sour or rancid belching. If you have indigestion and heartburn, whether it is due to eating a fatty, rich meal or even to eating too late in the evening, *Carbo vegetabilis* may help. It is the right remedy if your condition is accompanied by a sense of bloatedness and sluggish, indifferent mental processes that match your sluggish digestion. See "How to Use Homeopathic Remedies" in Chapter 2.

Essential Oils for Better Digestion

"The application of aromatherapy principles can help prevent many digestive problems, for many plant foods contain essential oils that stimulate the digestive system, so encouraging good digestion by galvanizing sluggish organs into activity," says Daniele Ryman, author of *Aromatherapy: The Encyclopedia of Plants and Oils and How They Can Help You*. "The smells of herbs while cooking foods can start the first part of the process—the production of saliva—and those same herbal oils can help break down the foods when in the gut. . . . The essential oils of aromatic herbs, fruits, vegetables, and spices should be incorporated in cooking and diet whenever possible."

Ryman and other aromatherapists frequently cite such essential oils as Clove (*Eugenia caryophyllata* or *Syzygium aromaticum*), Garlic, Ginger, Lavender, Cardamom (*Elettaria cardamomum*), Cinnamon (*Cinnamomum zeylanicum*), Fennel (*Foeniculum vulgare*), and Black Pepper (*Piper nigrum*) for their effects on the digestive system. Perhaps the most popular essential oils for stimulating digestion and relieving digestive complaints are those derived from mints, a species of plant whose properties were recognized by the ancient Egyptians, Chinese, and Romans. As the first-century Roman writer Pliny the Elder noted, "The smell of mint stirs up the mind and appetite, to a greedy desire for food."

Peppermint

Both herbalists and aromatherapists have long used the leaves and flowers of this garden perennial for its medicinal properties. The essential oil of Peppermint has become a popular flavoring agent in foods, candies, chewing gum, and toothpastes. Drinking a peppermint-leaf tea or using dilutions of the essential oil will help relieve upset stomach, nausea, diarrhea, and flatulence. The essential oil contains menthol, a medicinally active alcohol that exhibits significant antiseptic and anti-inflammatory powers, making it useful as a topical remedy for itchy skin, insect bites, and toothaches. Peppermint is somewhat stimulating (see Chapter 5), so you may choose not to use it late at night.

The oil may irritate some people's skin if applied undiluted or in high doses. Peppermint will negate the effects of homeopathic remedies, so use one or the other, but not both simultaneously.

Essential oils can be massaged into the stomach and abdomen to help relieve indigestion, heartburn, and flatulence, and into the lower abdomen to relieve constipation. Applying a warm compress of essential oils to the lower abdomen for 10 to 15 minutes is a good way to help treat diarrhea. Essential oils can be added to a bath to help relieve constipation (avoid using Peppermint in a bath, however). Vaporization is another method for using essential oils to enhance digestion. (See "How to Use Essential Oils" in Chapter 2.)

Though essential oils are extremely concentrated substances and are generally *not* taken orally, it is safe to make a tea by adding 2 to 3 drops of the essential oil of Peppermint to hot water. Many people find that peppermint tea benefits their digestion. In some cases, however, peppermint tea may actually contribute to heartburn.

Where to Start

Taking the following supplements will help you to revitalize an abused or poorly functioning digestive system.
- Beneficial live bacteria, such as acidophilus and bifidus ($\frac{1}{2}$ to 1 teaspoon of powder or liquid daily, or 2 to 3 billion viable organisms)
- Fiber supplements (1 teaspoon, or 4 to 5 g in capsules or tablets, once or twice daily with water)
- Herbal bitters (1 teaspoon three times a day, either undiluted or mixed with $\frac{1}{4}$ cup of warm water, carbonated spring water, or herbal tea, 15 to 30 minutes before meals)

Beyond Herbs and Supplements

Maintaining a healthy digestive system takes more than merely using natural substances to establish the proper intestinal flora. Digestion can be affected by individual foods and overall diet, attitudes and emotions, and exercise and fitness. Here are some of the basics to keep in mind:
- Eat a balanced, high-fiber, low-fat, primarily plant-based wholefoods diet. This is an essential first step in regulating your digestion and

preventing constipation and heartburn. Well-cooked grains, tofu, and complex carbohydrates may help to neutralize excess stomach acid.

• Chew your food thoroughly. Proper chewing is the first step in digestion and makes subsequent steps proceed more smoothly. Thorough chewing also improves nutrient assimilation.

• Avoid eating meals while you are anxious or emotionally upset. Digestion benefits immeasurably when you eat in a relaxed, unhurried manner. Eating while driving to work, watching a scary movie on TV, or arguing with your partner hampers proper digestion.

• If you suffer from such problems as heartburn, constipation, and peptic ulcers, avoid the foods that are most irritating to the digestive system. Fatty, greasy, and fried foods slow digestion; caffeine and chocolate can irritate the esophagus; and alcoholic beverages, refined sugar, and the drugs tobacco and aspirin increase stomach acids.

• Do something restful after a meal. Your body responds to food in the stomach by diverting blood and energy toward the digestive organs. Allow this natural process to happen rather than jogging, swimming, or doing something else that requires blood and energy in the major muscles of the legs and arms. On the other hand, you may find that your digestion benefits when you take a leisurely walk after a large meal.

• Get plenty of exercise or physical activity between meals; lack of exercise can lead to digestive sluggishness.

Attain Your Ideal Weight

The good news is that compared to Americans in the 1960s, Americans today have cut back somewhat on their total fat intake and are consuming no more calories overall. The bad news is that this has not been accompanied by an average weight reduction. Just the opposite is true: Recent national studies involving both children and adults show that growing numbers of Americans are considered overweight by their doctors. According to a study published in the *Journal of the American Medical Association* in 1994, 32 percent of adult men studied between 1988 and 1991 met the medical definition of overweight, compared to 23 percent of adult male Americans studied between 1960 and 1962. For women the corresponding numbers were 35 percent in 1988–1991 and 26 percent in 1960–1962. Researchers who compared children in 1991 to children in 1984 found that the percentage of those who were overweight increased from 24 percent to 34 percent during the seven-year span. Teens too are gaining weight. The percentage of those who were overweight rose from 15 percent in the 1970s to 21 percent in 1991. According to the Surgeon General, an estimated 34 million of these overweight Americans are actually obese, weighing at least 20 percent more than their desirable weight.

This dramatic national weight problem drives an industry in books, supplements, special foods, and other products that attracts in excess of $30 billion in consumer spending every year. Unfortunately, much of this money is wasted. Numerous studies have found that fad diets and calorie-deprivation schemes rarely result in long-term weight loss. All too frequently, individuals cannot sustain the continual hunger or the unpleasantness of eating only certain foods. Lost weight is quickly regained, and in many cases the lapsing dieter adds on pounds so readily that he or she flies right past the weight at which the diet began in the first place. There is a well-known reason for this yo-yo effect: your body thinks it is being starved and takes steps to protect itself. A lack of sufficient food causes the body to adjust its metabolism to a lower setpoint. As a result, you start to burn fewer calories, and weight loss becomes increasingly difficult. When you do begin to eat normal amounts of food, this reduced metabolic rate causes you to regain weight swiftly.

The tremendous national focus on body weight also obscures an equally important factor in the equation. The percentage of your body that is made up of fat relative to muscle and other tissue is crucial for overall health. Muscle tissue is denser and heavier than fat. A person with firm, well-toned muscles who weighs 180 pounds but has only 15 percent total body fat is likely to be much healthier than someone of the same height who weighs five pounds less but has 30 percent total body fat. Weight-loss schemes that cause you to lose weight by trimming muscle from your frame are ill-advised. If you reduce your weight by dropping mostly muscle mass, as many dieters do, you lose the many health benefits of toned muscle, from better cardiovascular function to attractive physical appearance. Because muscle tissue has a higher resting metabolic rate than fat tissue, you also make it more likely that you'll readily regain all your lost weight.

Thus, it can be misleading to rely on only the bathroom scale to tell you whether a weight-loss program is benefiting your health. Equally important are the tools necessary to determine whether you are adding, or at the least maintaining, lean body mass or muscle. Your eyes are one tool. Looking at yourself in the mirror is usually enough to tell you whether you have proper muscle tone or too much flabby fat. For those who want to be more precise, there are skin-fold calipers, underwater weighing, and other techniques for determining percentage of body fat.

Failure to maintain optimal body weight and body-fat percentage is a major factor in overall health and well-being. An estimated 300,000 American lives are lost each year from conditions related to obesity. Researchers have found that being overweight either causes or is associated with an increased risk of some types of cancer and various degenerative diseases, including heart disease, stroke, arthritis, and diabetes. A whole host of psychological difficulties is also common among overweight people, especially the clinically obese. These problems include guilt feelings, extreme shyness, and lack of self-esteem.

Health authorities believe that modern Americans' increasingly sedentary lifestyle is partly responsible for the spread of weight problems even while total fat intake falls. Attaining an ideal weight can thus be seen as a balancing of two principal opposing factors: what goes into the body versus how much the body burns up. For most people, weight is lost most readily when less food is consumed while at the same time more energy is expended. Focusing on only one of these factors and ignoring the other is a recipe for failure.

For those who are truly motivated to lose weight, the essence of weight loss is taking a long-term approach that involves eating healthful foods, increasing the routine physical activity in your everyday life as well as getting regular aerobic exercise, learning to love your body, and taking natural supplements that work with the body to enhance its natural appetite-regulating and calorie-burning processes.

Pathways to Weight Loss

The two main supplemental approaches to promoting weight loss are appetite suppressants that encourage you to take in less fuel and thermogenic agents that speed up your ability to burn off what you do consume.

Suppress appetite. Hunger results from a complex interplay of physical and emotional factors. Brain researchers have determined that appetite is affected by bodily levels of a variety of substances, including blood glucose, digestive hormones, water, protein, and certain neurotransmitters. Information on such hunger controllers is sent to the cerebral cortex and the small region of the brain known as the hypothalamus. The hypothalamus helps to regulate various bodily functions, from sleeping patterns to appetite. While some anorectics—drugs or natural substances that suppress appetite—have direct effects on the brain's appetite-control center, exactly how they promote weight loss is still being investigated.

Conventional over-the-counter weight-loss products such as Dexatrim and Acutrim (as well as cold and flu remedies such as Contac) contain up to 75 mg of the potent central nervous system stimulant phenylpropanolamine (PPA). Although PPA has garnered FDA approval as a weight-loss drug, many health practitioners dispute both its efficacy as an appetite suppressant and its safety. According to the

American Medical Association's *Drug Evaluations,* "Side effects may occur with any dose, but particularly when the amount exceeds 75 mg/day." Potential side effects include those common to nervous system stimulants, such as insomnia, restlessness, and elevated blood pressure. According to the *Physicians' Desk Reference for Nonprescription Drugs,* the maximum recommended daily dose (75 mg of PPA) should be taken by adults only. Also, "exceeding the recommended dose may cause serious health problems." Clearly, PPA has a lower ratio of recommended-to-toxic dosage than for most other OTC drugs. *Drug Evaluations* concludes, "Since serious adverse reactions occur and long-term effectiveness of the drug has not been demonstrated, the usefulness of phenylpropanolamine as an aid to weight reduction is limited."

Prescription forms of amphetamine (Dexedrine, Obetrol) are now rarely used for appetite suppression and weight loss because of their side effects and the potential for abuse. Other prescription appetite suppressants with amphetaminelike properties include diethylpropion (Tenuate), mazindol (Sanorex), and phentermine (Adipex-P, Fastin). The common side effects of these drugs include elevated blood pressure, impotence, insomnia, depression, and dependence. Physicians generally reserve use of such drugs for extreme obesity and then only for a limited time.

A more direct route to appetite suppression is applying to the tongue substances that inhibit its ability to taste foods. The theory is that people who can't taste their food will be less inclined to overindulge. Studies confirm this effect, to a degree. Even so, this approach remains a relatively unpopular one for the obvious reason that few people want to forgo for long the sensual pleasures of eating. The local anesthetic benzocaine is included in conventional OTC gums and lozenges that numb the tongue to inhibit taste. Topical application of a natural herb discussed below, gymnema, seems to block principally the taste buds responsible for the taste of sweetness.

Increase thermogenesis. Thermogenesis is the process of producing heat. Thermogenic substances are those that, when consumed, increase the body's ability to burn food calories before they get stored as body fat. The increased heat-producing effect from taking thermogenic supplements also promotes the body's ability to burn off stored fat. The overall impact from regular use of thermogenic substances is a boost in energy levels and a gradual loss of weight.

Taking supplements to increase the body's heat-producing and fat-burning capacity is a relatively new approach to weight loss. Until recently most weight-loss researchers believed that only a few potent drugs, such as thyroid hormones, could affect thermogenesis. Overeating was considered the primary cause of obesity, and most researchers focused on appetite suppressants to promote weight loss. Beginning with the pioneering work of the late Dr. Derek Miller in the early 1960s, researchers have gained a more complete understanding of the mechanics of weight loss and the importance of improved calorie-burning. Human and animal studies have shown that in many cases overweight subjects eat amounts of food similar to those eaten by people who are not overweight but who have greater capacities for preventing fat gain.

Thermogenesis and weight loss was the subject of an international scientific symposium in Geneva, Switzerland, in 1992, the proceedings of which were published in a 1993 issue of the *International Journal of Obesity*. The collective findings of this new generation of weight-loss researchers has spurred the development of an expanding line of thermogenic supplements, most of which are based on herbs and nutrients. Among the best thermogenic agents yet identified are the naturally occurring plant compounds known as xanthines, including caffeine, theophylline, and theobromine; ephedrine from the plant ephedra; aspirin; and minerals such as magnesium and potassium. Combinations of these are now widely used in natural thermogenic weight-loss products that go by names such as Thermo-Plex, Thermo-Lift, and Thermogenic Enhancer.

While suppressing appetite and increasing thermogenesis are distinct strategies for weight loss, in many cases the drugs and natural substances that help people to shed pounds have some effect on both of these actions. Increasingly natural-product companies are combining substances with multiple weight-loss functions in mind. In many cases these formula products are much more promising as long-term weight-loss aids than are the dated, one-dimensional pharmaceutical products such as PPA.

Herbs for Weight Loss

Herbal remedies for weight loss usually make use of a variety of herbs that have different potential effects on the body. Some of these herbs and their effects are more likely than others to be worthwhile for long-term weight loss.

Water-loss herbs. Various plant substances are known as mild diuretics, capable of promoting increased urination. The elimination of bodily fluids can lead to a quick weight loss of five to ten pounds or more. The diuretic herbs include parsley, juniper berries, dandelion, and those that contain caffeine. While this fluid-reducing action can benefit certain health conditions, such as high blood pressure and urinary infections, it results in only a temporary weight loss. It can come in handy if you're a boxer trying to meet a weight limit a few hours before a fight, but otherwise there is no particular benefit to taking diuretics for long-term weight loss.

Hot and spicy herbs. These are among the herbs that help to temporarily raise body temperature and thus promote weight loss. The ones most commonly found in combination weight-loss products include cayenne (capsicum), ginger, and cinnamon.

White willow. The bark of the white willow tree (*Salix alba*) is a natural source of salicin, a compound chemically related to synthetic aspirin (acetylsalicylic acid). Studies have found that aspirin works as a synergistic, heat-creating agent, as do caffeine and ephedrine. White willow bark, however, has not been similarly tested as a weight-loss agent. Also, it contains low levels of salicin (1 or 2 percent) compared to commercial aspirin products. Though the rationale is reasonable for including white willow bark in combination weight-loss products, it is yet to be proven that the low levels have the intended effect.

Gymnema. This ancient herb of India has shown promise in the treatment of diabetes (see Chapter 13). Its use as a weight-loss aid, however, is controversial. A number of prominent herbalists and naturopaths, including Rob McCaleb, president of the Herb Research Foundation in Boulder, Colorado, have criticized supplement producers for making misleading claims about gymnema. For example, some manufacturers selling gymnema in capsules or in combination weight-loss products promote the herb as a "sugar-blocker." Taking gymnema is said to promote weight loss by blocking the body's ability to absorb or be affected by dietary sugar. According to McCaleb, "There is *no* evidence that the plant reduces or prevents absorption of sugars, nor their calories."

Although gymnema can't magically block sugar in the body, extracts put on the tongue apparently do have the unusual ability to inhibit the taste of sweetness. Thus, gymnema can potentially act like the anesthetic benzocaine, reducing the inclination to eat. When such use has been put to the test, researchers have found that subjects do decrease their food consumption.

According to herbalist Christopher Hobbs, "While gymnema blocks the sweet taste on the tongue, it would not necessarily have the same effect when swallowed in capsule form. I would definitely use gymnema clinically for its proven anti-diabetic effects, but its use as a weight-loss herb remains unproven."

The Weight-Loss Stimulants

Many people find that the most powerful natural weight-loss products are those that contain two alkaloids with potent stimulant effects: caffeine and ephedrine. Sources of caffeine (and related xanthines, such as theophylline) include coffee, green tea, kola nut, guarana, and chocolate. The main source of ephedrine is ephedra, particularly the Chinese species known as ma huang. Caffeine and ephedrine boost the body's overall metabolic rate and promote the burning of body fat. A number of studies have found that the weight-loss effects of caffeine and ephedrine are up to twice as great when they are combined than when they are used singly. In fact, caffeine's weight-loss effects in the absence of ephedrine are minimal. An animal study published in 1986 in the *American Journal of Clinical Nutrition* found that using only ephedrine led to a 14 percent loss in weight and a 42 percent reduction in body fat, whereas combining ephedrine with caffeine or theophylline increased those figures to 25 and 75 percent, respectively.

Weight-loss supplement producers also often combine caffeine and ephedrine with chromium picolinate and white willow bark, cayenne, and other herbs. Look for products such as MetaboLift and DietMax.

Green Tea

One of the best sources of caffeine for those looking to lose a few pounds is green tea. Most of the research on green tea has concentrated on its anticancer and antioxidant effects, but it has also been tested for its ability to promote weight loss. While the mildly stimulating effects of the caffeine in green tea account for some of this herb's potential as a weight-loss agent, researchers have also found that its polyphenols and catechins can promote the burning of fat and help to regulate blood sugar and insulin. One placebo-controlled study found that overweight women who complemented their low-calorie diet by taking tea supplements lost three times more weight after a month than those who didn't take the supplement.

Weight-loss products containing green tea go by names like Thermo-Lift Powder and ThermoLoss. Read label contents carefully for caffeine content to avoid consuming excessive amounts of caffeine. Only 100 to 150 mg of caffeine per day is sufficient to boost the effects of ephedrine and other weight-loss factors. Some green-tea-extract products may have little or no caffeine, while others may have caffeine added from other sources.

Don't drink green tea scalding hot, which may reduce its health benefits or possibly even increase your risk of esophageal cancer.

HOW TO USE GREEN TEA: It comes mainly in teas and capsules. If you brew a tea, steeping for two to three minutes may yield approximately 20 to 30 mg of caffeine; thus an average daily dose is 4 to 6 cups. An average daily dosage of the capsules to obtain 50 to 100 mg of polyphenols is 300 to 600 mg for capsules standardized for 15 percent polyphenols, or 100 to 200 mg of the capsules standardized for 50 percent polyphenols.

Ephedra/Ma Huang

This ancient herb (see Chapter 5) contains a number of potent alkaloids, with ephedrine being the chief central nervous system stimulant. In addition to boosting the rate of metabolism, heartbeat, and breathing, ephedrine curbs appetite and increases the burning of fat, thus promoting weight loss.

Researchers have found that relatively low daily levels of ephedrine (40 to 50 mg) are sufficient to accelerate weight loss. Taken together, a single dose of 25 mg of ephedrine and 75 mg of caffeine stimulates the central nervous system about the same amount as does drinking 6 ounces of drip coffee (with 140 to 160 mg of caffeine). The body tends to build up a tolerance to ephedrine's effects on the nervous system but not to its heat-generating, fat-burning effects.

North American species of ephedra, such as Mormon tea (*Ephedra nevadensis*), have few alkaloids and are of no use in a weight-loss program. Look for products using Chinese ephedra/ma huang (*E. sinica*) that go by names like Thermo 'T'. Ephedra is also a popular ingredient in bodybuilding products such as Ripped Fuel. In addition to caffeine, other substances that can enhance the weight-loss effects of ephedrine include aspirin and mineral electrolytes such as potassium and magnesium.

As a potent nervous-system stimulant, ephedra is easily abused. Prolonged use may weaken the adrenal glands or cause nervousness, insomnia, and other side effects. Ephedra shouldn't be used by women who are pregnant or breast-feeding, children under 13, anyone taking MAO-inhibitor antidepressants, or people with high blood pressure, glaucoma, diabetes, thyroid conditions, difficulty in urination due to prostate enlargement, or heart disease.

How TO USE EPHEDRA/MA HUANG: Ephedra is sold dried and in capsules, concentrated drops, tinctures, and extracts. Extracts are often standardized for an alkaloid (mostly ephedrine) content of 5 to 10 percent. Thus, an average dosage for a 10 percent alkaloid content extract would be 200 to 250 mg of ma huang (yielding 20 to 25 mg ephedrine), taken twice daily. To maximize weight loss, take each dose of ephedra with 50 to 75 mg of caffeine from green tea or some other source. The ephedrine content of tinctures and concentrated drops varies considerably; an average dosage is $1/2$ to 1 dropperful. Stop taking ephedrine-caffeine combination products by early afternoon in order to avoid late-evening insomnia.

Taking It Off with Nutrients

People who are seriously overweight, as well as people following typical weight-loss diets, often suffer from vitamin and mineral deficiencies. Overweight people may be eating large volumes of foods, but they're usually foods high in calories and fat and low in nutrients. Dieters who limit their caloric intake to between 1,500 and 2,000 calories per day are unlikely to consume even the RDA of all twenty or so of the most essential vitamins and minerals. People on weight-loss programs also have higher-than-average requirements for antioxidants (to counter the adverse effects of fat-stored toxins released by fat-burning) and for the various nutrients that play a role in metabolism, digestion, and fat transport.

Vitamin and mineral deficiencies can also trigger feelings of hunger. "When foods are very low in vitamins and minerals," notes nutrition authority Jeffrey Bland, Ph.D., "the liver becomes depleted of these nutrients and signals to the brain that it is hungry for more nutrition. Therefore, lack of adequate vitamins and minerals can turn on the appetite mechanism."

Thus, as a starting point, anyone looking to lose weight should take an insurance level multivitamin-multimineral product. The following nutrients also have special benefits for those who want to shed a few extra pounds.

The major minerals. When dissolved in the blood and other bodily fluids, the minerals potassium, magnesium, calcium, and phosphate are known as electrolytes. In solution form, they allow the transmission of minute electrical currents that are crucial not only for proper functioning of the muscles and nerves but also for regulating body heat. Studies have found that optimal levels of these electrolytes boost metabolism and help to burn off fat. Most people get excessive amounts of phosphates from soft drinks and other food sources. Balanced multimineral supplements usually contain potassium, magnesium, and calcium.

Digestive enhancers. These include beneficial live bacteria such as acidophilus and bifidus, the complex carbohydrate inulin/FOS, and dietary enzymes such as papain and bromelain. Proper digestion leads to optimum absorption of nutrients, improved blood-glucose regulation, and more complete elimination of wastes. See Chapter 16 for more information and recommended dosages of digestive enhancers.

Coenzyme Q10. This vitaminlike substance helps the body's cells use oxygen and generate energy at the cellular level. To this date only a few studies have specifically examined its potential role in weight loss, though with some promise. For example, a study of 27 obese people found that those who had comparatively low coQ10 blood levels were able to lose weight more quickly when taking coQ10 supplements than those with normal blood levels of the nutrient. An average daily dosage of coQ10 is 15 to 30 mg.

The trace elements zinc and copper. Adequate daily levels of zinc (17 to 25 mg) and copper (2 to 4 mg), along with beta carotene (25,000 to 50,000 IU or 15 to 30 mg) and vitamin E (400 to 600 IU), promote optimum functioning of the thyroid. An endocrine gland located in the front of the neck, the thyroid plays a central role in setting the body's basal metabolic rate. If the thyroid gland is producing insufficient amounts of certain hormones, or if your body is lacking the nutrients necessary for tissues to use these hormones, you may gain weight easily and have difficulty taking it off. Tiredness and sensitivity to cold are further symptoms of poor thyroid function. A preliminary indication of an underactive thyroid is an average morning body temperature lower than 97.8°F, as measured for ten minutes in the armpit. Blood tests that measure for thyroid hormone levels can confirm an inactive thyroid. Health practitioners can also check for a deficiency of the trace element iodine, necessary for the production of thyroid hormones. (Most people don't need to take supplemental iodine because they get more-than-adequate levels from consuming iodized salt.)

Vitamin B complex. A number of the B vitamins have been linked with better thyroid function as well as improved fat metabolism. An average dosage is 25 to 50 mg twice daily.

Choline/phosphatidylcholine/lecithin. Choline in any of its various forms (see Chapter 2 for more information on the distinctions between choline, phosphatidylcholine, and lecithin) helps the body to break down fats and transport them in and out of cells. An average daily dose of choline is 100 to 200 mg; of phosphatidylcholine that is 90 percent pure, 1,100 to 2,200 mg; of lecithin that is 20 percent phosphatidylcholine, 5 to 10 g, or 1 to 2 tablespoons of granules.

Chromium

Chromium is a valuable addition to a weight-loss regimen for two reasons: it not only promotes the loss of fat but also increases lean body mass. As mentioned earlier, the percentage of body fat can be as important for overall health as total body weight. Because chromium helps you to add muscle while losing fat, the total weight loss in pounds tells only half the story. You may not shed the quantity of pounds you do using other supplements, but the pounds you do shed are quality ones in terms of permanent weight loss.

Chromium's dual effect is tied to its important role in the production and utilization of the hormone insulin. The pancreas secretes insulin in response to increases in blood-glucose levels. Insulin helps to regulate blood-sugar levels by promoting the ability of the liver and muscles to absorb glucose. Insulin is thus an important cog in the bodily mechanism that connects blood-sugar levels with the brain's center for appetite control and metabolism. When insulin secretion is working as it should, blood-sugar levels are regulated, and the brain properly signals satiety or hunger. Poor insulin activity can lead to reduced energy levels and increased cravings for sugar.

Not surprisingly, a lack of insulin or an inability to use the insulin the body produces, such as with diabetes, often leads to easy weight gain. By the same token, a dramatic increase in body fat hampers the functioning of insulin. Weight loss then becomes more difficult. Chromium is necessary not only for the production of insulin but for the ability of muscles and other tissues to properly use it.

A number of placebo-controlled studies using athletes, college students, overweight adults, and other test subjects indicate that average doses of chromium (200 to 400 mcg daily) taken for two to three months do indeed boost weight loss while adding muscle. For example, researchers recently did a double-blind study at a San Antonio weight-loss clinic. Even without making specific dietary and exercise recommendations, they found that overweight adults who took 200 to 400 mcg of chromium picolinate daily for two months lost over four pounds of fat while gaining nearly a pound and a half of muscle. Test subjects who took a placebo lost only 0.4 pounds of fat and gained only 0.2 pounds of lean body mass. Another study of men and women in a weight-training program at Louisiana State University found that those who took 200 mcg of chromium picolinate daily gained an average of over 40 percent in lean body mass and lost an average of over 20 percent in body fat.

Chromium's effects are enhanced when it is combined with a low-fat diet and regular exercise.

HOW TO USE CHROMIUM: Chromium supplements are widely available in tablets (usually 100 to 200 mcg), capsules, and liquids. An average daily dosage for adults is 200 to 400 mcg.

Fiber Supplements

Fiber has a number of positive effects on the body that combine to promote weight loss. Consumed as supplements shortly before meals, fiber in the stomach and intestines is bulky and promotes a sense of fullness, thus reducing the amount of food you're likely to want when you do sit down to eat. Fiber-rich foods need to be well chewed, so you tend to eat them more slowly and in smaller quantities. Fiber-rich foods also tend to be naturally low in calories and high in nutrients.

Whether from supplements or foods, fiber in the gastrointestinal system helps to balance blood-glucose levels and thus eliminate hunger pangs. Fiber promotes the transport of fats and calories through the digestive system, thus lowering the amounts absorbed by the blood and stored in the body. Fiber may also stimulate the release of hormones that suppress appetite.

The best way to increase your dietary fiber intake is to eat plenty of whole grains, fresh vegetables, fruits, and legumes. Though supplements can also help, they shouldn't be consumed as a substitute for healthful foods.

Don't overdo supplemental fiber. Start with up to 4 or 5 g per day and gradually increase your intake if necessary as your body adjusts. Some people who take excessive levels of supplementary fiber (usually over 30 g per day) may experience mineral deficiencies due to impaired absorption of nutrients. You should also drink healthy amounts of water (6 to 8 glasses per day) to prevent fiber supplements from leading to constipation.

Many supplement companies offer fiber-based weight-loss products featuring mainly soluble fiber from psyllium, guar gum, pectin, glucomannan, or other sources. Look for products such as Ever-Slender, Fiber-Trim, and Fiber-Slim.

HOW TO USE FIBER SUPPLEMENTS: These come in powders, tablets, liquids, and other forms. To boost weight loss, take 1 to 2 heaping teaspoons, or 4 to 8 g in tablets or capsules, 15 to 30 minutes before each meal with a large glass of water, juice, or tea.

Hydroxycitric Acid

Hydroxycitric acid (HCA) is a natural substance chemically similar to the citric acid found in oranges and other fruits. HCA is derived from an extract of the rind of the Malabar tamarind, or goraka. A tropical fruit that looks somewhat like a small pumpkin, the Malabar tamarind grows on a tree (*Garcinia cambogia*) native to South Asia. The native peoples of this area have long used the fruit as a food, condiment (devotees of Thai cooking may have tasted it in curried dishes), and herb (it is said to be a digestive aid). Though HCA is also found in a few other (mostly South Asian) plants, the Malabar tamarind is the richest known source.

Studies on both animals and people have found that HCA has the unusual effect of reducing the body's conversion of carbohydrates to fats. This tends to curb appetite and reduce food intake, thus leading to loss of weight. The mechanism has been traced to glucose metabolism. High blood-sugar levels cause the body to convert glucose to glycogen for storage in the liver and muscles. When these bodily stores have no room for additional glycogen, glucose is broken down and converted in a number of steps into fatty acids and cholesterol for storage elsewhere in the body. Researchers have found that HCA temporarily inhibits the enzyme (ATP-citrate lyase) necessary for this glucose-to-fat conversion. Two studies on animals determined that HCA reduces the synthesis of fats by 40 to 70 percent for between 8 and 12 hours following a meal. The liver takes the leftover glucose and synthesizes additional amounts of glycogen for storage, alerting the hypothalamus to signal a sense of fullness.

Human studies indicate that HCA reduces food consumption by about 10 percent. One human study of 22 obese subjects put on a low-fat diet found that after two months those who took 250 mg of HCA plus 100 mg of a chromium supplement three times daily lost an average of 11 pounds, compared to only 4 for those taking a placebo. The HCA subjects reported decreased appetite and fewer cravings for sweets in particular.

Popular Malabar tamarind extracts include Citrin and CitriMax, the latter a trademarked formulation used by more than a dozen producers. CitriMax is standardized for 50 percent HCA. The extract is found in products called CitriMax; in chromium products such as Citrilite, Trim Control, Garcinia Max Diet Systems, and CitriMax Plus ChromeMate; and in multiple-ingredient formulas such as CitriMax Plus, CitriMax Extra, and Thermo Tropic.

Though it has not been as widely tested as citric acid, HCA is thought to be similarly safe. Food and body-care companies use small amounts of citric acid as a preservative or flavoring in a wide variety of products, from shampoos to Pepsi. HCA is, however, used in larger doses, which can affect certain hormones. Thus it should not be used by pregnant or lactating women, or by children. In general, HCA is much safer than appetite suppressants, such as amphetamine, PPA, and ephedrine, that directly stimulate the central nervous system. HCA has no known potential for abuse.

Most of the animal studies involved high dosages of HCA, equivalent to 3 to 6 g per day for humans. Human studies such as the aforementioned trial with obese subjects indicate lower levels are also effective, particularly when HCA is combined with chromium. Researchers have also found that HCA is much more effective when taken two or three times daily, in divided doses, than when taken once daily.

According to Dallas Clouatre, Ph.D., coauthor of *The Diet and Health Benefits of HCA (Hydroxycitric Acid),* "Based upon what we know now, dieters using HCA can vary their intake to suit their own individuality. While the majority of dieters will see positive results using the minimum dosage of HCA, people who have not begun to see results after three weeks at this level should double their dosage for another three weeks. This amount of HCA—1,500 mg daily—in combination with niacin-bound chromium gives good results for roughly 80 percent of those using the product."

How to use hca: To aid a weight-loss program, an average beginning dosage is 250 mg of HCA plus 100 mcg chromium three times per day, 30 to 60 minutes before meals.

Carnitine

Increasing numbers of bodybuilders and athletes are taking carnitine supplements to enhance strength and endurance (see Chapter 4), and others are using it promote better heart function (see Chapter 8).

Another significant use for carnitine is to encourage weight loss. Currently, the scientific evidence for carnitine's effects on athletic performance and on heart function is much more substantial than the evidence for its presumed effect on body weight. Carnitine's role in the body, however, suggests that when studies are done, they will confirm that this vitaminlike compound deserves its reputation as a weight-loss aid.

Carnitine is crucial for proper fat burning. In the body carnitine is concentrated in the heart and muscles, where it plays a vital role in the transport of fatty acids into cells' mitochondria for combustion and energy production. Taking supplemental carnitine is thought to significantly increase the body's ability to create energy by metabolizing stored fat, allowing the person to shed a few extra pounds in the process.

The L- form of this amino acid derivative (the form used in virtually all supplement products) is safer and more effective than inactive D-carnitine or the mixed form DL-carnitine. Carnitine is frequently combined with other nutrients, such as chromium, in weight-loss products such as Chroma Slim.

How to use carnitine: It typically comes in capsules and tablets of 250 to 500 mg, and in liquid form. An average dosage for boosting weight loss is 250 to 500 mg once or twice daily with meals.

Amino Acids for Weight Loss

Amino acid levels in the bloodstream can have direct effects on certain neurotransmitters in the brain capable of affecting hunger and appetite. For example, tryptophan is thought to reduce appetite by increasing levels of serotonin, one of the neurotransmitters that helps the hypothalamus to signal a sense of fullness and thus reduce appetite.

Tryptophan and another amino acid, phenylalanine, can also potentially affect hunger and weight loss in an indirect way. When fatty foods enter the duodenum (the upper portion of the small intestine), it releases into the bloodstream a hormone called cholecystokinin (CCK). CCK causes digestive organs such as the gallbladder and pancreas to release substances (including bile and certain enzymes) that aid digestion. In addition, there is some evidence that CCK affects the pituitary (where it stimulates the release of fat-burning growth hormone) and the hypothalamus. Studies have found that obese people have lower levels of CCK, or reduced sensitivity to its effects.

In recent years a few manufacturers have offered CCK itself as a supplement. It is unclear, however, whether taking CCK orally has the same effect as promoting its secretion in the body. Scientists have discovered that tryptophan and phenylalanine release CCK in the gastrointestinal system and thus help to suppress appetite.

Prior to late 1989, when more than three dozen deaths associated with the use of contaminated tryptophan prompted the FDA to ban its sale as a supplement, some natural-health practitioners recommended tryptophan as an appetite suppressant. Some of the scientific studies done on tryptophan and weight loss confirm an effect.

As of early 1995, tryptophan remains off the market. It is possible to take advantage of its effects by eating certain foods (see Chapter 12). Until tryptophan gets a clean bill of health, phenylalanine and arginine remain the amino acids of choice for their weight-controlling effects.

Phenylalanine

In addition to its role in promoting secretion of CCK, phenylalanine helps to control weight through its role as a precursor in the body for the amino acid tyrosine. Among other functions, tyrosine is necessary for the thyroid to produce the hormones that regulate metabolism. Tyrosine is also the first link in the production of certain neurotransmitters, including dopamine, noradrenaline, and adrenaline, that are suspected of playing important roles in controlling appetite.

Phenylalanine should be avoided by pregnant women, people with high blood pressure, and anyone taking MAO-inhibitor antidepressants. It should also be avoided by people with phenylketonuria, a genetic disorder of phenylalanine metabolism. As with most other stimulants, its potential side effects include insomnia and anxiety.

L-phenylalanine is the preferred form of the amino acid for promoting weight loss. Both phenylalanine and tyrosine are sometimes found in combination weight-loss products such as Slimmer.

HOW TO USE PHENYLALANINE: L-phenylalanine typically comes in capsules of 375, 500, or 750 mg. An average dosage to promote weight loss is 375 to 500 mg two or three times daily, taken before meals to promote the secretion of CCK.

Arginine

Arginine is a favorite amino acid among bodybuilders because of its ability to promote the secretion of growth hormone from the pituitary gland (see Chapter 4). Because growth hormone increases the body's ability to metabolize fat and to build muscle tissue, arginine is also useful for those who want to lose a few pounds and reduce overall body fat percentage.

Pregnant women, anyone with kidney or liver diseases, and people under the age of 20 (whose bones are still growing) should not take supplemental arginine. Since it is possible that high levels of arginine can reactivate latent herpes viruses in some individuals, combining it with lysine (which may prevent herpes outbreaks) is a reasonable precaution for those with the virus. Even those who do not harbor the herpes virus may want to combine arginine with equal amounts of lysine, since one of the most noteworthy studies showing an increase in growth hormone secretion was done with subjects given 1,200 mg of arginine and 1,200 mg of lysine.

How TO USE ARGININE: Arginine is available as a single ingredient in capsule and powder form. It is also an ingredient in fat-burning and muscle-building products, where it is frequently combined with such nutrients as ornithine, methionine, and vitamin B_6. An average dosage for weight loss is 250 to 500 mg once or twice daily, with meals.

Scents That Help Weight Loss

The senses of smell and taste are intimately connected, as anyone who has held their nose while trying to distinguish the taste of an apple from that of an onion can attest. If you had to rely only on your tongue to provide your sense of taste, you'd be working with a mere four variables: sweet, sour, bitter, and salty. Your olfactory sense, on the other hand, can distinguish an estimated two to four thousand aromas. These aromas account for about 80 percent of the sensation of taste.

Anatomy also supports a major role for the sense of smell in eating and hunger. The olfactory bulb, in the roof of the nasal cavity, is linked with parts of the brain, including the hypothalamus, that control appetite. Researchers have also noted that the digestive system hormone cholecystokinin can function as a neurotransmitter in the olfactory bulb.

Some of the other interesting connections between smell, taste, and appetite include the following:

• Your nose's ability to smell is somewhat reduced when you've finished a meal and are no longer hungry.

• Food tastes blander in airplanes in part because cabin pressure reduces the dispersal of aromas.

• Perhaps most important, researchers have tied loss of the sense of smell with weight gain.

One of the few scientific studies to look at the relationship of smell to weight loss was done in 1993 at the Smell & Taste Treatment and Research Foundation in Chicago. Foundation director Alan R. Hirsch, M.D., and colleagues studied 3,193 overweight subjects, predominantly middle-aged women averaging five feet five inches in height and 217 pounds. The researchers found that subjects who frequently inhaled three times in each nostril a blend of banana, peppermint, and green-apple scents whenever they were hungry lost nearly five pounds per month over six months, without making any changes to their normal dietary and exercise habits. Some individuals lost up to 18 pounds per month. The researchers believe that inhaling foodlike odors somehow tricks the brain into equating the smell with the actual food, promoting a feeling of fullness and suppressing appetite.

Hirsch, a neurologist, says that the scents were more effective with people who had a good sense of smell. The researchers also determined that "the amount of weight the subjects lost directly correlated with the frequency of their use of the inhalers." They concluded that "it may be possible for individuals with good olfaction, by inhaling certain aromas, to induce and sustain loss of weight over a six-month period." Hirsch and his staff are now conducting a similar 12,000-person, 13-month follow-up study to see if weight loss can be sustained over a longer term. The researchers are also testing new scents, including Oreo cookie, cola, cranberry, and vanilla.

Another researcher who has found close connections between smell and weight loss is Dr. Susan Schiffman of Duke University. She has promoted weight loss in obese people by spraying test subjects' favorite dishes with special fragrances that enhance the strength of the foods' intrinsic aromas, allowing the subjects to satisfy their appetite while consuming fewer calories.

At this point the research on using scents to promote weight loss is too preliminary to provide the basis for recommending any single essential oil used in the traditional manner of dispersing it throughout the room. It is possible that such a use could actually stimulate appetite rather than substitute for it. Most aromatherapists don't consider weight loss to be among the potential benefits of using essential oils. On the other hand, there are a few combination aromatherapy products, with names such as Slender Essence, targeting the weight-loss market. The large essential-oil producer Aroma Vera, in Los Angeles, offers Slimming/Body Contour, a blend of Cypress, Lemon, and

Thyme that is said to promote circulation and encourage elimination of excess fluids. It is sold in the form of a liquid for room dispersal and as a cleansing bar, shower gel, and massage oil.

When asked whether a scent diffused into the air rather than sniffed from a test tube would reduce hunger or increase metabolism, Hirsch says, "It's a good question, but we haven't studied that." He also notes that in its clinical trials the foundation uses artificial odors because it is easier to get approval to use them in a scientific study than to get approval for natural oils.

If you want to experiment, however, with using natural essential oils and the direct-sniffing technique used in the scientific studies, it is certainly safe to do so and may also be effective. The one fragrance researchers used that is widely available as an essential oil is Peppermint, a sweet-smelling oil that is slightly stimulating (see Chapter 5). Keep a bottle handy, and whenever you feel hungry, sniff three times with each nostril. The evidence suggests that the more frequently you use this method, the more likely you will eat less and lose some weight.

Homeopathic Remedies for Slimming

Practitioners of homeopathy use a number of remedies to help promote weight loss, depending upon the specific characteristics of the person. Is he or she more often chilly or warm? Craving hot foods or sweets? Passive or restless? and so forth. For long-term treatment of a serious weight problem, it is worthwhile to see a homeopathic practitioner who can help you determine the right remedies and develop an integrated approach encompassing dietary and lifestyle changes as well. For those looking for help in shedding a few pounds, there are homeopathic combination remedies for weight loss. These often include such single remedies as *Calcarea carbonica, Hepar sulph, Pulsatilla,* and *Graphites.* Look for products with names such as Appetite. The single homeopathic remedy most frequently associated with weight loss is *Calcarea carbonica.*

Calcarea carbonica

Calcarea carbonica is calcium carbonate, usually derived from oyster shells. The person who is most likely to benefit from *Calcarea carbonica* is on the tubby side and frequently suffers from indigestion. He or she often feels chilly from a slow metabolism and has a pale complexion and hands that are cold and clammy. He or she also commonly has cravings for sweets. See "How to Use Homeopathic Remedies" in Chapter 2.

Where to Start

If you're new to using herbs and nutrients to complement a weight-loss program, a simple and basic approach is to take the recommended doses of the following three types of supplements:

- A combination thermogenic formula, such as any of the widely available ones that contain moderate levels of caffeine and ephedrine; look for a formula that also has additional useful nutrients such as vitamins, minerals, coenzyme Q10, carnitine, or tyrosine
- An HCA and chromium combination product (250 mg of HCA plus 100 mcg chromium three times per day, 30 to 60 minutes before meals)
- Fiber supplements (1 to 2 heaping teaspoons, or 4 to 8 g in tablets or capsules, 15 to 30 minutes before each meal, with a large glass of water, juice, or tea)

Depending upon how much weight you need to lose, you may need to take these for a few weeks or a few months. After you've reached your ideal weight, you can discontinue the thermogenic formula and the HCA; chromium and fiber have many important health benefits beyond weight loss and can be taken indefinitely.

Beyond Herbs and Supplements

Attaining your ideal body weight and body-fat level requires more than merely downing some useful supplements on a daily basis. When you can fight the battle of the bulge on more than one front, your chances for ultimate victory are considerably enhanced. As millions of dieters who have seen their weight yo-yo up and down can attest, liquid-protein diets and other fads rarely work for very long. Dietary changes are most effective when they are accompanied by steps such as developing a positive attitude toward your body and increasing your physical activity.

A long-term or even lifelong program for controlling weight is more likely to succeed than those that promise a quick fix. Keep in mind that many people find that their body weight naturally fluctuates by a few pounds according to the seasons, monthly hormonal cycles, and other factors. Jumping onto the scales three times a day is a waste of time, notes Dr. James Rippe, an exercise authority and the director of the Center for Clinical and Lifestyle Research in Shrewsbury, Massachusetts. Daily intake of calories or weight changes are irrelevant to long-term weight loss, he says, which really is determined by "slow regulation processes that occur over months and years."

Some of the most important factors to consider for long-term weight regulation include the following:

• Don't diet. Rather, change your regular eating pattern to one that emphasizes low-fat, high-fiber foods, particularly complex carbohydrates. A growing number of doctors and nutritionists, including Dean Ornish, M.D., author of *Eat More, Weigh Less,* and Neal Barnard, M.D., author of *Food for Life,* contend that the primary consideration is not total calories but the fat content of your diet. "The answer for permanent weight loss," Barnard states, "is to base your diet on grains, beans, vegetables, and fruits. These foods are more powerful in controlling weight than any weight-loss scheme. Most people can eat all they want, anytime they want, and stay slim."

• Stay physically active. Exercising regularly or physically exerting yourself in your everyday life has multiple positive effects on body weight. Exercise increases your metabolic rate not only while you work out but also while you're resting. It builds muscle tissue, which at rest burns more calories than does fat. Physical activity also helps control appetite, since it stimulates the release of endorphins, hormones that help to reduce your urge to eat.

• Drink plenty of water or diluted fruit juice. Liquids can help make you feel full and reduce your tendency to overeat at mealtimes. Sorry, but alcoholic beverages don't count—they're often high in calories and can actually inhibit your body's fat-burning mechanisms.

• Avoid extremes in blood-sugar levels (see Chapter 13). Consuming excessive amounts of highly refined, sugary foods or caffeinated beverages can cause large swings in blood-glucose levels and a surge in hunger when blood sugar reaches its lowest levels.

• Fast for twelve hours every day. This may sound difficult, but what it means is not eating between the time you finish dinner in the early evening and the next morning's breakfast. Evening snacks eaten while lounging in front of the TV are often fatty, and this fat gets stored more easily because of the lack of activity.

• Cut back on your TV watching. A number of studies have found an association between body weight and the number of hours spent watching the tube.

THREE

Putting It All Together

Combine Natural Substances with a Healthful Lifestyle

The appeal of using natural substances to stay well is seductively simple: take this pill and you'll feel better, look more attractive, live longer. Compared to sweating through a workout on the StairMaster, preparing a tasty but low-fat dinner, or sitting still in silent meditation for an hour, taking a supplement is fast and easy. It is, of course, this same fast-and-easy appeal that supplies practitioners of conventional modern medicine with most of their patients. Who wants to bother with wholesale changes in one's diet to lower a high cholesterol level when your doctor says that instead you can just pop a few of these lovastatin tablets each day?

The fast-and-easy nature of such an approach to health has a significant drawback, one that applies both to the remedies promoted by practitioners of natural medicine and to the pharmaceuticals promoted by doctors of modern medicine. Simply put, pill-popping encourages a tendency to rely on the substance as *the* tool for effecting the desired change, as opposed to considering the substance as *one* of the tools that need to be used for long-term success. No substance should be expected to substitute for addressing the direct causes of the physical condition, whether that condition is chronically low energy levels or elevated total blood cholesterol. Though garlic may be safer than lovastatin for lowering cholesterol, and may offer many other important health benefits as well, popping a garlic capsule every day while continuing to eat a high-cholesterol, 50-percent-of-calories-from-saturated-fat, low-fiber diet, and while also leading a stressful, sedentary life, is unlikely to have much positive effect.

Supplements are supplements, not substitutes, for better health. They work best as a synergistic element of the healthful lifestyle, one that includes attention to diet, emotions, attitudes, fitness, and other factors.

Simple Steps to Natural Health

In my previous book, *52 Simple Steps to Natural Health,* I detailed the many diverse elements—relating to diet, work, personal relations, relaxation, and more—that support a lifestyle resulting in long-term health, happiness, and longevity. Many of these simple steps are contained in the "Beyond Herbs and Supplements" sections in most of the chapters of this book. As important as it is to supplement your diet with the right herbs and nutrients, you multiply these substances' healthful benefits by paying attention to the many other elements of health. What follows are some of the most essential components of a well-rounded program for optimal health and longevity.

• Eat a healthful diet. The standard American diet (appropriately abbreviated SAD) is high in animal foods, saturated fat, and refined carbohydrates, and low in fiber and complex carbohydrates. The SAD diet needs to be stood on its head. The U.S. Surgeon General, the USDA, the American Heart Association, and virtually every progressive nutritionist in the country now agree that the best diet for long-term health is primarily plant-based and made up of mostly fresh vegetables and fruits, whole grains, legumes, breads and cereals, and fish. Such a diet is low in saturated fat, refined sugars, meats, and processed foods. It is rich in fiber, complex carbohydrates, and nutrient-dense foods. Adopting a healthful diet will substantially reduce your risk of almost all of the killer diseases of industrialized societies, including heart disease, cancer, diabetes, and osteoporosis.

• Drink sufficient water to stay hydrated. Many people are marginally dehydrated without realizing it. This reduces the functioning capacity of various bodily organs such as the skin and increases the risk of kidney stones and other conditions. Six to eight glasses of fluid per day, primarily in the form of water but also including diluted fruit juice or noncaffeinated herbal teas, should be your norm.

• Don't diet to lose weight—change your diet permanently. Focus on reducing saturated fat rather than the number of calories, and on attaining an appropriate level of body fat rather than an arbitrary weight in pounds. Make junk foods and fast foods an occasional treat, not a daily routine.

• Fast every day for twelve hours, by not eating between when you finish dinner and the next morning's breakfast. Your digestive system gets a much-needed rest, and you'll probably be cutting out those foods that you least need, anyway.

• Stay physically active, not only by exercising regularly at the health club or by playing tennis, but by taking the available opportunities to use your body in everyday life. Walking, bicycling, climbing stairs, raking leaves, gardening—these are the everyday activities that should complement scheduled exercise time.

• Balance your exercise-and-fitness program to include each of the four distinct elements of physical health: building muscles, increasing flexibility, improving endurance, and enhancing balance and coordination. Tailor your exercise to your capabilities, interests, budget, and personality.

• Avoid the daily habits that are most destructive to overall health, particularly smoking cigarettes, drinking alcohol to excess, and leading a totally sedentary lifestyle. These three elements themselves account for hundreds of thousands of premature deaths in the United States today.

• Pay attention to how you move your body and to your posture when your body is still. Back pain, much of it posture-related, is endemic in American society. By sitting on the two arches of bone at the bottom of the pelvis when you sit, and carrying yourself in an erect manner when you walk and move, you'll look and feel stronger and more graceful. Exercise and stretch to keep your back supple and strong.

• Create a natural, nontoxic environment where you live and work. Limit your everyday exposure to household, industrial, and urban pollutants, including secondhand cigarette smoke, strong electromagnetic fields, and toxins off-gassed from carpets and other sources.

• Get some regular sun without overdoing it. Sunburns are hazardous to your skin's long-term health, but a total avoidance of sun, whether from never getting outside or overuse of suntan lotions, can also lead to health problems.

• Develop a better sense of how your body works and how you can diagnose it and treat it with natural remedies when it becomes sick. Learn how to substitute safe and effective natural remedies for the conventional pain-killers, anti-inflammatories, cold remedies, and other drugs used most frequently for minor conditions.

• Find a health practitioner who shares your overall beliefs and can be a partner in your journey to wellness.

• Learn how to breathe correctly—through the nose with the abdomen rising on the inhalation—rather than breathing "backwards" (sucking in the stomach to inhale), as many people do. You'll breathe more slowly and evenly and increase your lungs' oxygen intake.

• Get enough sleep. Individual needs vary, but many people are walking around in a constant state of sleep deprivation. Sufficient sleep is as important to your overall health as sufficient exercise.

• Avoid time fixations. Rushing through life with your eyes glued to the clock is a sure way to develop "hurry sickness," a condition characterized by such stress-inducing qualities as quickness to anger, extreme competitiveness, and hostility. An increased risk of heart disease may result.

• Learn to laugh at yourself and with others, seeing humor wherever possible. As a seventeenth-century physician once said, "The arrival of a good clown exercises more beneficial influence upon the health of a town than that of twenty asses laden with drugs." Laughter benefits circulation, digestion, and immunity.

• Recognize harmful addictive traits in your work and play and seek to overcome them. Ask yourself, are you in control when you gamble, have sex, spend money, drink alcohol, exercise, eat? Question and change your habits and routines to be more open to the unusual or the revealing.

• Develop positive outlooks that keep your mind and spirit constantly refreshed. Affirm your ability to remain basically hopeful, optimistic, and purposeful even while recognizing that loneliness, sadness, and fear are common human emotions.

• Consciously relax. Whether you prefer biofeedback, meditation, or a quiet walk in the woods, find some technique for attaining that elusive state of being calm yet alert, relaxed yet focused, resting yet awake.

• Communicate heart to heart with friends, coworkers, lovers, and family members. Learn how to express your true self to them and receive in turn their expressions of themselves to you.

• Enjoy life's simple pleasures, from making love to playing with children to connecting with nature.

Using herbs and supplements to stay well should enhance all of these important steps to natural health, not substitute for them.

The Off-the-Shelf Natural Health Medicine Chest

You're heading out the door for the local natural-food store and hoping to remember your favorite natural relaxant or digestive aid? The following summary list of the top twenty natural substances may help.

Herbs

Garlic: immune booster, heart protector, cancer preventive, life extender, system balancer, digestive revitalizer

Ginkgo: energizer, mood elevator, sexual stimulant, heart protector, life extender, brain booster, sense developer

Ginseng: strength and endurance enhancer, energizer, sexual stimulant, heart protector, life extender, brain booster, system balancer

Siberian Ginseng: immune booster, mood elevator, system balancer

Vitamins and Minerals

Vitamin A/beta carotene: immune booster, cancer preventive, life extender, sense developer, skin beautifier

Vitamin C: immune booster, strength and endurance enhancer, mood elevator, heart protector, cancer preventive, life extender, brain booster, sense developer, skin beautifier

Vitamin E: immune booster, strength and endurance enhancer, sexual stimulant, heart protector, cancer preventive, life extender, sense developer, skin beautifier

Calcium and magnesium: strength and endurance enhancer, energizer, mood elevator, heart protector, cancer preventive, brain booster, relaxant, skin beautifier

Chromium: strength and endurance enhancer, heart protector, system balancer, sense developer, weight-loss promoter

Zinc: immune booster, sexual stimulant, cancer preventive, brain booster, system balancer, sense developer, skin beautifier, weight-loss promoter

Nutritional Substances

Choline: mood elevator, sexual stimulant, brain booster, weight-loss promoter

Coenzyme Q10: strength and endurance enhancer, energizer, heart protector, weight-loss promoter

Essential fatty acids: heart protector, cancer preventive, skin beautifier

Polyphenols and flavonoids: heart protector, cancer preventive, life extender, system balancer, sense developer

Beneficial live bacteria: cancer preventive, digestive revitalizer, weight-loss aid

Melatonin: mood elevator, life extender, relaxant

Amino Acids

Phenylalanine: energizer, mood elevator, sexual stimulant, brain booster, weight-loss promoter

Tyrosine: mood elevator, sexual stimulant

Medicinal Mushrooms

Reishi: immune booster, cancer preventive, system balancer

Shiitake: immune booster, cancer preventive

Remember, even if you embrace only a few of these healthful natural substances, the result may well be a longer, happier life.

19

Resources

Chapter 1: Natural Health and Natural Medicines

To learn more about the treatment of arthritis, allergies, PMS, heart disease, indigestion, and other conditions using natural remedies, refer to any of the following titles.

Better Health Through Natural Healing by Dr. Ross Trattler (New York: McGraw-Hill, 1988)

The Complete Medicinal Herbal by Penelope Ody (New York: Dorling Kindersley, 1993)

The Doctors' Book of Home Remedies by the editors of *Prevention Magazine* Health Books (Emmaus, Penn.: Rodale Press, 1990)

An Encyclopedia of Natural Medicine by Michael Murray, N.D., and Joseph Pizzorno, N.D. (Rocklin, Calif.: Prima Publishing, 1991)

Healing Through Nutrition by Melvyn Werbach, M.D. (New York: HarperCollins, 1993)

The Natural Family Doctor by Dr. Andrew Stanway with Richard Grossman (New York: Simon & Schuster, 1987)

Chapter 2: The Top Twenty Natural Substances

Some useful books and booklets on specific herbs and other topics include:

Garlic: Nature's Original Remedy by Stephen Fulder and John Blackwood (Rochester, Vt.: Healing Arts Press, 1991)

Ginkgo by Steven Foster (Austin, Tx.: American Botanical Council, 1991)

Ginkgo: Elixir of Youth by Christopher Hobbs (Capitola, Calif.: Botanica Press, 1991)

Folk Medicine: The Art and the Science edited by Richard P. Steiner (Washington, D.C.: American Chemical Society, 1986)

Medicinal Mushrooms by Christopher Hobbs (Capitola, Calif.: Botanica Press, 1986)
The following is the producer of hemp oil, rich in essential fatty acids:
Ohio Hempery
7002 State Route 329
Guysville, OH 45735
(614) 662–4367
(800) 289–4367

The following mail-order supplement catalog contains a variety of pill dispensers, crushers, splitters, and organizers:

Star Professional Pharmaceuticals
1500 New Horizons Blvd.
Amityville, NY 11701
(800) 274–6400

Chapter 3: Boost Your Immunity

Some useful books with more information on enhancing your immune system include:
Echinacea: The Immune Herb! by Christopher Hobbs (Capitola, Calif.: Botanica Press, 1990)
Echinacea: Nature's Immune Enhancer by Steven Foster (Rochester, Vt.: Healing Arts Press, 1991)
Immune Power by Jon D. Kaiser, M.D. (New York: St. Martin's Press, 1993)

Chapter 4: Enhance Your Strength and Endurance

The following book has an up-to-date discussion of nutrients for muscular development as well as mental enhancement and other functions.
Eat Smart, Think Smart by Robert Haas (New York: HarperCollins, 1994)

Chapter 5: Increase Your Energy Levels

A useful book that summarizes the stimulant effects of various herbs and nutrients is:
Natural Energy Boosters by Carlson Wade (West Nyack, N.Y.: Parker Publishing Company, 1993)
The following is a fascinating history of Coca-Cola:
Secret Formula: How Brilliant Marketing and Relentless Salesmanship Made Coca-Cola the Best-Known Product in the World by Frederick Allen (New York: HarperCollins, 1994)

Chapter 6: Elevate Your Mood

An excellent discussion of the biogenic amine theory of mood development can be found in the following book:
Listening to Prozac by Peter D. Kramer (New York: Viking, 1992)

Chapter 7: Stimulate Your Sexuality

Books with useful information on sexual stimulants and strengtheners include:
Love Potions: A Guide to Aphrodisiacs and Sexual Pleasures by Cynthia Mervis Watson, M.D., with Angela Hynes (New York: Jeremy P. Tarcher/Perigee, 1993)
The Magical and Ritual Use of Aphrodisiacs by Richard Alan Miller (Rochester, Vt.: Destiny Books, 1993)
Male Sexual Vitality by Michael T. Murray, N.D. (Rocklin, Calif.: Prima Publishing, 1994)
Vitex: The Women's Herb by Christopher Hobbs (Capitola, Calif.: Botanica Press, 1990)
See the notes for Chapter 11 for how to obtain liquid deprenyl.
You can order muira puama (quantities only) from:

The Natural and Tropical Source
530 E. 8th St., Suite 204
Oakland, CA 94606
(510) 451–7862

See "For Further Information," below, for mail-order sources of bulk deer antler, eucommia bark, and other Chinese herbs to boost sex drive. The following company sells an herbal aphrodisiac in caplet and chocolate candy form.

Love Potions
31255 Cedar Valley Dr., Suite 317
Westlake Village, CA 91362
(800) 856–8380

Chapter 8: Prevent Heart Disease

The following books have useful discussions of herbs and supplements for preventing heart disease:
Natural Alternatives to Over-the-Counter and Prescription Drugs by Michael T. Murray, N.D. (New York: William Morrow, 1994)
Natural Prescriptions by Robert M. Giller, M.D., and Kathy Mathews (New York: Carol Southern Books, 1994)

Chapter 9: Lower Your Cancer Risk

Two excellent books on alternative approaches to cancer, both treatment and prevention, are:
Choices in Healing: Integrating the Best of Conventional and Complementary Approaches
  to Cancer by Michael Lerner (Cambridge, Mass.: MIT Press, 1994)
Cancer Therapy: The Independent Consumer's Guide to Non-Toxic Treatment & Preven-
  tion by Ralph W. Moss, Ph.D. (New York: Equinox Press, 1992)

Chapter 10: Extend Your Life

Some useful books on antioxidants, nutritional substances, and other factors relating to
longevity include:
The Antioxidants by Richard Passwater, Ph.D. (New Canaan, Conn.: Keats Pub-
  lishing, 1985)
The Complete Guide to Anti-Aging Nutrients by Sheldon Saul Hendler, M.D.,
  Ph.D. (New York: Simon and Schuster, 1985)
Longevity: Fulfilling Our Biological Potential by Kenneth R. Pelletier (New York:
  Delacorte and Delta/Seymour Lawrence, 1981)
Milk Thistle: The Liver Herb by Christopher Hobbs (Capitola, Calif.: Botanica
  Press, 1984)
The Natural Health Guide to Antioxidants by Nancy Bruning and the Editors of
  Natural Health Magazine (New York: Bantam Books, 1994)
The 120-Year Diet: How to Double Your Vital Years by Roy L. Walford, M.D. (New
  York: Pocket Books, 1988)
Reverse the Aging Process Naturally by Gary Null, Ph.D. and Marvin Feldman,
  M.D. (New York: Villard Books, 1993)

Chapter 11: Boost Your Brain Power

More detailed discussions of brain-boosting nutrients and "smart drugs," and extensive lists
of suppliers, can be found in the following books:
Brain Boosters: Foods & Drugs That Make You Smarter by Beverly A. Potter, Ph.D.,
  and Sebastian Orfali (Berkeley, Calif.: Ronin Publishing, 1993)
Smart Drugs II: The Next Generation by Ward Dean, M.D., John Morganthaler,
  and Steven Wm. Fowkes (Menlo Park, Calif.: Health Freedom Publications,
  1993)
Smart Nutrients by Abram Hoffer, Ph.D., and Morton Walker, D.P.M. (Garden
  City Park, N.Y.: Avery Publishing Group, 1994)
The following company is an excellent resource for further information on brain boosters.
Send $2 for an up-to-date instruction sheet on how to order liquid deprenyl and other
"smart" pharmaceuticals from overseas. (Note that although FDA policy is to allow
consumers to order from foreign sources small quantities of unapproved drugs for personal
use, on occasion FDA's field officers may arbitrarily detain such shipments.) CERI can also

help you to locate medical practitioners knowledgeable about these products. It publishes Smart Drug News *($44 for ten issues).*

Cognitive Enhancement Research Institute
P. O. Box 4029
Menlo Park, CA 94026
(415) 321–2374

The following are mail-order suppliers of nutrient-based smart products:

Smart Products
870 Market St., Suite 1262
San Francisco, CA 94102
(415) 989–2500

NutriGuard Research
P. O. Box 865-A
Encinitas, CA 92023
(800) 433–2402

Wholesale Nutrition
Box 3345
Saratoga, CA 95070
(800) 325–2664

Chapter 12: Calm Your Nervous System

A useful book on herbs and supplements for relaxation is:
An Herbal Guide to Stress Relief by David Hoffman (Rochester, Vt: Healing Arts
   Press, 1991)

The following company offers dream pillows filled with hop, chamomile, and other herbs; a
"dream balm" containing lavender and other herbs to apply to your temples and forehead; a
"dream tea"; and a wide assortment of herbs, essential oils, natural cosmetics, books, and
other products:
Mountain Rose Herbs
P. O. Box 2000
Redway, CA 95560
(707) 923–7867
(800) 879–3337

Chapter 13: Strengthen and Balance Your System

A short but informative book on adaptogens is the following:
Adaptogens: Nature's Key to Well-Being by Mikael Wahlström (Göteborg, Sweden:
   Skandinavisk Bok, 1987)

All of the balancing herbs and supplements are widely available in natural-food stores and by mail order, with the possible exception of Swedish roseroot. For it, contact:

Swedish Herbal Institute
P. O. Box 99
York Harbor, ME 03911
(207) 351–1084
(800) 619–1199

An excellent discussion of natural approaches to controlling blood-sugar levels is contained in:

Diabetes and Hypoglycemia: How You Can Benefit from Diet, Vitamins, Minerals, Herbs, Exercise and Other Natural Methods by Michael Murray, N.D. (Rocklin, Calif.: Prima Publishing, 1994)

Chapter 14: Develop Your Senses

Some excellent books on natural vision improvement include:
Natural Vision Improvement by Janet Goodrich, Ph.D. (Berkeley, Calif.: Celestial Arts, 1985)
Seeing Beyond 20/20 by Robert-Michael Kaplan, O.D. (Vancouver, B.C.: Beyond Words Publishing, 1987)
Seven Steps to Better Vision by Richard Leviton (Brookline, Mass.: East West/ Natural Health Books, 1992)
For an interesting cross-cultural perspective on how different medical systems view the senses, consult:

World Medicine: The East West Guide to Healing Your Body by Tom Monte and the editors of *East/West Natural Health* (New York: Jeremy P. Tarcher/Perigee, 1993)

The following organization promotes natural methods for vision improvement:

Optometric Extension Program Foundation
1921 E. Carnegie Av., Suite 3L
Santa Ana, CA 92705
(714) 250–8070

Chapter 15: Keep Your Skin Smooth and Supple

The following are useful reference works for evaluating conventional and natural body-care products:
A Consumer's Dictionary of Cosmetic Ingredients, 3rd ed., by Ruth Winter (New York: Crown Publishers, 1989)

Natural Organic Hair and Skin Care by Aubrey Hampton (Tampa, Fla.: Organica Press, 1987)

Chapter 16: Revitalize Your Digestive System

See the following book for an excellent discussion of beneficial live bacteria and their role in health.
Probiotics by Leon Chaitow, N.D., and N. Trenev (London: Thorsons, 1990)
The following company specializes in probiotic products.

Natren
3105 Willow Ln.
Westlake Village, CA 91361
(800) 992–3323 (national)
(800) 992–9393 (in Calif.)

Chapter 17: Attain Your Ideal Weight

A useful summary of research on hydroxycitric acid can be found in:
The Diet and Health Benefits of HCA (Hydroxycitric Acid) by Dallas Clouatra, Ph.D., and Michael Rosenbaum, M.D. (New Canaan, Ct.: Keats Publishing, 1994)
Contact the following organization for further information on its research linking scents and weight loss:

Smell & Taste Treatment and Research Foundation
Water Tower Place, Suite 990W
845 No. Michigan Ave.
Chicago, IL 60611
(312) 938–1047

Chapter 18: Combine Natural Substances with a Healthful Lifestyle

Some useful guides to a wide range of natural health steps include:
52 Simple Steps to Natural Health: A Week-by-Week Guide to More Healthful Living by Mark Mayell and the editors of *Natural Health* (New York: Pocket Books, 1995)
Natural Health, Natural Medicine: A Comprehensive Manual for Wellness and Self-Care by Andrew Weil, M.D. (Boston: Houghton Mifflin, 1990)

Acknowledgements

I owe a debt of gratitude to the many thousands of researchers and writers who have dedicated their lives to studying the effects of herbs, nutrients, and other natural substances on the human body. Their work provides the foundation for much of what I've collected here. I'd also like to thank the following people for their guidance, insights, and answers to questions large and small: Christopher Hobbs, Carol J. Corio, Georg Wikman, Alan Hirsch, M.D., Mark Blumenthal, Bob Bonanno, M.D., Bill Thomson, and Bob Felt. Agents Judith Weber and Nat Sobel of Sobel Weber Associates ably assisted my efforts from proposal to finished manuscript. Executive Editor Leslie Meredith of Bantam Books offered many valuable suggestions for focusing the book and making it as practical as possible. Brian Tart of Bantam made sure that all of the various elements necessary for a finished book were paid attention to at the right time. Family members who have been especially supportive and helpful throughout this project include Hillary Mayell White, Dick White, and my wife, Jeanne Mayell.

Index

About the Author

Mark Mayell is the coauthor, with the editors of *Natural Health* magazine, of *The Natural Health First-Aid Guide* and *52 Simple Steps to Natural Health*. His experience includes a seven-year stint as the editor of *Natural Health* and two years as the editor of the magazine's book publishing division. He has also served as the editor of *Nutrition Action,* the monthly newsletter of the Washington, D.C., nutrition advocacy group Center for Science in the Public Interest. Mark has written extensively on alternative approaches to health for *Natural Health* and other magazines. He serves on the advisory boards of the American Holistic Health Association and Food & Water, Inc. Mark has a master's degree in philosophy and social policy from George Washington University. He currently lives with his wife and two children in the Boston area.